Study Guide for

Perry's Maternal Child Nursing Care in Canada

Study Guide for

Perry's Maternal Child Nursing Care in Canada

Third Edition

Lisa Keenan-Lindsay, RN, MN, PNC(C)
Cheryl A. Sams, RN, BScN, MSN
Constance (Connie) O'Connor, MN, RN(EC)

US Editors:

Maternity
Shannon E. Perry, RN, PhD, FAAN
Deitra Leonard Lowdermilk, RNC, PhD, FAAN
Mary Catherine (Kitty) Cashion, RN-BC, MSN
Kathy Rhodes Alden, EdD, MSN, RN, IBCLC

Associate Editor
Ellen F. Olshansky, PhD, RN, WHNP-BC, NC-BC, FAAN

Pediatric
Marilyn J. Hockenberry, PhD, RN, PPCNP-BC, FAAN
David Wilson, MS, RNC-NIC (deceased)
Cheryl C. Rodgers, PhD, RN, CPNP, CPON

Study Guide prepared by:
Lisa Keenan-Lindsay, RN, MN, PNC(C)
Professor, School of Nursing
Seneca College of Applied Arts and Technology
Toronto, Ontario

Jennifer Young, MN, RN(EC) NP-Pediatrics, NNP-BC
Professor, Sally Horsfall Eaton School of Nursing
George Brown College
Neonatal Nurse Practitioner, SickKids® Hospital
Toronto, Ontario

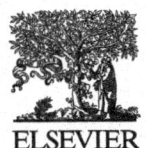

ELSEVIER

STUDY GUIDE FOR PERRY'S MATERNAL CHILD NURSING CARE IN CANADA, THIRD EDITION

ISBN: 978-0-323-79901-0

Notice

Practitioners and researchers must always rely on their own experience and knowledge in evaluating and using any information, methods, compounds, or experiments described herein. Because of the rapid advances in the medical sciences, in particular, independent verification of diagnoses and drug dosages should be made. To the fullest extent of the law, no responsibility is assumed by Elsevier, authors, editors, or contributors for any injury and/or damage to persons or property as a matter of products liability, negligence or otherwise, or from any use or operation of any methods, products, instructions, or ideas contained in the material herein.

Managing Director, Global ERC: Kevonne Holloway
Senior Content Strategist (Acquisitions, Canada): Roberta A. Spinosa-Millman
Director, Content Development Manager: Laurie Gower
Content Development Specialist: Lenore Gray Spence
Publishing Services Manager: Deepthi Unni
Project Manager: Radjan Lourde Selvanadin

We are honoured to have received permission to reproduce the work, "A Mother's Love", by Order of Canada award-winning Indigenous artist, Maxine Noel (Ioyan Mani), for this third Canadian edition, maternity and pediatric nursing text's cover.

Maxine has lent her voice and art to projects to improve the health and well-being of Indigenous women and girls; in projects related to maternal and infant health and, in collaboration with the NWAC in their work to raise awareness of the brutal dangers facing Indigenous women.

"A Mother's Love" is Copyright © MAXINE NOEL, ARTIST, COURTESY OF CANADIAN ART PRINTS AND WINN DEVON ART GROUP, INC

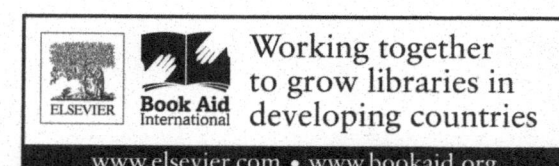

Last digit is the print number: 9 8 7 6 5 4 3 2 1

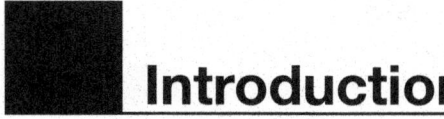 Introduction

Perry's Maternal Child Nursing Care in Canada, Third Edition, is a comprehensive textbook of maternity and pediatric nursing. This *Study Guide* is designed to help students use the textbook more effectively. In addition to reviewing content of the text, this *Study Guide* encourages students to think critically in applying their knowledge.

ORGANIZATION

Each chapter in this *Study Guide* is designed to incorporate learning activities that will help students meet the objectives of the corresponding textbook chapter. The content is organized as follows:

■ **Learning Key Terms**—Matching or fill-in-the-blank questions give students the opportunity to test their ability to define all key terms in the corresponding textbook chapter.

■ **Reviewing Key Concepts**—A variety of questions (matching, fill-in-the-blank, true/false, short answer, and multiple choice) are used to provide students with ample opportunity to assess their knowledge and comprehension of the information covered in the text. These activities are specifically designed to help students identify the important content of the chapter and test their level of knowledge and understanding after reading the chapter.

■ **Thinking Critically**—Students are required to apply concepts found in the chapter to solve problems, make clinical judgement decisions, and provide responses to patients' questions and concerns. Case studies are used for this application of knowledge.

■ **Answer Key**—Answers to all questions are provided at the end of this *Study Guide*.

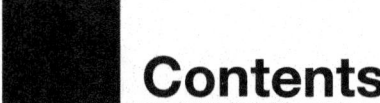

Contents

Contents

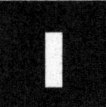# Maternal Child Nursing

1 Contemporary Perinatal and Pediatric Nursing in Canada

I. LEARNING KEY TERMS

MATCHING: Match each term with its corresponding description.

1. _____ Provides temporary health coverage for certain groups of refugees before they are covered under provincial or territorial health insurance plans.

2. _____ Social and economic factors that influence people's health, either positively or negatively.

3. _____ Approach that recognizes the connections between violence, trauma, negative health outcomes and behaviours

4. _____ The absence of unfair systems and policies that cause health inequalities.

5. _____ Result from a lack of access to the social determinants of health, which creates conditions of vulnerability.

6. _____ Social and cultural deprivation, such as limited employment opportunities, inferior educational opportunities, or a lack of or inferior medical services and health care facilities.

7. _____ A major cause of homelessness.

8. _____ Negative, stressful, traumatising events that occur before the age of 18 and the effects this can have on health risk across the lifespan

a. Health equity

b. Family violence

c. Social determinants of health

d. Adverse childhood events

e. Health inequities

f. Invisible poverty

g. Interim federal health program

h. Trauma-informed care

FILL IN THE BLANKS: Insert the term that corresponds to each of the following definitions or descriptions.

9. _____ Specialty area of nursing practice that focuses on the care of child-bearing women and their families through preconception throughout the child-bearing year.

10. _____ Organisation that focuses on population health, health promotion, and pandemic planning.

11. _____ A set of 17 goals to be achieved by 2030 that respond to the world's main development challenges and are replacing the previous Millennium Development Goals.

12. _____ Approach to health care that encompasses complementary and alternative therapies in combination with conventional Western modalities of treatment.

13. _____ An umbrella term for the use of communication technologies and electronic information to provide or support health care when the participants are separated by distance.

14. _____ Term that refers to a spectrum of abilities, ranging from reading an appointment slip to interpreting medication instructions.

15. _____ Health care that is based on information gained through research and clinical trials.

16. _____ Guidelines for nursing practice that reflect current knowledge, represent levels of practice agreed on by leaders in the specialty, and can be used for clinical benchmarking.

II. REVIEWING KEY CONCEPTS

1. Briefly discuss the impact of technology on the growing number of ethical concerns and debates related to maternal-child nursing care.

2. An integrative health care approach implies which of the following? (Circle all that apply.)
   a. The focus is on the whole person.
   b. Conventional Western modalities of treatment are not included.
   c. The beliefs, values, and desires of the patient in terms of health and health care are respected.
   d. Patient autonomy is limited in terms of choosing alternative therapies.
   e. The patient's disease complex is the primary consideration when choosing treatment approaches.

3. Explain why each of the groups listed below have been identified as vulnerable populations:
   a. Homeless families
   b. Adolescent girls and older women
   c. Children
   d. Indigenous people
   e. Refugees and immigrants

4. A nurse would like to obtain certification in community health. Which organisation would provide this certification?
   a. CAPWHN
   b. RNAO
   c. CNA
   d. NANN

III. THINKING CRITICALLY

1. Explain how a nurse could use social media to improve the health care provided to a child-bearing family. Identify the precautions the nurse must take to ensure that patient confidentiality and privacy are respected.

2. Discuss some of the health inequities that face Indigenous people. What can health care providers do to decrease some of these inequities?

3. Many barriers interfere with a person's participation in health care. Describe the significance of some of the barriers.

4. A homeless woman presents for routine health care. She is extremely anxious about having a Pap test done. Explain how the nurse could approach this person.

5. Discuss measures that can be taken to ensure that the health literacy needs of patients are met.

6. Explain the significance to a child of exposure to forms of physical and emotional abuse, neglect, or household dysfunction.

7. Develop a strategy to ensure that LGBTQ2 people are provided care that is inclusive.

2 The Family and Culture

LEARNING KEY TERMS

MATCHING: Match the family described with the appropriate family category.

1. _____ Miss M. lives with her 4-year-old adopted daughter, Kim.

2. _____ Anne and Duane are married and live with their daughter, Susan, and Duane's parents.

3. _____ Gloria and Andy are a married couple living with their new baby girl, Annie.

4. _____ Carl and Allan are a gay couple living with Carl's daughter, Sally, whom they are raising together.

5. _____ The S. family consists of Jim; his second wife, Jane; and Jim's two daughters by a previous marriage.

a. Multigenerational family

b. Lone-parent family

c. Same-sex parent family

d. Nuclear family

e. Blended family

f. No-parent family

MATCHING: Match the description with the appropriate cultural concept.

6. _____ Mrs. M., an Asian patient who just gave birth, tells the nurse not to include certain foods on their meal tray because their mother told them to avoid those foods while breastfeeding. The nurse tells the patient that they do not have to avoid any foods and should eat whatever they desire.

7. _____ Ms. P., an immigrant from Vietnam, has lived in Canada for 1 year. She tells you that while she enjoys the comfort of wearing blue jeans and sneakers for casual occasions, like shopping, she still wears traditional or "conservative" clothing for family gatherings.

8. _____ A Somalian family immigrated to Canada 1 year ago. Their child is ill and they are hesitant to see a doctor. The nurse sits with the family and asks questions about the health beliefs of the family in order to understand their concerns.

9. _____ The nurse is preparing to provide health teaching for a postpartum patient who is Cree and lives on reserve in Northern Ontario. In doing so, the nurse takes the time to include information from elders in the community.

a. Cultural humility

b. Ethnocentrism

c. Cultural safety

d. Acculturation

FILL IN THE BLANKS: Insert the concept that corresponds to each of the following definitions.

1. _____ An ongoing process that influences a person throughout their. It provides an individual with beliefs and values about each facet of life that are passed from one generation to the next.

2. _____ Recognising that people from different cultural backgrounds comprehend the same objects and situations differently; that a culture determines a person's viewpoint.

3. _____ Changes that occur within one group or among several groups when people from different cultures come in contact with one another and exchange and adopt each other's mannerisms, styles, and practices.

5

4. _____ A belief that one's cultural way of doing things is the right way, supporting the notion that "My group is the best."

5. _____ Approach that involves the ability to think, feel, and act in ways that acknowledge, respect, and build upon ethnic, cultural, and linguistic diversity; to act in ways that meet the needs of the patient and are respectful of ways and traditions that may be different from one's own.

6. _____ Type of time orientation that maintains a focus on achieving long-term goals; families or people who practice this time orientation are more likely to return for follow-up visits related to health care and to participate in primary prevention activities.

7. _____ Type of time orientation of families or people who are more likely to strive to maintain tradition or the status quo and have little motivation for formulating future goals.

8. _____ Type of time orientation of families or people who may have difficulty adhering to strict schedules and are often described as living for the moment.

9. _____ Cultural concept that reflects dimensions of personal comfort zones. Actions such as touching, placing the woman in proximity to others, taking away personal possessions, and making decisions for the woman can decrease personal security and heighten anxiety.

10. _____ A unit of socialisation and nurturing within a community that preserves and transmits culture. It is a social network that acts as a potent support system for its members.

11. _____ Family category in which husband and wife and their children live as an independent unit, sharing roles, responsibilities, and economic resources.

12. _____ Family category in which an unmarried biological or adoptive parent heads the household; it is becoming an increasingly recognised structure in our society. These families tend to be vulnerable both socially and economically.

13. _____ Family category that forms as a result of divorce and remarriage. It includes stepparents, stepchildren, and stepsiblings who join to create a new household.

14. _____ Family category comprised of gay, lesbian, bisexual, and transgender couples who live together with or without children.

15. _____ Family category consisting of grandparents, children, and grandchildren. This family form is becoming increasingly common.

16. _____ Term for members of a family that are related by blood.

17. _____ Term for the family tree format that depicts relationships of family members over at least three generations; it provides valuable information about a family and its health.

18. _____ Term for a graphic portrayal of social relationships of the patient and family including school, work, religious affiliations, and club memberships.

19. _____ An aspect of humans that is above and beyond the mind and body, ultimately giving meaning and purpose to one's life.

20. _____ Questions asked to patients related to spirituality and religion.

II. REVIEWING KEY CONCEPTS

1. Discuss why the nurse should take each of the following "products of culture" into consideration when providing care within a cultural context:

   a. Communication

   b. Personal space

   c. Time orientation

   d. Family roles

2. Which one of the following nursing actions is most likely to reduce a patient's anxiety and enhance the patient's personal security as it relates to the concept of personal space needs?
   a. Touching the patient before and during procedures
   b. Providing explanations when performing tasks
   c. Making eye contact as much as possible
   d. Reducing the need for the patient to make decisions

3. An Asian patient gave birth to a baby girl 12 hours ago. The nurse notes that the postpartum patient keeps their baby in the bassinet except for feeding and states that they will wait until they get home to begin breastfeeding. The nurse recognises that this behaviour is most likely a reflection of:
   a. embarrassment.
   b. delayed attachment.
   c. disappointment that the baby is a girl.
   d. cultural beliefs regarding the care of newborns.

4. A student nurse is planning to communicate with their postpartum patient using an interpreter. The instructor should provide further guidance if the student does which of the following?
   a. Chooses a female interpreter from the woman's country of origin.
   b. Stops periodically during the interaction to ask the interpreter how things are going.
   c. Asks questions while looking at the interpreter.
   d. Gathers culturally appropriate learning aids and reading materials to use during the interaction.

5. Which of the following strategies are used to deliver culturally appropriate care (Circle all that apply.)
   a. Ask about traditional beliefs such as the role of hot and cold
   b. Ask about patient's fears and those of the family regarding an unfamiliar care setting
   c. Provide hospital menu for meals and let the patient know the set meals
   d. Be sensitive regarding interpreters and language barriers
   e. Ask about group practices and beliefs

6. A student nurse is planning a presentation on Spiritual Wellness. Which of the following questions would help the student cover this topic? Select all that apply
   a. What does suffering mean to the patient?
   b. Who or what provides the patient with strength and hope?
   c. When was the last time you attended church?
   d. How does your faith help you patient cope

III. THINKING CRITICALLY

1. Imagine that you are a nurse working in a clinic that provides prenatal services to a multicultural community. Describe how you would provide culturally safe care to patients from different cultures.

2. Pamela is a 20-year-old Indigenous woman who is 3 months pregnant. She lives in a remote Northern British Columbia community and attends the prenatal clinic on reserve for her first prenatal visit. State factors related to equity that may ultimately negatively impact the outcome of Pamela's pregnancy.

3. The nurse at a prenatal clinic has been assigned to care for a refugee couple from Thailand who recently immigrated to Canada. The woman is 2 months pregnant. Neither she nor her partner speaks English. Outline the process that this nurse should use when working with a translator to facilitate communication with this couple to enhance care.

4. A nurse is calling a hospital chaplain to assist in spiritual care for a patient in preterm labour.

   a. Discuss what spiritual care encompasses.

   b. How does spirituality affect the family?

   c. Identify ways a nurse could include spirituality in their care.

3 Community Care

I. LEARNING KEY TERMS

MATCHING: Match each term with its corresponding description.

1. _____ Group of people who have shared characteristics

2. _____ The study of population characteristics

3. _____ Increased probability of developing a disease, injury, or illness

4. _____ The science of population health applied to the detection of morbidity and mortality in a population.

5. _____ Measures the occurrence of new events in a population during a period of time.

6. _____ Measures existing events in a population during a period of time.

7. _____ Preventing disability through restoration of optimal functioning

8. _____ Those who are knowledgeable about the social and health care needs of the population

a. demography

b. aggregate

c. incidence

d. epidemiology

e. community gate keepers

f. prevalence

g. tertiary prevention

h. risk

FILL IN THE BLANKS: Insert the term that corresponds to each of the following definitions or descriptions.

1. _____, _____, _____ Three factors that make up the epidemiological triangle.

2. _____ includes efforts made before the development of illness to promote general health and well-being.

3. _____ involves early detection of health problems so that treatment can begin before significant disability occurs. This includes various

   methods of _____

4. _____, _____,

   _____, _____,

   _____ Different methods of assessing a community.

5. Involves being actively part of the community to understand the community more fully and to validate observations.

6. _____, _____,

   _____, _____,

   _____, _____,

   _____, _____ Data is provided through the census.

II. REVIEWING KEY CONCEPTS

1. State the rationale for the increasing emphasis on home- and community-based health care. How has this trend changed the demands placed on the community-based nurse?

2. Community health promotion requires the collaborative efforts of many individuals and groups within a community. Cite several programs that could be established to promote the health of a community's childbearing and child-rearing families.

3. Describe the ways that nurses can provide care to using the telephone.

4. When making a home visit, it is essential that the nurse use appropriate infection control measures. Of the measures listed below, which one is the most important?
   a. Including personal protective equipment in the home care bag
   b. Designating a dirty area with a trash bag to collect soiled equipment and supplies
   c. Wearing clean vinyl gloves for procedures that involve touching the patient
   d. Performing hand hygiene using either soap and running water or a self-drying antiseptic solution.

5. T F Childhood immunization is an example of primary prevention

6. T F Newborn screening is an example of tertiary prevention.

7. T F Mortality or death rates are calculated on the number of deaths attributed to a particular health problem, such as lung cancer per 10 000 population.

8. T F Infection control measures are less important when care is given in the patient's home.

9. T F When documenting a home visit, a nurse should avoid statements, such as "no change" or "same as last visit."

10

III. THINKING CRITICALLY

1. Imagine that you are a nurse who has just been hired to provide in-home health care. Before you begin seeing your patients, you realise that it would be helpful for you to become familiar with the neighbourhood and resources in the community where your patients live. You decide to conduct a walking survey of this community.

   a. Describe how you would go about conducting this survey and gathering data.

   b. List the data you believe it would be essential to gather.

   c. Discuss how you would use the findings from your walking survey when providing health care to the patients you will be visiting.

2. Eileen gave birth to a son 36 hours ago. A home care nurse has been assigned to visit Eileen and her partner in their home to assess the progress of her recovery after birth, the health status of her newborn son, and the adaptation of family processes to the responsibilities of newborn care.

   a. Outline the approach the nurse should take in preparing for this visit.

   b. Describe the nurse's actions during the visit using the care management process as a format.

   c. Discuss how the nurse should end the visit.

d. Identify interventions the nurse should implement at the conclusion of the visit with Eileen and her partner.

e. Specify how the nurse should protect their personal safety both outside and inside Eileen's home.

f. Cite the infection control measures the nurse should use when conducting the visit and providing care in Eileen's home.

3. Angela has recently been diagnosed with hyperemesis gravidarum and has been hospitalized to stabilize her fluid and electrolyte balance. The hospital-based nurse must evaluate Angela for referral to home care.

a. State the criteria that this nurse should follow to determine Angela's readiness for discharge from hospital to home care.

b. Angela has been discharged and will be receiving parenteral nutrition in her home. Discuss the additional information required related to high technology home care.

c. Identify specific home environment criteria that must be met to ensure the safety and effectiveness of Angela's treatment.

II Perinatal Nursing

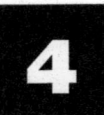

4 Perinatal Nursing in Canada

I. LEARNING KEY TERMS

MATCHING: Match each term with its corresponding description.

1. _____ Number of live births in 1 year per 1 000 population.

2. _____ Number of deaths of infants younger than 28 days of age per 1 000 live births.

3. _____ Number of maternal deaths from births and complications of pregnancy, childbirth, and puerperium (the first 42 days after termination of the pregnancy) per 100 000 live births.

4. _____ A newborn who, at birth, demonstrates no signs of life, such as breathing, heartbeat, or voluntary muscle movements.

5. _____ Number of stillbirths and number of neonatal deaths per 1 000 live births.

6. _____ Number of births per 1 000 women between the ages of 15 and 44 years (inclusive), calculated on an annual basis.

7. _____ Number of deaths of infants younger than 1 year of age per 1 000 live births.

a. Fertility rate

b. Infant mortality rate

c. Birth rate

d. Maternal mortality rate

e. Neonatal mortality rate

f. Perinatal mortality rate

g. Stillbirth

II. REVIEWING KEY CONCEPTS

1. When assessing pregnant patients, what factors would you recognise as having the potential to contribute to the rate of maternal mortality in Canada?

2. A nurse manager of a prenatal clinic should recognize that the following barriers encountered by pregnant patients may impact their ability to access health care? (Select all that apply)
   a. Lack of transportation to the clinic
   b. Child care responsibilities
   c. Inability to pay
   d. Deficient knowledge related to the benefits of prenatal care

3. In Canada, one of the leading causes of maternal mortality is which one of the following?
   a. Unsafe abortion
   b. Infection
   c. Hypertension
   d. Diabetes

4. Although the rates of teen pregnancy have decreased in Canada, what are some of the health risks associated with teen pregnancy?

5. Which of the following accounts for a significant number of small-for-gestational age (SGA) babies?
   a. Malnutrition
   b. Geographical location
   c. Maternal diabetes
   d. Maternal cigarette smoking

6. What is the role of the Canadian Perinatal Surveillance System? How can this data improve outcome for childbearing families?

III. THINKING CRITICALLY

1. Imagine that you are a nurse in a prenatal clinic on a remote reserve in Northern Saskatchewan. Your goal is to ensure healthy mothers and healthy babies. Describe three nursing services you could provide for these patients that considers the social determinants of health.

2. Marie is a single parent of two young children ages 4 years and 1 year. She and her children have been homeless for 3 months because she lost her job as she had no one to help her care for her children.

   a. Discuss the basis for the types of health problems to which Marie and her children are most vulnerable.

   b. What factors related to being homeless could increase Marie's risk for becoming pregnant? If she did become pregnant, explain why it would be considered a high risk pregnancy.

   c. How would you, as a nurse, provide health care services to Marie and her children?

3. Imagine that you are a nurse working in a clinic that provides prenatal services to a multicultural community. Describe how you would adapt care measures to reflect the cultural beliefs and practices of pregnant patients and their families from different cultural groups.

4. Discuss two international concerns that have serious detrimental effects on the health and safety of women. Explain how nurses can address these concerns.

5. A patient is 12 weeks pregnant and is considering a home birth with a registered midwife. What information can a nurse provide about this option?

5 Health Promotion

I. LEARNING KEY TERMS

FILL IN THE BLANKS: Insert the term that corresponds to each of the following definitions or descriptions related to women's health care.

1. _____Central nervous system stimulus that creates a sense of euphoria and is addictive

2. _____ Recommended opioid to use in pregnancy, which is metabolized more rapidly

3. _____ A relatively cheap and highly addictive stimulant that makes many users feel hypersexual and uninhibited

4. _____ Use of illicit drugs and inappropriate use of prescription medications

5. _____ Biopsychosocial disease that has persons behaviour seeking out drugs.

6. _____ Exercise that is used to strengthen the muscles that support the pelvic floor

7. _____ Type of health care that provides child-bearing persons and their partners with information that is needed to make decisions about their reproductive future.

8. _____ Term that describes a body mass index (BMI) of 30 or greater.

9. _____ Term that describes a chronic eating disorder in which patients undertake strict and severe diets and rigorous, extreme exercise as a result of a distorted view of their bodies as being much too heavy.

10. _____ Term that describes an eating disorder characterised by secret, uncontrolled binge eating alternating with practices that prevent weight gain, which can include self-induced vomiting, laxatives or diuretics, strict diets, fasting, and rigorous exercise.

11. _____ Term applied to a pattern of assaultive and coercive behaviours inflicted by a spouse, partner, or someone who has an intimate relationship with the person being battered.

12. _____ According to the cycle of violence theory, battering occurs in cycles. The three-phase cyclic pattern that occurs begins with a

period of _____ leading to

the _____, which is then followed

by a period of _____ known

as the _____ phase.

13. _____ Surgical closure of the labia minora

14. _____ People are forced into becoming part of the unpaid labour force, usually in sweatshops or in domestic work, or in order to serve as sex slaves.

FILL IN THE BLANKS: Insert the term that corresponds to each of the following definitions or descriptions related to teaching and learning.

1. _____ involves the acquiring of knowledge and development of intellectual skills, including the recall of specific facts

2. _____ Learning that involves feelings, emotions, and values

3. _____ Acquisition of a new motor skill.

4. _____ Best to facilitate discussion of personal, sensitive topics of interest or concern

5. _____ May be used as opportunity to practice a desired behaviour

6. _____ Often done through use of lecture or group discussion.

7. _____ Best method to learn a new skill

8. _____ Requires the ability to solve problems, evaluate information, and know when to take action

II. REVIEWING KEY CONCEPTS

1. Although patients may recognise the need for reproductive health care, they may encounter barriers to accessing this type of care. Identify one barrier represented by each of the following issues and describe a solution you would propose for helping patients overcome the barrier identified.

   ■ Financial issues

   ■ Cultural issues

   ■ Gender issues

2. What are the essential questions that should be asked when providing health care to patients to assess them for abuse?

3. Eating disorder screening tools can be used to determine whether a person is experiencing an eating disorder and to what degree. Explain the SCOFF tool and how you would use it when providing well woman care.

4. Using and misusing some substances while pregnant can increase the risk for adverse outcomes for the patient. Identify the effects for each of the substances listed below.

   ■ Alcohol

   ■ Tobacco

   ■ Caffeine

   ■ Cocaine

   ■ Marijuana

   ■ Opiates

   ■ Methamphetamines

5. When assessing patients, it is important for the nurse to keep in mind the possibility that they are victims of violence. The nurse should:
   a. use an abuse assessment screen during the assessment of every patient.
   b. recognize that abuse rarely occurs during pregnancy.
   c. assess a patient's legs and back as the most commonly injured areas.
   d. notify the police immediately if abuse is suspected.

6. A 52-year-old woman asks the nurse practitioner about how often she should be assessed for the common health problems women of her age could experience. The nurse would recommend which of the following screening measures? (Circle all that apply.)
   a. A Pap test every 3 years
   b. A fecal occult blood test every year
   c. A mammogram every 2-3 years
   d. Clinical breast examination every year
   e. Bone mineral density testing every year beginning when she is 55
   f. Vision examination every 5 years

7. Which of the following group descriptions is most accurate regarding those persons who should participate in preconception counselling?
   a. All patients and their partners as they make decisions about their reproductive future, including becoming parents
   b. All patients during their childbearing years
   c. Sexually active patients who do not use birth control
   d. Patients with chronic illnesses such as diabetes who are planning to get pregnant

8. A newly married 25-year-old woman has been smoking since she was a teenager. She has come to the women's health clinic for a checkup before she begins trying to get pregnant. The woman demonstrates a need for further instruction about the effects of smoking on reproduction and health when she makes which of the following statements? (Circle all that apply.)
   a. "Smoking can interfere with my ability to get pregnant."
   b. "My husband also needs to stop smoking because secondhand smoke can have an adverse effect on my pregnancy and the development of the baby."
   c. "Smoking can make my pregnancy last longer than it should."
   d. "Smoking can reduce the amount of calcium in my bones."
   e. "Smoking will mean I will experience menopause at an older age than my friends who do not smoke."

9. When communicating with a woman who is a victim of intimate partner violence, which of the following statements should be avoided? (Circle all that apply.)
   a. "Why do you think your partner hits you even though you are pregnant?"
   b. "I cannot believe how terrible your partner is being to you."
   c. "The violence you are experiencing now is likely to continue and to get even worse as your pregnancy progresses."
   d. "Tell me why you did not go to the shelter I recommended to you; they are very helpful and you would have avoided this beating if you had gone."
   e. "Next time you come in for care, I want you to be sure to bring your partner so I can talk to him myself."
   f. "I am afraid for your safety and the safety of your other children."

10. A women's health nurse practitioner is preparing an education presentation on the topic of intimate partner violence (IPV) to a group of women who come to the clinic where she practices. As part of the presentation, she plans to dispel commonly held myths regarding IPV. Which of the following statements represent the facts related to IPV? (Circle all that apply.)
   a. Battering almost always affects women who are poor.
   b. Approximately one-third of people experience violence in their life.
   c. Women usually are safe from battering while they are pregnant, although the battering will resume after they have the baby.
   d. Women tend to leave the relationship if the battering is bad.
   e. Counselling may be successful in helping the batterer stop his behaviour.
   f. Women do not like to be beaten and will often do anything to avoid a confrontation.

III. THINKING CRITICALLY

1. An inner-city women's health clinic serves a diverse population in terms of age, ethnic background, and health problems. Describe how each of the following factors should influence a women's health nurse practitioner's approach when assessing the health of the women who come to the clinic for care.

   a. Culture

   b. Age

   c. Abuse

   d. Gender identify

2. Nurses working in women's health care must be aware of the growing problem of intimate partner violence. All patients should be screened when being assessed during health care for the possibility of abuse.

   a. Describe how you as a nurse would adjust the environment and your communication style when conducting the health history interview and physical examination in order to elicit a patient's confidence and trust.

   b. Identify indicators of possible abuse that you would look for before the appointment and then during the health history interview and physical examination.

   c. State the questions you would ask to screen for abuse.

   d. Discuss the approach you would take if abuse is confirmed during the assessment.

3. A nurse is teaching a group of young adult women about health promotion activities. As part of the discussion, the nurse identifies preconception care and counselling as an important health promotion activity. One woman in the class asks, "I know you need to go for checkups once you are pregnant, but why would you need to see a doctor before you get pregnant? Isn't that a big waste of time and money?" Explain how the nurse should respond to this woman's question.

4. During a routine checkup for her annual Pap smear, Julie, a 26-year-old woman, asks the nurse for advice regarding exercise and stress reduction. Discuss the advice the nurse should give to Julie.

5. You are a nurse working in a community clinic. As part of your role, you need to teach teenagers about the importance of well-person care. What topics would you include in your teaching?

6. Alice, a 30-year-old woman, comes to the women's health clinic stating symptoms of fatigue, insomnia, and feeling anxious. She works as a stockbroker for a major brokerage firm. Alice states that, although she enjoys the challenge of her job, she never can seem to find time for herself or to socialize with her friends. Alice tells the nurse practitioner that she has been drinking more and started to smoke again to help her relax. She is glad that she has lost some weight, attributing this occurrence to her diminished appetite.

   a. State the physical and psychological manifestations of stress that the nurse should take note of when assessing Alice.

   b. Discuss how the nurse can help Alice cope with stress and its consequences in a healthy manner.

   c. Alice expresses interest in attempting to stop smoking. "I felt so much better when I stopped the first time. That was over 2 years ago, and now here I am back at it again." Describe an approach the nurse could use to help Alice achieve a desired change in health behaviour that is long lasting.

7. As a nurse working in a prenatal health clinic you must be alert to cues indicative of intimate partner violence committed against patients when they are pregnant.

   a. Carol, a 24-year-old woman, comes to the clinic to confirm her belief that she is pregnant. During the assessment phase of the visit, you note cues that lead you to suspect that Carol is being abused by her partner. Discuss the approach you would take to confirm your suspicion that Carol is being abused.

b. Carol admits to you that her partner "beats her sometimes and it has been increasing." Now she is afraid it will get worse since she "was not supposed to get pregnant." Discuss the nursing actions that you could take to help Carol.

c. List the possible reasons why Carol, now that she is pregnant, is experiencing an escalation of IPV from her partner.

d. Discuss how Carol's pregnancy could be adversely affected by the abuse she is experiencing.

e. Describe the activities in which the nurse can become involved in order to prevent the escalating incidence of intimate partner violence.

6 Health Assessment

I. LEARNING KEY TERMS

MATCHING: Match the communication strategy described with the appropriate definition.

1. _____ Using a word or posture that communicates interest.

2. _____ Repeating a word or phrase that a person has used.

3. _____ Putting into words what the nurse infers about the person's feelings or about the meaning of their symptoms, events, or other matters

4. _____ Asking the person what is meant by a stated work or phrase

5. _____ Identifying something about the person's behaviour or feelings not expressed verbally or apparently inconsistent with their history.

6. _____ Acknowledging the feelings of a person through statements.

a. Empathic responses

b. Interpretation

c. Reflection

d. Confrontation

e. Clarification

f. Facilitation

II. REVIEWING KEY CONCEPTS

1. It is essential that guidelines for laboratory and diagnostic procedures be followed exactly in order to ensure the accuracy of the results obtained. Outline the guidelines that should be followed when performing a Papanicolaou test in terms of each of the following:

   a. Patient preparation

   b. Timing during examination when the specimen is obtained

   c. Sites for specimen collection

   d. Handling of specimens

   e. Frequency of performance

2. A 48-year-old woman asks the nurse about whether she should perform breast self-examination (BSE) on a regular basis. What should the nurse teach the patient?

3. A women's health nurse practitioner is going to perform a pelvic examination on a female patient. Which of the following nursing actions would be least effective in enhancing the patient's comfort and relaxation during the examination?
   a. Encourage the patient to ask questions and express feelings and concerns before and after the examination.
   b. Ask the patient questions as the examination is performed.
   c. Allow the patient to keep her shoes and socks on when placing her feet in the stirrups.
   d. Instruct the patient to place her hands over her diaphragm and take deep, slow breaths.

4. To enhance the accuracy of the Papanicolaou (Pap) test, the nurse should instruct the patient to do which of the following?
   a. Schedule the test just prior to the onset of menses.
   b. Stop taking birth control pills for 2 days before the test.
   c. Avoid intercourse for 24 to 48 hours before the test.
   d. Douche with a specially prepared antiseptic solution the night before the test.

23

III. THINKING CRITICALLY

1. Imagine that you are a nurse working at a clinic that provides health care to women. Describe how you would respond to each of the following concerns or questions of women who have come to the clinic for care.

   a. Serena, a 17-year-old woman, has just been scheduled for her first women's health checkup, which will include a pelvic examination and Pap smear. She nervously asks if there is anything she needs to do to get ready for the examination.

   b. Anne, a 24-year-old woman, asks the nurse about a recommended douche prior to her pap test.

2. Julie, a 24-year-old woman, has come to the women's health clinic for a women's health checkup. During the health history interview she becomes very anxious and states, "I have to tell you this is my first examination. I am very scared; my friends told me that it hurts a lot to have this examination." Describe how the nurse should respond in an effort to reduce Julie's anxiety.

3. As a nurse working in a women's health clinic, you have been assigned to interview Angie, a 25-year-old new patient, to obtain her health history.

   a. List the components that should be emphasised in gathering Angie's history.

   b. Write a series of questions that you would ask to obtain data related to Angie's reproductive and sexual health and practices.

   c. Give an example of how you would use each of the following therapeutic communication techniques to develop trust, to facilitate the collection of data, and to provide support during the assessment process.

   Facilitation

   Reflection

Clarification

Empathy

Confrontation

Interpretation

Open-ended questions and statements

4. Lu is a 25-year-old exchange student from China who has been living in Canada for 3 months. This is the first time that she is away from home. She comes to the university women's health clinic for a checkup and to obtain birth control. Describe how the nurse assigned to Lu would approach and communicate with her in a culturally sensitive manner.

5. Nurses working in women's health care must be aware of the growing problem of intimate partner violence. All patients should be screened when being assessed during health care for the possibility of abuse.

a. Describe how you as a nurse would adjust the environment and your communication style when conducting the health history interview and physical examination in order to elicit a patient's confidence and trust.

b. Identify indicators of possible abuse that you would look for before the appointment and then during the health history interview and physical examination.

c. State the questions you would ask to screen for abuse.

d. Discuss the approach you would take if abuse is confirmed during the assessment.

6. As a student you may be assigned to assist a health care provider during the performance of a pelvic examination for one of your patients.

   a. Describe how you would do each of the following:
      Prepare your patient for the examination

      Support your patient during the examination

      Assist your patient after the examination

   b. Describe how you would assist the health care provider who is performing the examination.

7. A 45-year old trans-man who has just begun transitioning, visits a clinic for a wellness visit. Discuss the health counselling that would be important to provide for this patient.

7 Reproductive Health

I. LEARNING KEY TERMS

FILL IN THE BLANKS: Insert the term that corresponds to each of the following definitions related to the female reproductive system and breasts. Use the anatomical drawings (Figs. 7-1, 7-2, 7-4, 7-5, and 7-6 in your textbook) to visualize each of the structures as you are inserting the terms.

1. _____ Fatty pad that lies over the anterior surface of the symphysis pubis.

2. _____ Two rounded folds of fatty tissue covered with skin that extend downward and backward from the mons pubis; their purpose is to protect the inner vulvar structures.

3. _____ Two flat, reddish folds composed of connective tissue and smooth muscle, which are supplied with nerve endings that are extremely sensitive.

4. _____ Hood-like covering of the clitoris.

5. _____ Fold of tissue under the clitoris.

6. _____ Thin flat tissue formed by the joining of the labia minora; it lies underneath the vaginal opening at the midline.

7. _____ Small structure underneath the prepuce composed of erectile tissue with numerous sensory nerve endings; it increases in size during sexual arousal.

8. _____ Almond-shaped area enclosed by the labia minora that contains openings to the urethra, Skene's glands, vagina, and Bartholin's glands.

9. _____ Bladder opening found between the clitoris and the vagina.

10. _____ Skin-covered muscular area between the fourchette and the anus that covers the pelvic structures.

11. _____ Fibromuscular, collapsible tubular structure that extends from the vulva to the uterus and lies between the bladder and rectum. Its mucosal lining is arranged in transverse folds called _____.

    _____ glands (located on each side of the urethra), and _____ glands (located on each side of the vagina) secrete mucus that lubricates the vagina. The _____ is a connective tissue membrane that surrounds the vaginal opening and can be perforated during strenuous exercise, insertion of tampons, masturbation, and vaginal intercourse.

12. _____ Anterior, posterior, and lateral pockets that surround the cervix.

13. _____ Muscular pelvic organ located between the bladder and the rectum and just above the vagina. The _____ is a deep pouch, or recess, posterior to the cervix formed by the posterior ligament.

14. _____ Upper triangular portion of the uterus.

15. _____ Also known as the lower uterine segment, it is the short constricted portion that separates the corpus of the uterus from the cervix.

16. _____ Dome-shaped top of the uterus.

17. _____ Highly vascular lining of the uterus.

18. _____ Layer of the uterus composed of smooth muscles that extend in three different directions.

19. _____ Lower cylindric portion of the uterus composed of fibrous connective tissue and elastic tissue.

20. _____ Canal connecting the uterine cavity to the vagina. The opening between the uterus and this canal is the _____. The opening between the canal and the vagina is the _____.

21. _____ Location in the cervix where the squamous and columnar epithelium meet; it is also known as the _____ zone; it is the most common site for neoplastic changes; cells from this site are scraped for the Pap smear.

22. _____ Passageways between the ovaries and the uterus; they are attached at each side of the dome-shaped uterine fundus.

23. _____ Almond-shaped organs located on each side of the uterus; their two functions are _____ and the production of the hormones _____, _____, and _____.

24. _____ Structure that protects the bladder, uterus, and rectum; accommodates the growing foetus during pregnancy; and anchors support structures.

25. _____ The paired mammary glands.

26. _____ Segment of mammary tissue that extends into the axilla.

27. _____ Mammary papilla.

28. _____ Pigmented section of the breast that surrounds the nipple.

29. _____ Sebaceous glands that secrete a fatty substance to lubricate the nipple and cause the areola to appear rough.

FILL IN THE BLANKS: Insert the term that corresponds to each of the following definitions related to the menstrual cycle. Use the illustration of the Menstrual Cycle (Fig. 7-8 in your textbook) to visualise the cycle as you are inserting the terms.

30. _____ The first menstruation.

31. _____ Transitional stage between childhood and sexual maturity.

32. _____ Transitional phase during which ovarian function and hormone production decline.

33. _____ The last menstrual period dated with certainty once one year has passed after menstruation ceases.

34. _____ Period preceding the last menstrual period that lasts about 4 years; during this time ovarian function declines, ova diminish, more menstrual cycles become anovulatory, and irregular bleeding occurs.

35. _____ Periodic uterine bleeding that begins approximately 14 days after ovulation. It is controlled by the feedback system of three cycles, namely _____, _____, and _____. The average length of each menstrual cycle is _____ but variations are normal. Day one of the cycle is considered to be _____ _____. The average duration of menstrual flow is _____ with a range of _____.

36. _____ Cycle that involves cyclic changes in the lining of the uterus. It consists of four phases, namely _____, _____, _____, and _____.

37. _____ Cycle that involves secretion of hormones required to stimulate ovulation.

38. _____ Cycle that involves the changes in the ovary leading to ovulation. It consists of two phases, namely _____ and _____.

39. _____ Hormone secreted by the hypothalamus when ovarian hormones are reduced to a low level. It stimulates the pituitary gland to secrete two critical hormones for the menstrual cycle, namely _____ and _____.

40. _____ Pituitary hormone that stimulates the development of graafian follicles in the ovary.

41. _____ Pituitary hormone that stimulates the expulsion of the ovum from the graafian follicle and formation of the corpus luteum.

42. _____ Ovarian hormone that stimulates the thickening of the endometrium that occurs after menstruation and prior to ovulation; it is also responsible for changes in the cervix and the stretchable quality of the cervical mucus called _____.

43. _____ Ovarian hormone that is responsible for the changes in the endometrium that occur after ovulation to facilitate implantation should fertilisation occur; it is also responsible for the rise in _____ temperature that occurs after ovulation.

44. _____ Localised, lower abdominal pain that coincides with ovulation. Some vaginal spotting may occur.

45. _____ Oxygenated fatty acids classified as hormones. They are thought to play an essential role in ovulation, transport of sperm, regression of the corpus luteum, and menstruation. By increasing the myometrial response to oxytocin, they also play a role in labour and dysmenorrhea.

FILL IN THE BLANKS: Insert the term that corresponds to each of the following descriptions related to menstrual concerns.

46. _____ Absence of menstrual flow.

47. _____ Cessation of menstruation related to a problem in the central hypothalamic–pituitary axis.

48. _____ Syndrome characterized by the interrelation of disordered eating, absence of menstrual flow, and premature osteoporosis.

49. _____ Painful menstruation; one of the most common gynecological problems for patients during their childbearing years.

50. _____ Type of painful menstruation associated with ovulatory cycles; it has a biochemical basis arising from the release of prostaglandins.

51. _____ Type of painful menstruation that occurs later in life, typically after age 25, and is associated with pelvic pathology.

52. _____ A cluster of physical and psychological symptoms that begins in the luteal phase of the menstrual cycle and is followed by a symptom-free follicular phase.

53. _____ Diagnostic term for a disorder that affects a smaller percentage of women who suffer from severe PMS with an emphasis on symptoms related to mood disturbances.

54. _____ A menstrual disorder that is characterised by the presence and growth of endometrial tissue outside of the uterus.

55. _____ Infrequent menstrual periods.

56. _____ Scanty menstruation at normal intervals.

57. _____ Excessive bleeding during menstruation.

58. _____ Bleeding between menstrual periods.

59. _____ Any form of uterine bleeding that is irregular in amount, duration, or timing and is not related to regular menstrual bleeding; it can have organic causes such as systemic or reproductive tract disease.

FILL IN THE BLANKS: Insert the term that corresponds to each of the following descriptions related to infection.

60. _____ Infections or infectious disease syndromes primarily transmitted by sexual contact.

61. _____ Bacterial infection that is reportable in Canada and the rate has been increasing steadily in both males and females. This infection is often silent and is associated with an increased risk of ectopic pregnancy and tubal factor infertility.

62. _____ The second most common STI in Canada. Because it is a reportable communicable disease, health care providers are legally responsible for reporting all cases to health authorities.

63. _____ One of the earliest sexually transmitted infections (STIs). It is caused by Treponema pallidum, a spirochete. During the primary stage a characteristic lesion called a _____ appears 3 to 90 days after infection. During the second stage, a widespread _____ appears on the palms and soles along with generalised _____. _____ (broad, painless, pink-gray, wartlike infectious lesions) may develop on the vulva, perineum, or anus.

64. _____ Infectious process that most commonly involves the uterine tubes, uterus, and more rarely, ovaries and peritoneal surfaces.

65. _____ Infection also named condylomatata acuminate, or genital warts. It is now the most common viral STI seen in ambulatory health care settings.

66. _____ A viral infection that is transmitted sexually and is characterized by painful recurrent ulcers.

67. _____ Viral infection acquired primarily through a fecal-oral route by ingestion of contaminated food and fluids and through person-to-person contact.

68. _____ Viral infection involving the liver that is transmitted parenterally, perinatally, and through intimate contact. A vaccine is available to protect infants, children, and adults.

69. _____ A blood-borne infection that is an important cause of chronic liver disease. It is transmitted parenterally and through intimate contact. No vaccine is available to provide protection against this infection.

70. _____ A virus that is transmitted primarily through exchange of body fluids. _____ Severe depression of the cellular immune system associated with this infection.

71. _____ A virus that is spread via mosquitos and sexual contact through semen. There is an increased risk for giving birth to an infant with microcephaly if infected with virus.

72. _____ Vaginal infection formerly called *nonspecific vaginitis, Haemophilus vaginitis*, or *Gardnerella*; it is the most common type of vaginitis and is characterised by a profuse, thin, and white, gray, or milky discharge that has a characteristic "fishy" odour.

73. _____ Yeast infection that is a common type of vaginal infection in Canada. It is characterised by a thick, white, lumpy discharge.

74. _____ A vaginal infection caused by an anaerobic one-celled protozoan with characteristic flagella. The typically copious discharge is yellowish green, frothy, mucopurulent, and malodorous. It is almost always sexually transmitted.

II. REVIEWING KEY CONCEPTS

MATCHING: Match the description with the appropriate breast disorder.

1. _____ Lumpiness with or without tenderness in both breasts; nipple discharge may occur.

2. _____ Fatty unilateral breast tumor that is soft, nontender, and mobile with discrete borders; no nipple discharge occurs.

3. _____ Unilateral, firm, occasional tenderness, discrete benign breast mass; it increases in size during pregnancy but decreases in size with aging.

4. _____ Rare, benign condition that develops in the terminal nipple ducts and is usually too small to palpate; a unilateral spontaneous serous, serosanguineous, or bloody nipple discharge can also occur.

5. _____ Spontaneous, bilateral milky sticky breast discharge unrelated to malignancy.

6. _____ Inflammatory process in the breast characterized by a thick, sticky, white or coloured discharge. Burning pain and itching may be experienced. A mass may be palpated behind the nipple.

a. Fibroadenoma

b. Fibrocystic changes

c. Mammary duct ectasia

d. Lipoma

e. Galactorrhea

f. Intraductal papilloma

7. Cite several common risk factors for sexually transmitted infections.

9. Describe the how the Zika virus is transmitted.

   a. List information that should be given to patients regarding the risks during pregnancy.

8. a. What behaviours increase a person's risk for HIV infection?

10. Breast cancer is a major health problem facing women in Canada. Nurses are often responsible for educating patients about breast cancer.

   a. Outline the information the nurse should give patients about the risk factors associated with breast cancer.

   b. List the clinical manifestations that may be exhibited during seroconversion to HIV positivity.

   b. List the clinical manifestations that are strongly suggestive of breast cancer.

   c. Outline line counselling tips for a nurse for a HIV positive patient.

11. Which of the following patients is at greatest risk for developing hypogonadotropic amenorrhea?
    a. 48-year-old patient experiencing perimenopausal changes
    b. 13-year-old figure skater
    c. 18-year-old softball player
    d. 30-year-old (G3 T3 P0 A0 L3) person who is breastfeeding

12. Pharmacological preparations can be used to treat primary dysmenorrhea. Which preparation would be least effective in relieving the symptoms of primary dysmenorrhea?
    a. Oral contraceptive pill (OCP)
    b. Naproxen sodium
    c. Acetaminophen (Tylenol)
    d. Ibuprofen (Motrin)

13. Women experiencing PMS should be advised to avoid use of which of the following?
    a. Chamomile tea
    b. Coffee
    c. Whole-grain cereals
    d. Parsley to season food

14. The nurse counselling a 30-year-old patient regarding effective measures to use to relieve the discomfort associated with dysmenorrhea could suggest which of the following? (Circle all that apply.)
    a. Decrease intake of fruits, especially peaches and watermelon.
    b. Use back massages and heat application to abdomen to enhance relaxation and circulation.
    c. Avoid exercise just before and during menstruation when discomfort is at its peak.
    d. Add ginger to diet.
    e. Perform guided imagery for relaxation and distraction.
    f. Limit intake of salty and fatty foods.

15. A 28-year-old patient has been diagnosed with endometriosis. They have been placed on a course of treatment with danazol (Cyclomen). The patient exhibits understanding of this treatment when they say which of the following? (Circle all that apply.)
    a. "Because this medication stops ovulation, I do not need to use birth control."
    b. "I will experience more frequent and heavier menstrual periods when I take this medication."
    c. "I should follow a low-fat diet because this medication can increase the level of cholesterol in my blood."
    d. "I can experience a decrease in my breast size, oily skin, and hair growth on my face as a result of taking this medication."
    e. "I will need to spray this medication into my nose twice a day."
    f. "I may need to use a lubricant during intercourse to reduce discomfort."

16. A 55-year-old woman tells the nurse that she has started to experience pain when she and her partner have intercourse. The nurse would record that this woman is experiencing:
    a. dyspareunia.
    b. dysmenorrhea.
    c. dysuria.
    d. dyspnea.

17. Infections of the female mid reproductive tract, such as chlamydia, are dangerous primarily because these infections:
    a. are asymptomatic.
    b. cause infertility.
    c. lead to PID.
    d. are difficult to treat effectively.

18. A finding associated with HPV infection would include which of the following?
    a. White, curd-like, adherent discharge
    b. Soft papillary swelling occurring singly or in clusters
    c. Vesicles progressing to pustules and then to ulcers
    d. Yellow to green frothy malodorous discharge

19. A recommended medication effective in the treatment of vulvovaginal candidiasis would be which of the following?
    a. Metronidazole (Flagyl)
    b. Miconazole (Monistat)
    c. Ampicillin
    d. Acyclovir

20. When providing a patient recovering from primary herpes with information regarding the recurrence of herpes infection of the genital tract, the nurse would tell them which of the following?
    a. Fever and flulike symptoms will precede each recurrent infection.
    b. Little can be done to control the recurrence of infection.
    c. Cortisone-based ointments should be used to decrease discomfort.
    d. Itching and tingling often occur before the appearance of vesicles.

21. When teaching women about breast cancer, the nurse should emphasise which of the following facts? (Circle all that apply.)
    a. The incidence of breast cancer is highest among Black patients.
    b. One in ten Canadian women will develop breast cancer in her lifetime.
    c. The mortality rate from breast cancer decreases with early detection.
    d. Most women diagnosed with breast cancer report a family history of breast cancer.
    e. Maintaining a normal weight and reducing alcohol intake could have an effect on reducing a woman's chances of developing breast cancer.
    f. The majority of breast lumps found by women are not malignant.

22. A 26-year-old patient has just been diagnosed with fibrocystic change in their breasts. Which of the following nursing concerns would be a priority for this patient?
    a. Acute pain related to cyclical enlargement of breast cysts or lumps
    b. Risk for infection related to altered integrity of the areola associated with accumulation of thick, sticky discharge from nipples
    c. Anxiety related to anticipated surgery to remove the cysts in her breasts
    d. Fear related to high risk for breast cancer

23. When assessing a patient with a diagnosis of fibroadenoma, the nurse would expect to find which of the following characteristics?
    a. Bilateral tender lumps behind the nipple
    b. Milky discharge from one or both nipples
    c. Soft and nonmoveable lumps
    d. Well-delineated, firm moveable lump in one breast

24. Herbal preparations can be used as part of the treatment for a variety of menstrual disorders. Which of the following herbs would be beneficial for a patient experiencing menorrhagia? (Circle all that apply.)
    a. Ginger
    b. Shepherd's purse
    c. Black cohosh root
    d. Black haw

III. THINKING CRITICALLY

1. Marie is a 16-year-old gymnast who has been training vigorously for a placement on Olympic team. She has been experiencing amenorrhea, and the development of her secondary sexual characteristics has been limited. Marie expresses concern because her nonathletic friends have all been menstruating for at least 1 year and have well-developed breasts. After a health assessment, Marie was diagnosed with hypogonadotropic amenorrhea.

   a. State the risk factors and assessment findings for this disorder that Marie most likely exhibited during the assessment process.

   b. Outline a typical care management plan for Marie that will address the issues associated with hypogonadotropic amenorrhea.

   c. At Marie's all female high school there is a large athletic department that emphasizes participation and excellence in a wide variety of sports. You are concerned that there are other students like Marie who may be exhibiting signs of the female athlete triad. The nurse has decided to institute an education program aimed at prevention and early detection of the triad.

      (1) What is the meaning of the female athlete triad?

      (2) Which sports should the nurse emphasise with her program?

      (3) What measures should this nurse include in her program as a means of prevention and early detection of the female athlete triad?

2. Mary, a 17-year-old who experienced menarche at age 16, comes to the women's health clinic for a routine checkup. She tells the nurse that her last few periods have been very painful. "I have missed a few days of school because of it. What can I do to reduce the pain that I feel during my periods?" Physical examination and testing reveal normal structure and function of Mary's reproductive system. A medical diagnosis of primary dysmenorrhea is made.

   a. What questions should the nurse ask Mary to get a full description of her pain?

   b. What should the nurse tell Mary about the likely cause for the type of pain she is experiencing?

   c. Identify appropriate relief measures for primary dysmenorrhea that the nurse could suggest to Mary.

   d. What alternative therapies could the nurse suggest to Mary to help relieve her discomfort?

3. A patient experiences physical and psychological signs and symptoms associated with PMS during every ovulatory menstrual cycle.

   a. List the signs and symptoms most likely described by the patient that led to the diagnosis of PMS.

   b. Describe the approach the nurse would use in helping the patient deal with this menstrual disorder.

   c. What symptoms would the patient describe that would indicate they are also experiencing PMDD?

4. A 26-year-old patient has been diagnosed recently with endometriosis.

   a. List the signs and symptoms the patient most likely exhibited that led to this medical diagnosis.

   b. The patient asks, "What is happening to my body as a result of this disease?" Describe the nurse's response.

c. The patient asks about treatment options. "Are there medications I can take to make me feel better?" Describe the action/effect and potential side effects for each of the following pharmacological approaches to treatment.

Oral contraceptive pills

Gonadotropin-releasing hormone agonists

Androgenic synthetic steroids

d. Identify support measures the nurse can suggest to assist the patient to cope with the effects of endometriosis.

5. A 20-year-old woman, comes to a women's health clinic for her first visit.

a. During the health history interview, it is imperative that the nurse practitioner determine the patient's risk for contracting an STI, including HIV. Write one question for each of the following risk categories.

Sexual risk

Drug use–related risk

Blood-related risk

HIV concerns

b. The patient asks the nurse about measures she could use to protect herself from STIs. Cite the major points that the nurse practitioner should emphasise when teaching the patient about prevention measures.

c. The patient tells the nurse that she does not know if she could ever tell a partner that he must wear a condom. Describe the approach the nurse can take to enhance the patient's assertiveness and communication skills.

6. Suzanne is a 20-year-old patient, is admitted for suspected severe, acute PID.

 a Identify the risk factors for PID that the nurse would be looking for in the patient's health history.

 b A complete physical examination is performed to determine whether the criteria for PID are met. Specify the criteria that the patient's health care provider would be alert for during the examination.

 c The patient is hospitalized when the diagnosis of PID secondary to chlamydial infection is confirmed. Intravenous antibiotics will be used as the primary medical treatment followed by oral antibiotics at the time of discharge. Outline a nursing management plan for Suzanne in terms of each of the following:

 Position and activity

 Comfort measures

 Support measures

 Health education in preparation for discharge

 d List the recommendations for the patient's self-care during the recovery phase.

 e Identify the reproductive health risks that the patient may face as a result of the pelvic infection experienced.

7. Laura has just been diagnosed with gonorrhea, a sexually transmitted infection. Outline a management plan that will assist Laura in taking control of her self-care and prevent future infections.

8. Cheryl, a 27-year-old woman, is being treated for HPV. A primary diagnosis identified for Cheryl is "pain related to lesions on the vulva and around the anus secondary to HPV infection." State the measures the nurse could suggest to Cheryl to reduce the pain from the condylomata and enhance their healing.

9. Mary, a 20-year-old woman, has just been diagnosed with a primary herpes simplex 2 infection. In addition to the typical systemic symptoms, Mary exhibits multiple painful genital lesions.

   a Relief of pain and healing without the development of a secondary infection are two expected outcomes for care. Identify several measures that the nurse can suggest to Mary in an effort to help her achieve the expected outcomes of care.

   b Mary asks the nurse if there is anything she can do so that this infection does not return. Discuss what the nurse should tell Mary about the recurrence of HSV-2 infection and the influence of self-care measures.

10. Sonya is concerned that she has been exposed to HIV and has come to the women's health clinic for testing.

   a During the health history the nurse questions Sonya about behaviours that could have placed her at risk for HIV transmission. Cite the behaviours that the nurse would be looking for.

   b Explain the testing procedure that will most likely be followed to determine Sonya's HIV status.

   c Outline the counselling protocol that should guide the nurse when caring for Sonya before and after the test.

   d Sonya's test result is negative. Discuss the instructions the nurse should give Sonya regarding guidelines she should follow to reduce her risk for the transmission of HIV with future sexual partners.

11. Mary Anne comes to the women's health clinic stating that her breasts feel lumpy.

   a Outline the assessment process that should be used to determine the basis for Mary Anne's concern.

   b A diagnosis of fibrocystic breast changes is made. Describe the signs and symptoms Mary Anne most likely exhibited to support this diagnosis.

   c State one nursing diagnosis that the nurse would identify as a priority when preparing a plan of care for Mary Anne.

   d Identify measures the nurse could suggest to Mary Anne for lessening the symptoms she experiences related to fibrocystic changes.

8 Infertility, Contraception, and Abortion

I. LEARNING KEY TERMS

FILL IN THE BLANKS: Insert the term that corresponds to each of the following descriptions related to alterations in fertility.

1. _____ Diagnosis made when a couple has not achieved pregnancy after 1 year of regular, unprotected intercourse when the woman is less than 35 years of age or after 6 months when the woman is older than 35 years.

2. _____ Term used to describe the chances of achieving pregnancy and subsequent live birth within one menstrual cycle.

3. _____ Fertility treatments in which both eggs, sperm or both are handled outside the human body.

4. _____ Assisted human reproduction that involves collection of a woman's eggs, then fertilising them in the laboratory with sperm, and transferring the resultant embryo into her uterus.

5. _____ Assisted human reproduction that involves selection of one sperm cell that is injected directly into the egg to achieve fertilisation; it is used with in vitro fertilisation (IVF).

6. _____ Assisted human reproduction that involves retrieval of oocytes from the ovary, placing them in a catheter with washed motile sperm, and immediately transferring the gametes into the fimbriated end of the uterine tube. Fertilisation occurs in the uterine tube.

7. _____ Assisted human reproduction that involves placing ova after IVF into one uterine tube during the zygote stage.

8. _____ Assisted human reproduction that involves using sperm from a person other than the male partner to inseminate the female partner.

9. _____ Assisted human reproduction that involves transferring IVF embryo(s) from one couple into the uterus of another person who has contracted with the couple to carry the baby to term although the person cannot be paid for this service. This person has no genetic connection with the child.

10. _____ Assisted human reproduction that involves inseminating a woman with the semen from the infertile woman's partner; she then carries the baby until birth.

11. _____ Assisted human reproduction that involves penetrating the zona pellucida chemically or manually to create an opening for the dividing embryo to hatch and to implant into the uterine wall.

12. _____ Assisted human reproduction that involves donating eggs by an IVF procedure; the eggs are then inseminated and transferred into the recipient's uterus, which has been hormonally prepared with estrogen-progesterone therapy.

13. _____ Assisted human reproduction that involves transferring another woman's embryo into the uterus of an infertile woman at the appropriate time.

14. _____ Using the sperm of a donor to inseminate the woman.

15. _____ Procedure used to freeze embryos for later implantation.

16. _____ Basic test for male infertility; detects ability of sperm to fertilise an ovum.

17. _____ Examination of uterine cavity and tubes using radiopaque contrast material instilled through the cervix. It is often used to determine tubal patency and to release a blockage if present.

18. _____ Test used to detect the timing of lutein hormone surge before ovulation.

19. _____ Test performed to evaluate tubal patency, uterine cavity, and myometrium; it will not disrupt a fertilised ovum.

FILL IN THE BLANKS: Insert the term that corresponds to each of the following descriptions regarding methods to prevent or plan pregnancy.

20. _____ Intentional prevention of pregnancy during sexual intercourse.

21. _____ Device and/or practice used to decrease the risk of conceiving or bearing offspring.

22. _____ Conscious decision regarding when to conceive or to avoid pregnancy throughout the reproductive years.

23. _____ Term that refers to the percentage of contraceptive users expected to have an unplanned pregnancy during the first year of using a birth control method even when they use the method consistently and correctly.

24. _____ The most effective reversible contraceptive methods used to prevent pregnancy. They include contraceptive implants and intrauterine contraception.

25. _____ Contraceptive method that requires the male partner to withdraw his penis from the woman's vagina before ejaculation.

26. _____ Group of contraceptive methods that rely on avoidance of intercourse during fertile days.

27. _____ Method that combines the charting of signs and symptoms of the menstrual cycle with the use of abstinence or other contraceptive methods during fertile periods.

28. _____ Method based on the number of days in each cycle counting from the first day of menses. The fertile period is determined after accurately recording lengths of menstrual cycles for 6 months.

29. _____ A modified form of the calendar rhythm method that has a "fixed" number of days of fertility for each cycle; cycle beads can be used to track fertility, with day 1 of the menstrual flow as the first day to begin counting.

30. _____ Method based on variations in a woman's lowest body temperature, which is determined after waking and before getting out of bed.

31. _____ Method that requires the woman to recognise and interpret the cyclical changes in the amount and consistency of cervical mucus that characterise her own unique pattern of changes.

32. _____ Term that refers to the stretchiness of cervical mucus.

33. _____ Method that uses the physiological and psychological changes that occur during each phase of the menstrual cycle to determine the occurrence of ovulation and the fertile period.

34. _____ Method that requires the woman to ask herself two questions every day: (1) "Did I note secretions today?" and (2) "Did I note secretions yesterday?" An answer of "yes" requires the use of a backup method of birth control or avoidance of coitus.

35. _____ Temporary method of birth control that is based on the suppression of ovulation, which occurs with breastfeeding.

36. _____ Chemical that destroys or limits the mobility of sperm. When inserted into the vagina it acts as both a chemical and a physical barrier to sperm. It is also an effective lubricant.

37. _____ Thin, stretchable sheath that covers the penis or is inserted into the vagina.

38. _____ Shallow, dome-shaped rubber device with a flexible rim that covers the cervix.

39. _____ A soft natural rubber dome with a firm but pliable rim that fits snugly around the base of the cervix close to the junction of the cervix and vaginal fornices.

40. _____ A small round polyurethane device that contains a spermicide. It fits over the cervix and has a woven polyester loop to facilitate its removal.

41. _____ Birth control method that is taken orally; it contains a combination of estrogen and progesterone that inhibits the maturation of follicles and ovulation.

42. _____ Combined estrogen-progesterone birth control method that involves application of the hormones to the skin of the lower abdomen, upper outer arms, buttocks, or upper torso where the hormones are absorbed; it is applied once a week for 3 weeks.

43. _____ Combined estrogen-progesterone birth control method that involves insertion of the hormones into the vagina for 3 weeks.

44. _____ Form of contraception that involves administration of a progestin-only pill, which should be taken as soon as possible after but within 60 hours of unprotected intercourse or birth control mishap to prevent unintended pregnancy

45. _____ Small, T-shaped object inserted into the uterine cavity. It can be loaded with copper or a progestational agent such as Levonorgestrel.

46. _____ Surgical procedures intended to render the person infertile.

_____ Method used to render a female infertile. _____ Method that is the easiest and most commonly used method for males; it involves ligating and then severing the vas deferens of each testicle.

47. _____ Purposeful interruption of a pregnancy before 20 weeks of gestation. If it is performed at the patient's request, it is termed an _____. If it is performed for reasons of maternal or fetal health or disease, it is termed a _____.

II. REVIEWING KEY CONCEPTS

1. A woman is a little uncomfortable about checking her cervical mucus and asks the nurse what she could possibly find out about doing this assessment. State the useful purpose of self-evaluation of cervical mucus.

2. Joyce has chosen the diaphragm as her method of contraception. Which of the following actions would indicate that Joyce is using the diaphragm effectively? (Select all that apply.)
   a. Joyce came to be refitted after healing was complete following a term vaginal birth.
   b. Joyce applies a spermicide only to the rim of the diaphragm just before insertion because she dislikes the stickiness of the spermicide.
   c. Joyce empties her bladder before inserting the diaphragm.
   d. Joyce inserts the diaphragm about 3 to 4 hours before intercourse to increase spontaneity.
   e. Joyce applies more spermicide for each act of intercourse.
   f. Joyce removes the diaphragm within 1 hour of intercourse.
   g. After removal, Joyce washes the diaphragm with warm water and an antiseptic-type soap, dries it, and then applies baby powder.
   h. Joyce always uses the diaphragm during her menstrual periods.

3. A woman must assess herself for signs that ovulation is occurring. Which of the following is a sign associated with ovulation?
   a. Reduction in level of LH in the urine 12 to 24 hours before ovulation
   b. Spinnbarkeit
   c. Drop in BBT during the luteal phase of her menstrual cycle
   d. Increase in amount and thickness of cervical mucus

4. A young adult woman received instructions from the nurse regarding the use of an oral contraceptive. The woman would demonstrate a need for further instruction if she does which of the following?
   a. Stops asking her sexual partners to use condoms with spermicide
   b. States that her menstrual periods should be shorter with decreased blood loss
   c. Takes a pill every morning
   d. Uses a barrier method of birth control if she misses three or more pills

5. The most common, and for some patients the most distressing, side effect of progestin-only contraceptives such as the minipill would be which of the following?
   a. Irregular vaginal bleeding
   b. Headache
   c. Nervousness
   d. Nausea

6. Patients using DMPA should be carefully screened for which of the following possible adverse reactions to its use?
   a. Diabetes mellitus—type 2
   b. Reproductive tract infection
   c. Decrease in bone mineral density
   d. Weight loss

7. A woman has had a copper IUD inserted. The nurse should recognize that the woman needs further teaching if she makes which of the following statements? (Select all that apply.)
   a. "I should check the string before each menstrual period."
   b. "The IUD cam remain effective for up to 10 years."
   c. "It is normal to experience an increase in bleeding and cramping within the first year after it has been inserted."
   d. "My IUD works by releasing progesterone."
   e. "I should avoid using NSAIDs like Motrin if I have cramping."
   f. "I must use safer sex measures to prevent infections in my uterus."

8. A woman experiencing infertility will begin taking clomiphene citrate (Clomid). In order to ensure she takes this medication safely and effectively, the nurse should do which of the following?
   a. Teach the patient's partner how to the patient an IM injection.
   b. Show the woman how to spray the medication into one of her nostrils, emphasizing that she use a different nostril for each dose.
   c. Tell her to inject one dose of human chorionic gonadotropin subcutaneously the day after she takes the last does of the clomiphene citrate.
   d. Tell her to begin taking her tablet daily beginning on the 3rd day of menstruation.

III. THINKING CRITICALLY

1. Mark and his partner, Mary, are undergoing testing for impaired fertility.

   a. Describe the nursing support measures that should be used when working with this couple.

   b. Mark must provide a specimen of semen for analysis. Describe the procedure he should follow to ensure accuracy of the test.

   c. State the semen characteristics that will be assessed.

   d. Mark and Mary tell the nurse that they would like to solve their problem by getting pregnant using nonmedical measures if possible and ask the nurse about the use of alternative measures including the use of herbs to promote fertility. What types of measures could the nurse suggest they try?

2. Assisted human reproduction (AHRs) are being developed and perfected, creating a variety of ethical, legal, financial, and psychosocial concerns. Discuss the issues and concerns engendered by these technologies.

3. Kathy, an 18-year-old, has come to Planned Parenthood for information on birth control methods and assistance with making her choice. She tells the nurse that she is planning to become sexually active with her boyfriend of 6 months and is worried about getting pregnant. "I know I should know more about all of this, but I just don't." Outline the approach the nurse should use to help Kathy make an informed decision in choosing contraception that is right for her.

4. June plans to use a combination estrogen-progestin oral contraceptive.

   a. Describe the mode of action for this type of contraception.

   b. List the advantages of using oral contraception.

   c. Using the acronym ACHES, identify the signs and symptoms that would require June to stop taking the pill and notify her health care provider.

      A

      C

      H

      E

      S

   d. Specify the instructions the nurse should give June about taking the pill to ensure maximum effectiveness.

43

5. Anita has just had a levonorgestrel-releasing intrauterine system (IUS) inserted as her contraceptive method of choice. Specify the instructions that the nurse should give Anita before she leaves the women's health clinic after the insertion.

6. Judy (G6 T4 P0 A2 L4) and Allen, both age 36, are contemplating sterilization now that their family is complete. They are seeking counselling regarding this decision.

   a. Describe the approach a nurse should use in helping Judy and Allen make the right decision for them.

   b. They decide that Allen will have a vasectomy. Discuss the preoperative and postoperative care and instructions required by Allen.

7. Anne and her partner, Ian, will be using the symptothermal method of fertility awareness.

   a. List the assessment components of this method that would indicate that ovulation is occurring and a period of fertility is present requiring abstinence or protected intercourse if pregnancy is not desired.

   b. Outline the points the nurse should emphasize when teaching Anne and Ian to ensure that they will accurately perform the following:

   Measure BBT

   Assess urine for LH

44

Evaluate cervical mucus characteristics

c. State the effectiveness of the symptothermal fertility awareness method of contraception.

8. Edna is a 20-year-old woman who is 9 weeks pregnant and is unsure about what to do. She comes to the women's health clinic and asks for the nurse's help in making her decision, stating, "I just cannot support a baby right now. I am alone and trying to finish my education. What can I do?"

a. Describe the approach the nurse should take in helping Edna make a decision that is right for her.

b. Edna elects to have an abortion. A vacuum aspiration will be performed in the morning. Edna asks what will happen to her as part of the abortion procedure. Describe how the nurse should respond to Edna's question.

c. Identify the nursing measures related to the physical care and emotional support that Edna will require as part of this procedure.

d. Outline the discharge instructions that Edna should receive.

9. Felicia is 7 weeks pregnant and is scheduled for a medically induced abortion using mifepristone and misoprostol (MIFE/MISO). What should the nurse tell Felicia about how these medications work, the method of their administration, and what adverse reactions she could experience?

10. Marlee comes to the women's health clinic to report that she had unprotected intercourse last night. She is worried about getting pregnant because she is at midcycle and has already noticed signs of ovulation. Marlee tells the nurse that she hardly knows her partner and that her emotions just got the best of her. She is very anxious and asks the nurse what her options are. Describe the approach this nurse should use to assist Marlee with her concerns.

9 Genetics, Conception, and Fetal Development

FILL IN THE BLANKS: Insert the term that corresponds to each of the following descriptions related to conception and foetal development.

1. _____ Union of a single egg and sperm. It marks the beginning of a pregnancy.

2. _____ Male and female germ cell. The male germ cell is a _____ and the female germ cell is an _____.

3. _____ Process whereby gametes are formed and mature. For the male, the process is called _____ and for the female, the process is called _____ _____.

4. _____ Process of penetration of the membrane surrounding the ovum by a sperm. It takes place in the _____ _____ of the uterine tube. The membrane becomes impenetrable to other sperm, a process termed _____.
The _____ number of chromosomes is restored when this union of sperm and ovum occurs.

5. _____ The first cell of the new individual. Within 3 days, it becomes a 16-cell solid ball of cells called a _____ _____. This developing structure becomes known as the _____ when a cavity becomes recognisable within it. The outer layer of cells surrounding this cavity is called the _____.

6. _____ Attachment process whereby the blastocyst burrows into the endometrium. _____ or finger-like projections develop out of the trophoblast and extend into the blood-filled spaces of the uterine lining. The uterine lining is now called the _____. The portion of this lining directly under the blastocyst is called the _____ and the portion of this lining that covers the blastocyst is called the _____.

7. _____ The term that refers to the developing baby from day 15 until about 8 weeks after conception.

8. _____ The term that refers to the developing baby from 9 weeks of gestation to the end of pregnancy.

9. _____ Membranes that surround the developing baby and the fluid. The _____ is the outer layer of these membranes and becomes the covering of the foetal side of the placenta. The _____ _____ is the inner layer.

10. _____ Fluid that surrounds the developing baby in the amniotic cavity.

11. _____ Structure that connects the developing baby to the placenta. It contains three vessels, namely two _____ and one _____.

12. _____ The connective tissue that prevents compression of the blood vessels ensuring continued nourishment of the developing baby.

47

13. _____ Structure composed of 15 to 20 lobes called cotyledons. It produces _____ essential to maintain the pregnancy, supplies the _____ _____, and _____ needed by the developing foetus for survival and growth, and removes _____ and _____.

14. _____ Capability of foetus to survive outside the uterus.

15. _____ Surface-active phospholipid that needs to be present in foetal/newborn lungs to facilitate breathing after birth. A _____ ratio can be performed using amniotic fluid as one means of determining the degree to which this phospholipid is present in foetal lungs.

16. _____ Special circulatory pathway that allows foetal blood to bypass the lungs.

17. _____ Shunt that allows most of the foetal blood to bypass the liver and pass into the inferior vena cava.

18. _____ Opening between the foetal atria.

19. _____ Formation of blood that occurs in the _____

20. _____ Dark green to black tarry substance that contains foetal waste products. It accumulates in the foetal intestines.

21. _____ Twins that are formed from two zygotes. They are also called _____ twins.

22. _____ Twins that are formed from one fertilised ovum that then divides. They are also called _____ twins.

MATCHING: Match the description with the appropriate genetic concept.

1. _____ The hereditary material carried in the nucleus of each somatic (body) cell; it determines an individual's characteristics.

2. _____ The process by which germ cells divide, producing gametes that each contain 23 chromosomes.

3. _____ Failure of a pair of chromosomes to separate.

4. _____ Basic physical units of inheritance that are passed from parents to offspring and contain the information needed to specify traits.

5. _____ Abnormality in chromosome number; the numeric deviation is not an exact multiple of the haploid number of chromosomes.

6. _____ Cells that contain half of the genetic material of a normal somatic cell.

7. _____ Union of a normal gamete with a gamete containing an extra chromosome resulting in a cell with 47 chromosomes.

8. _____ X, Y

9. _____ Genes at corresponding loci on homologous chromosomes that code for different forms or variations of the same trait.

10. _____ Process whereby body (somatic) cells replicate to yield two cells with the same genetic makeup as the parent cell.

11. _____ Term that denotes the correct number of chromosomes.

12. _____ The complete set of genetic inheritance in the nucleus of each human cell.

a. Mitosis

b. Meiosis

c. Haploid

d. Diploid

e. Teratogen

f. Human genome

g. Chromosome

h. Genes

i. Sex chromosomes

j. DNA

k. Aneuploidy

l. Trisomy

m. Nondisjunction

n. Monosomy

o. Translocation

p. Mutation

13. _____ Process by which genetic material is transferred from one chromosome to another different chromosome.

14. _____ Threadlike packages of genes and other DNA in the nucleus of a cell.

15. _____ Abnormality in chromosome number in which the deviation is an exact multiple of the haploid number of chromosomes.

16. _____ Somatic cell containing the full number of 46 chromosomes.

17. _____ Union of a normal gamete with a gamete missing a chromosome, resulting in a cell with only 45 chromosomes.

18. _____ A spontaneous and permanent change in normal gene structure.

19. _____ A mixture of cells, some with the normal number of chromosomes and others either missing a chromosome or containing an extra chromosome.

20. _____ Environmental substance or exposure that results in functional or structural disability of the embryo/fetus.

q. Alleles

r. Euploidy

s. Polyploidy

t. Mosaicism

FILL IN THE BLANKS: Insert the term that corresponds to each of the following descriptions related to genetics.

1. _____ Analysis of human DNA, ribonucleic acid (RNA), chromosomes, or proteins to detect abnormalities related to an inherited condition.

2. _____ Direct examination of the DNA and RNA that make up a gene.

3. _____ Examination of the markers that are coinherited with a gene that causes a genetic condition.

4. _____ Examination of the protein products of genes.

5. _____ Examination of chromosomes.

6. _____ Genetic testing that is used to clarify the genetic status of asymptomatic family members. _____ Genetic testing used to detect a disorder that is certain to appear if the defective gene is present and the individual lives long enough. _____ Genetic testing used to detect susceptibility to a disorder if the defective gene is present.

7. _____ Test used to identify individuals who have a gene mutation for a genetic condition but do not show symptoms of the condition because it is a condition that is inherited in an autosomal recessive form.

8. _____ Matched chromosomes.

9. _____ Term that denotes an individual with two copies of the same allele for a given trait. If the two alleles are different, the person is said to be _____ for the trait.

10. _____ The genetic makeup of an individual; an individual's entire genetic makeup or all the genes that the person can pass on to future generations.

11. _____ Observable expression of an individual's genetic makeup.

12. _____ Pictorial analysis of the number, form, and size of an individual's chromosomes.

13. _____ Pattern of inheritance involving a combination of genetic and environmental factors.

14. _____ Pattern of inheritance in which a single gene controls a particular trait, disorder, or defect.

15. _____ Genetic disorder in which only one copy of a variant allele is needed for phenotypic expression.

16. _____ Genetic disorder in which both genes of a pair must be abnormal for the disorder to be expressed.

17 _____ Disorder reflecting absent or defective enzymes leading to abnormal metabolism.

II. REVIEWING KEY CONCEPTS

1. Each of the following structures plays a critical role in foetal growth and development. List the functions of each of the structures listed.

   a. Yolk sac

   b. Amnion, chorion, and amniotic fluid

   c. Umbilical cord

   d. Placenta

2. Identify the tissues or organs that develop from each of the following primary germ layers.

   Ectoderm

   Mesoderm

   Endoderm

3. Angela has come for her first prenatal visit. Identify the questions the nurse should ask during the health history interview to determine whether factors are present that would place Angela at risk for giving birth to a baby with an inheritable disorder.

4. Couples referred for genetic counselling receive an estimation of risk for the genetic disorder of concern. Explain the difference between an estimate of occurrence risk and an estimation of recurrence risk.

5. Based on genetic testing of a newborn, a diagnosis of achondroplasia (dwarfism) was made. The parents ask the nurse if this could happen to future children. Because this is an example of autosomal dominant inheritance, the nurse would tell the parents:
   a. "For each pregnancy, there is a 50–50 chance the child will be affected by dwarfism."
   b. "This will not happen again because the dwarfism was caused by the harmful genetic effects of the infection you had during pregnancy."
   c. "For each pregnancy, there is a 25% chance the child will be a carrier of the defective gene but unaffected by the disorder."
   d. "Because you already have had an affected child, there is a decreased chance for this to happen in future pregnancies."

6. A female carries the gene for haemophilia on one of her X chromosomes. Now that she is pregnant, she asks the nurse how this might affect her baby. The nurse should tell her:
   a. "A female baby has a 50% chance of being a carrier."
   b. "Haemophilia is always expressed if a male inherits the defective gene."
   c. "Female babies are never affected by this disorder."
   d. "A male baby can be a carrier or have haemophilia."

7. A pregnant woman carries a single gene for cystic fibrosis. The father of her baby does not. Which of the following is true concerning the genetic pattern of cystic fibrosis as it applies to this family?
   a. The pregnant woman has cystic fibrosis herself.
   b. There is a 50% chance her baby will have the disorder.
   c. There is a 25% chance her baby will be a carrier.
   d. There is no chance her baby will be affected by the disorder.

8. When teaching a class of first time pregnant patients about foetal development, the nurse would include which of the following statements? (Select all that apply.)
   a. "The sex of your baby is determined by the 9th week of pregnancy."
   b. "The baby's heart begins to pump blood during the 10th week of your pregnancy."
   c. "You should be able to feel your baby move by weeks 16 to 20 of pregnancy."
   d. "We will begin to hear your baby's heartbeat using an ultrasound stethoscope by the 18th week of your pregnancy."
   e. "Your baby will be able to suck, swallow, and hiccup while in your uterus."
   f. "By the 24th week of your pregnancy, you will notice your baby responding to sounds in the environment such as your voice and music."

III. THINKING CRITICALLY

1. Imagine that you are a nurse working in a prenatal clinic. Formulate a response to each of the following concerns or questions directed to you from some of your prenatal patients.

   a. Harjit (2 months pregnant), Mary (5 months pregnant), and Roberta (7 months pregnant) all ask for descriptions of their foetuses at the present time.

   Harjit

   Mary

   Roberta

   b. Shanique states that a friend told her that babies born after about 35 weeks have a better chance to survive because they can breathe easier. She asks if this is true.

   c. Beth, who is 1 month pregnant, states that she heard that people who are pregnant experience quickening. She wants to know what that could mean and if it hurts.

   d. Sabrina, who is 6 months pregnant, states that she read in a magazine that a foetus can actually hear and see. She feels that this is totally unbelievable.

   e. Alexa is 2 months pregnant. She asks how the sex of her baby was determined and whether a sonogram could tell whether she is having a boy or a girl.

   f. Jaclyn is pregnant for the first time. She reveals that she has a history of twins in her family. She wants to know what causes twin pregnancies to occur and what the difference is between identical and fraternal twins.

2. A Jewish couple, are newly married and are planning for pregnancy. They express to the nurse their concern that the woman has a history of Tay-Sachs disease in her family. The husband has never investigated his family history.

   a. Describe the nurse's role in the process of assisting this couple to determine their genetic risk.

   b. The husband and wife are found to be carriers of the disorder. Discuss the estimation of risk and interpretation of risk as it applies to the couple for giving birth to a child who is normal, is a carrier, or is affected by the disorder.

   c. Outline the nurse's role in the education and emotional support of the couple now that a diagnosis and estimation of risk have been made.

10 Anatomy and Physiology of Pregnancy

I. LEARNING KEY CONCEPTS

FILL IN THE BLANKS: Insert the term that corresponds to each of the following descriptions related to pregnancy.

1. _____ Pregnancy.

2. _____ The number of pregnancies in which the foetus or foetuses have reached 20 weeks of gestation, not the number of foetuses (e.g., twins) born. The numeric designation is not affected by whether the foetus is born alive or is stillborn (i.e., showing no signs of life at birth).

3. _____ A woman who is pregnant.

4. _____ A woman who has never been pregnant.

5. _____ A woman who has not completed a pregnancy with a foetus or foetuses beyond 20 weeks of gestation.

6. _____ A woman who is pregnant for the first time.

7. _____ A woman who has completed one pregnancy with a foetus or foetuses who have reached 20 weeks of gestation or more.

8. _____ A woman who has had two or more pregnancies.

9. _____ A woman who has completed two or more pregnancies to 20 weeks of gestation or more.

10. _____ Capacity to live outside the uterus; usually between 22 and 25 weeks are considered on the threshold of viability.

11. _____ Designation given to a pregnancy that has reached 20 weeks of gestation but ends before completion of 36 weeks of gestation.

12. _____ Designation given to a pregnancy from 39 weeks 0 days to 40 weeks 6 days of gestation.

13. _____ Designation given to a pregnancy that goes beyond 42 weeks 0 days of gestation.

14. _____ The biological marker on which pregnancy tests are based. Its presence in urine or serum results in a positive pregnancy test result.

15. _____ Pregnancy-related changes felt by the pregnant patient.

16. _____ Pregnancy-related changes that can be observed by an examiner.

17. _____ Objective signs that can be attributed only to the presence of the foetus.

18. _____ Irregular, painless uterine contractions that can be felt through the abdominal wall soon after the fourth month of pregnancy.

19. _____ A rushing or blowing sound of maternal blood flow through the uterine arteries to the placenta that is synchronous with the maternal pulse.

20. _____ Sound of foetal blood coursing through the umbilical cord; it is synchronous with the foetal heart rate.

21. _____ Foetal movements first felt by the first time pregnant patient as early as 16 to 20 weeks of gestation.

22. _____ Change in blood pressure as a result of compression of abdominal blood vessels and decrease in cardiac output when a pregnant patient lies down on their back.

23. _____ Severe itching of the skin that occurs during pregnancy as a result of retention and accumulation of bile in the liver.

24. _____ Nonfood cravings for substances such as ice, clay, and laundry starch.

MATCHING

Match the assessment finding with the appropriate descriptive term.

25. _____ Subjective symptoms reported by patients that may be the result of pregnancy or another condition.

26. _____ Fundal height decreased, foetal head in pelvic inlet.

27. _____ Cervix and vagina violet-bluish in colour.

28. _____ Swelling of ankles and feet at the end of the day.

29. _____ Cervical tip softened.

30. _____ Lower uterine segment is soft and compressible.

31. _____ Foetal head rebounds with gentle upward tapping through the vagina.

32. _____ White or slightly gray mucoid vaginal discharge with faint, musty odour.

33. _____ Enlarged sebaceous glands in areola on both breasts.

34. _____ Plug of mucus fills endocervical canal.

35. _____ Pink stretch marks or depressed streaks on breasts and abdomen.

36. _____ The anterior pituitary stimulates production of this in the breasts by the end of the first trimester.

37. _____ Cheeks, nose, and forehead blotchy, brownish hyper-pigmentation.

38. _____ Pigmented line extending up abdominal midline to the top of the fundus.

39. _____ A decrease in cardiac output followed by reflex brady-cardia caused by compression of the vena cava in the second half of pregnancy

40. _____ Heartburn.

41. _____ Lumbosacral curve accentuated.

42. _____ Paresthesia and pain in hand radiating to elbow.

43. _____ Responsible for slight spotting following cervical pal-pation or intercourse.

44. _____ State of haemodilution caused by a haematocrit de-creased to 0.32 and haemoglobin to 110 g/L.

45. _____ Vascular spiders on neck and thorax.

46. _____ Palms pinkish red, mottled.

47. _____ Abdominal wall muscles separated.

48. _____ Red raised nodule on gums; bleeds after brushing teeth.

a. Colostrum

b. Operculum

c. Presumptive signs of pregnancy

d. Angiomata

e. Pyrosis

f. Friability

g. Striae gravidarum

h. Physiological anaemia

i. Linea nigra

j. Ballottement

k. Chadwick sign

l. Diastasis recti abdominis

m. Lordosis

n. Leukorrhea

o. Melasma (chloasma)

p. Lightening

q. Supine hypotension

r. Palmar erythema

s. Goodell sign

t. Physiological (dependent) oedema

u. Hegar sign

v. Montgomery tubercles

w. Carpal tunnel syndrome

x. Epulis (gingival granuloma gravidarum)

II. REVIEWING KEY CONCEPTS

1. Describe the obstetric history for each of the following person, using the 5-digit system.

   a. Manjit is pregnant. Her first pregnancy resulted in a stillbirth at 36 weeks of gestation and her second pregnancy resulted in the birth of her daughter at 42 weeks of gestation.

   b. Marsha is 6 weeks pregnant. Her previous pregnancies resulted in the live birth of a daughter at 40 weeks of gestation, the live birth of a son at 38 weeks of gestation, and a spontaneous abortion at 10 weeks of gestation.

   c. Alana is experiencing her fourth pregnancy. Her first pregnancy ended in a spontaneous abortion at 12 weeks, the second resulted in the live birth of twin boys at 32 weeks, and the third resulted in the live birth of a daughter at 39 weeks.

2. When assessing the pregnant patient, the nurse should keep in mind that baseline vital sign values will change as they progress through their pregnancy. Describe how each of the following would change:

   a. Blood pressure (BP)

   b. Heart rate and patterns

   c. Respiratory rate and patterns

3. Identify criteria that must be taken into consideration prior to counselling a woman regarding a positive home pregnancy test.

4. Specify the expected changes that occur in the following laboratory tests as a result of physiological adaptations to pregnancy:

   a. CBC: haematocrit, haemoglobin, white blood cell count

   b. Clotting activity

   c. Acid/base balance

   d. Urinalysis

5. Explain the expected adaptations in elimination that occur during pregnancy. Include in your answer the basis for the changes that occur.

   a. Renal

   b. Bowel

6. A pregnant woman at 10 weeks of gestation exhibits the following signs of pregnancy during a routine prenatal checkup. Which ones would be categorised as probable signs of pregnancy? (Select all that apply.)
   a. hCG in the urine
   b. Breast tenderness
   c. Ballottement
   d. Foetal heart sounds
   e. Hegar sign
   f. Amenorrhea

7. A pregnant patient with four children reports the following obstetrical history: a stillbirth at 32 weeks of gestation, triplets (two sons and one daughter) born via caesarean birth at 30 weeks of gestation, a spontaneous abortion at 8 weeks of gestation, and a daughter born vaginally at 39 weeks of gestation. Which of the following accurately expresses this woman's current obstetrical history using the 5-digit system?
   a. 5-1-4-1-4
   b. 4-1-3-1-4
   c. 5-2-2-0-3
   d. 5-1-4-1-4

8. An essential component of prenatal health assessment of pregnant women is the determination of vital signs. Which of the following would be an expected change in vital sign findings as a result of pregnancy?
   a. Increase in systolic blood pressure by 30 mm Hg or more after assuming a supine position
   b. Increase in diastolic BP by 5 to 10 mm Hg beginning in the first trimester
   c. Chest breathing replaces abdominal breathing with upward displacement of the diaphragm
   d. Gradual decrease in baseline pulse rate of approximately 20 beats per minute

9. During an examination of a pregnant patient the nurse notes that the cervix is soft on its tip. The nurse would document this finding as:
   a. friability.
   b. Goodell sign.
   c. Chadwick sign.
   d. Hegar sign.

10. A nurse is assessing a pregnant patient during a prenatal visit. Several presumptive indicators of pregnancy are documented. Which of the following are presumptive indicators? (Circle all that apply.)
   a. Nausea and vomiting
   b. Quickening
   c. Ballottement
   d. Palpation of foetal movement by the nurse
   e. Hegar's sign
   f. Amenorrhea

III. THINKING CRITICALLY

1. Describe how the nurse should respond to each of the following patient concerns and questions.

   a. Sabrina is 14 weeks pregnant. She calls the prenatal clinic to report that she noticed slight, painless spotting this morning. She reveals that she did have intercourse with her partner the night before.

   b. Preet suspects she is pregnant because her menstrual period is already 3 weeks late. She asks her friend, who is a nurse, how to use the pregnancy test that she just bought so that she obtains the most accurate results.

   c. Dina is 3 months pregnant. She tells the nurse that she is worried because a friend told her that vaginal and bladder infections are more common during pregnancy. She wants to know if this could be true and if so, why.

d. Tammy, who is 20 weeks pregnant, tells the nurse that she has noted some "problems" with her breasts: there are "little pimples" near her nipples and her breasts feel "lumpy and bumpy" and "leak a little."

e. Tamara is concerned because she read in a book about pregnancy that a pregnant patient's position could affect her circulation, especially to the baby. She asks what positions are good for her circulation now that she is pregnant.

f. Beth, a pregnant woman, calls to tell the nurse that she had a nosebleed this morning and has noticed occasional feelings of fullness in her ears. She asks if these occurrences are anything to worry about.

g. Vanessa is 7 months pregnant and works as an office receptionist full time. She asks the nurse if she should take a "water pill" that a friend gave her because she has noticed that her ankles "swell up" at the end of the day.

h. Jan is in her third trimester of pregnancy. She tells the nurse that her posture seems to have changed and that she occasionally experiences low back pain.

i. Monica, who is 36 weeks pregnant with her first baby, calls the clinic stating that she knows the baby is coming because she felt some uterine contractions before getting out of bed in the morning. Monica confirms that they seem to have decreased in intensity and frequency since she has gotten out of bed and walked around.

2. Accurate blood pressure readings are critical, if significant changes in the cardiovascular system are to be detected as a person adapts to pregnancy during the prenatal period. Write a protocol for blood pressure assessment that can be used by nurses working in a prenatal clinic to ensure accuracy of the results obtained during blood pressure assessment.

11 Nursing Care of the Family During Pregnancy

I. LEARNING KEY TERMS

FILL IN THE BLANKS: Insert the term that corresponds to each of the following descriptions.

1. _____ Rule used to determine the estimated day of birth by subtracting _____ months from _____, adding _____ days, and 1 year.

2. _____ The three 3-month periods into which pregnancy is divided.

3. _____ Measurement performed beginning in the second trimester as one indicator of the progress of fetal growth.

4. _____ Tasks accomplished by pregnant persons and their partners as they adapt to the changes of pregnancy; these tasks include _____, _____, _____ , _____ , and _____ .

5. _____ Rapid unpredictable changes in mood that are common in pregnancy.

6. _____ Having conflicting feelings about the pregnancy at the same time.

7. _____ Change in blood pressure that can occur when a pregnant patient lies on their back for an examination of the abdomen. The _____ and the _____ are compressed by the weight of the abdominal contents, including the uterus.

8. _____ Change in blood pressure that can occur if a pregnant woman changes her position rapidly from supine to upright.

9. _____ Pregnancy-related phenomenon in which partners experience pregnancy-like symptoms, such as nausea, weight gain, and other physical symptoms.

10. _____ Cultural directives that tell a pregnant person what to do during pregnancy. _____ Cultural directives that tell a pregnant person what not to do during pregnancy; they establish _____ .

11. _____ Professionally trained person who provides physical, emotional, and informational support to patients and their partners during labour and birth and in the postpartum period.

12. _____ Tool that can be used by expectant couples to explore their childbirth options and choose those that are most important to them; it serves as a tool for communication between the family and the health care providers.

II. REVIEWING KEY CONCEPTS

1. Calculate the expected date of birth (EDB) for each of the following pregnant patients using Nägele's rule.

   a. Diane's last menses began on May 5, 2020, and its last day occurred on May 10, 2020.
   b. Sara had intercourse on February 4, 2020. She has not had a menstrual period since the one that began on January 19, 2020, and ended 5 days later.

   c. Beth's last period began on July 4, 2020, and ended on July 10, 2020. She noted that her basal body temperature (BBT) began to rise on July 28, 2020.

2. Cultural beliefs and practices are important influencing factors during the prenatal period.

a. Describe how cultural beliefs can affect a woman's participation in prenatal care as it is defined by the Western biomedical model of care.

b. Identify one prescription and one proscription for each of the following areas:

Emotional responses

Clothing

Physical activity and rest

Sexual activity

Nutrition

3. Outline the assessment measures that should be used and the data that should be collected during each component of the initial prenatal visit and the follow-up prenatal visits.

INITIAL PRENATAL VISIT

Health History Interview

Physical Examination

Laboratory Testing

FOLLOW-UP PRENATAL VISITS

Updating History

Physical Examination

Foetal Assessment

Laboratory Testing

4. Nurses responsible for the care of pregnant patients must be alert for warning signs of potential complications that patient could develop as pregnancy progresses from trimester to trimester.

a. List the clinical manifestations (warning signs) for each of the following potential complications of pregnancy.

Hyperemesis gravidarum

Infection

Miscarriage

Hypertension conditions including preeclampsia

59

Premature rupture of the membranes (PROM)

Placental disorders (placenta previa; placental abruption)

Foetal demise

b. Describe the approach a nurse should take when discussing potential complications with a pregnant patient and their family.

5. Create a protocol for fundal measurement that will facilitate accuracy.

6. Prevention of injury is an important goal for nurses as they teach pregnant patients about how to care for themselves during pregnancy.

a. Describe three principles of body mechanics that a pregnant patient should be taught to prevent injury.

b. Identify five safety guidelines that the nurse should include in a pamphlet titled "Safety During Pregnancy" that will be distributed to pregnant patients during a prenatal visit.

7. During the third trimester, parents often make a decision concerning the method they will use to feed their newborn. Identify factors that may influence a pregnant patient to choose formula feeding rather than breastfeeding. How would you overcome this reluctance during a prenatal breastfeeding class?

8. Men experience pregnancy in many different ways. Three phases have been identified as characterising the developmental tasks experienced by expectant fathers. Briefly, discuss each phase and how the nurse can help the father to progress through each phase.

Announcement Phase

Moratorium Phase

Focusing Phase

9. A patient's last menstrual period (LMP) began on September 10, 2020, and it ended on September 15, 2020. Using Nägele's rule, the estimated date of birth would be:
a. June 17, 2021.
b. June 22, 2021.
c. August 17, 2021.
d. December 3, 2021.

10. A patient at 30 weeks of gestation assumes a supine position for a fundal measurement and Leopold manoeuvres. They state they are beginning to feel dizzy and nauseated. Their skin feels damp and cool. The nurse's first action would be to:
a. assess the patient's respiratory rate and effort.
b. provide the patient with an emesis basin.
c. elevate the patient's legs 20 degrees from the hips.
d. turn the patient on their side.

11. During an early bird prenatal class a nurse teaches a group of newly diagnosed pregnant patients about their emotional reactions during pregnancy. Which of the following should the nurse discuss with the pregnant patients? (Circle all that apply.)
    a. Sexual desire (libido) may be increased during the second trimester of pregnancy.
    b. A referral for counselling should be sought if a pregnant patient experiences ambivalence in the first trimester.
    c. Rapid, unpredictable mood swings reflect gestational bipolar disorder.
    d. The need to seek safe passage and prepare for birth begins early in the third trimester.
    e. A pregnant patient's own mother will be their greatest source of emotional support during pregnancy.
    f. Attachment to the infant begins late in the third trimester when they begin preparing for birth by attending childbirth preparation classes

12. The nurse evaluates a pregnant person's knowledge about prevention of urinary tract infections at the prenatal visit following a class on infection prevention that the patient attended. The nurse would recognize that the pregnant person needs further instruction when they tell the nurse about which one of the following measures that they now use to prevent urinary tract infections? (Circle all that apply.)
    a. "I drink about 1 litre of fluid a day."
    b. "I have stopped using bubble baths and bath oils."
    c. "I have started wearing panty hose and underpants with a cotton crotch."
    d. "I have yogurt for lunch or as an evening snack."
    e. "I should stop having intercourse with my partner since it increases my risk for urinary tract infections."
    f. "If I drink cranberry juice during breakfast and dinner I will not get a bladder infection."

13. Doulas are important members of a labouring person's health care team. Which of the following activities should be expected as part of the doula's role responsibilities?
    a. Monitoring hydration of the labouring patient, including adjusting IV flow rates
    b. Interpreting electronic foetal monitoring tracings to determine the well-being of the maternal-fetal unit
    c. Eliminating the need for the partner to be present during labour and birth
    d. Providing continuous support throughout labour and birth, including explanations of labour progress

14. A pregnant patient is concerned about what they should do if they notice signs of preterm labour such as uterine contractions. After reviewing the signs of preterm labour with the patient, the nurse reviews measures the patient should implement should the signs occur. The nurse should discuss which of the following measures with the patient? (Circle all that apply.)
    a. Empty bladder
    b. Drink 3 to 4 glasses of water to ensure adequate hydration
    c. Assume a supine position
    d. Assess contractions for 2 or more hours
    e. Report contractions that occur every 10 minutes or more often for 1 hour
    f. Recognise that uterine contractions may be perceived as a tightening in the abdomen or as a backache

III. THINKING CRITICALLY

1. A health history interview of the pregnant patient by the nurse is included as part of the initial prenatal visit.

    a. State the purpose of the health history interview.

    b. Write two questions for each component that is included in the initial health history interview. Questions should be clear, concise, and understandable. Most of the questions should be open ended to elicit the most complete response from the patient.

c. Write four questions that should be included in the interview when updating the health history during follow-up visits.

2. Imagine that you are a nurse working in a prenatal clinic. You have been assigned to be the primary nurse for Martha, an 18-year-old who has come to the clinic for confirmation of pregnancy. She tells you that she knows she is pregnant because she has already missed three periods and a home pregnancy test that she did last week was positive. Martha states that she has had very little contact with the health care system, and the only reason she came today is because her boyfriend insisted that she "make sure" she is really pregnant. Describe the approach that you would take regarding data collection and nursing interventions appropriate for this woman.

3. Terry is a primigravida in her first trimester of pregnancy. She is accompanied by her partner, Tim, to her second prenatal visit. Answer each of the following questions asked by Terry and Tim:

   a. "At the last visit I was told that my estimated date of birth is December 25, 2021. Can I really count on my baby being born on Christmas Day?"

   b. "Before I became pregnant my friend told me I should be doing Kegel exercises. I was too embarrassed to ask her about them. What are they and is it safe for me to do them while I am pregnant?"

   c. "What effect will pregnancy have on our sex life? We are willing to abstain during pregnancy, if we have to keep our baby safe."

   d. "This morning sickness I am experiencing is driving me crazy. I become nauseated in the morning and again late in the afternoon. Occasionally I vomit or have the dry heaves. Will this last for my entire pregnancy? Is there anything I can do to feel better?"

4. Tara is 2 months pregnant. She tells the nurse, at the prenatal clinic, that she is used to being active and exercises every day. Now that she is pregnant she wonders if she should reduce or stop her exercise routine. Discuss what information the nurse's response to Tara should include.

5. Write one nursing diagnosis for each of the following situations. State one expected outcome, and list appropriate nursing measures for the nursing diagnosis you identified.

a. Beth is 6 weeks pregnant. During the health history interview, she tells you that she has limited her intake of fluids and tries to hold her urine as long as she can because, "I just hate having to go to the bathroom so frequently."

Nursing diagnosis   Expected outcome   Nursing measures

b. Doris, who is 23 weeks pregnant, tells you that she is beginning to experience more frequent lower back pain. You note that when she walked into the examining room her posture exhibited a moderate degree of lordosis and neck flexion. She was wearing shoes with 2-inch narrow heels.

Nursing diagnosis   Expected outcome   Nursing measures

c. Lisa, a primigravida at 32 weeks of gestation, comes for a prenatal visit accompanied by her partner, the father of the baby. They both express anxiety about the impending birth of the baby and how they will handle the experience of labour. Lisa is especially concerned about how she will survive the pain, and her partner is primarily concerned about how he will help Lisa cope with labour and make sure she and the baby are safe.

Nursing diagnosis   Expected outcome   Nursing measures

6. Jane is a primigravida in her second trimester of pregnancy. Answer each of the following questions asked by Jane during a prenatal visit.

a. "Why do you measure my abdomen every time I come in for a checkup?"

b. "I am going to start changing the way that I dress now that I am beginning to show. Do you have any suggestions I could follow, especially since I have a limited amount of money to spend?"

c. "What can I do about gas and constipation? I never had much of a problem before I was pregnant."

d. "Since yesterday I have started to feel itchy all over. Do you think I am coming down with some sort of infection?"

63

e. "I will be flying out to Vancouver to visit my father in 1 month. Is airline travel safe for me when I am 5 months pregnant?"

7. While a nurse is measuring a pregnant patient's fundus, the patient becomes pale and diaphoretic. The patient, who is at 23 weeks of gestation, states that they feels dizzy and lightheaded.

   a. State the most likely explanation for the assessment findings exhibited by this patient.

   b. Describe what the nurse's immediate action should be.

8. Kelly is a primigravida in her third trimester of pregnancy. Answer each of the following questions asked by Kelly during a prenatal visit.

   a. "My husband and I have decided that I will breastfeed our baby but friends told me it is very difficult if my nipples do not come out. Is there any way I can tell now if my nipples are okay for breastfeeding?"

   b. "My ankles are swollen by the time I get home from work late in the afternoon [Kelly teaches second grade]. I have been trying to drink about 3 litres of fluid every day. Should I reduce the amount of liquid I am drinking or ask my doctor for a water pill?"

   c. "I woke up last night with a terrible cramp in my leg. It finally went away but my partner and I just did not know what to do. What if this happens again tonight?"

9. Ravneet, a pregnant patient (G2-T0-P0-A1-L0) beginning her third trimester, expresses concern about preterm birth. "I already had one miscarriage, and my sister's baby died after being born too early. I am so worried that this will happen to me."

   a. Identify one nursing diagnosis with an expected outcome that reflects Ravneet's concern.

   b. Indicate what the nurse can teach Ravneet about the signs of preterm labour.

   c. Describe the actions Ravneet should take if she experiences signs of preterm labour.

10. Carol is 4 months pregnant and is beginning to "show." She asks the nurse what she should expect as a reaction from her 13-year-old daughter and 3-year-old son. Describe the teaching the nurse would provide.

11. Your neighbour, Jane, is in her second month of pregnancy. Knowing that you are a nurse, her partner, Tom, confides to you, "I just can't figure out Jane. One minute she is happy and the next minute she is crying for no reason at all! I do not know how I will be able to cope with this for 7 more months." Discuss how you would respond to his concern.

12. Jennifer (G2-T1-P0-A0-L1) and her partner, Dan, are beginning their third trimester of a low-risk pregnancy. As you work with them on their birth plan, they tell you that they are having trouble making a decision about their choice of a birth setting. They experienced a delivery room birth with their first child. Jennifer states, "My first pregnancy was perfectly normal, just like this one, but the birth was disappointing, so medically focused with monitors, IVs, and staying in bed." They ask you for your advice about the different birth settings they have heard and read about, namely labour, delivery, recovery, and postpartum (LDRP) rooms at their local hospital, the birthing centre a few miles from their home, and even their own home. Describe the approach that you would take to guide Jennifer and Dan in their decision regarding a birth setting.

13. Nancy, a pregnant patient (G3-T2-P0-A0-L2) at 26 weeks of gestation, asks the nurse about doulas. "My friend had a doula and she said that she was amazing. My first two birth experiences were difficult—my husband and I really needed someone to help us. Do you think a doula could be that person?"

    a. Explain the role of the doula so that Nancy will have the information she will need to make an informed decision.

    b. Specify questions that Nancy should ask if she decides to hire a doula for her labour.

14. Tony and Andrea are considering the possibility of giving birth to their second baby at home. They have been receiving prenatal care from a registered midwife who has experience with home birth. Their 5-year-old son and both sets of grandparents want to be present for the birth. Discuss the decision-making process that Tony and Andrea should follow to ensure that they make an informed decision that is right for them and their family.

15. A 32-week pregnant patient attends a regular prenatal appointment. On assessment of the patient, a nurse discovers the following findings. Identify whether the findings are normal or abnormal and what would be the appropriate nursing action for each find.

Nursing actions include: (a) document the findings, (b) education, or (c) further assessment.

	Significance	Nursing Action
a. Lower back pain		
b. HR = 90		
c. BP 136/85		
d. Fundal height = 34 cm		
e. FHR = 170		
f. Constipation		
g. Voiding every 1-2 hours with burning sensation		
h. States they are anxious and are crying at appointment		
i. Dyspnea when climbing stairs		
j. Leukorrhea		
k. Nonpitting ankle oedema		

12 Maternal Nutrition

I. LEARNING KEY TERMS

FILL IN THE BLANKS: Insert the term that corresponds to each of the following descriptions.

1. _____ Birth weight of 2500 g or less.

2. _____ Nutrient, particularly important during the preconception period. Adequate intake is important for decreasing risk for _____ or failures in the closure of the neural tube. An intake of _____ _____ daily is recommended for low-risk persons capable of becoming pregnant.

3. _____ Recommendations for nutritional intake that meets the needs of almost all healthy members of the population.

4. _____ Method used to evaluate the appropriateness of weight for height. If the calculated value is less than 18.5, the person is considered to be _____. If the calculated value is between 18.5 and 24.9, the person is considered to be _____. If the calculated value is between 25 and 29.9, the person is considered to be _____, and if greater than 30 the person is considered to be _____.

5. _____ Presence of ketones in the urine as a result of catabolism of fat stores; it has been found to correlate with the occurrence of preterm labour.

6. _____ Normal adaptation that occurs during pregnancy when the plasma volume increases more rapidly than RBC mass.

7. _____ Inability to digest milk sugar because of the absence of the lactase enzyme in the small intestine.

8. _____ Practice of consuming nonfood substances or excessive amounts of food stuffs low in nutritional value.

9. _____ Guide that can be used to make daily food choices during pregnancy and lactation, just as during other stages of the life cycle.

10. _____ A discomfort most commonly experienced in the first trimester of pregnancy; it usually causes only mild-to-moderate nutritional problems but may be a source of substantial discomfort.

11. _____ Severe and persistent vomiting during pregnancy causing weight loss, dehydration, and electrolyte abnormalities.

12. _____ Discomfort of pregnancy that is often related to iron supplement intake and may be relieved with increased water and fibre intake.

13. _____ Discomfort of pregnancy that is usually caused by reflux of gastric contents into the esophagus.

1. Indicate the importance of each of the following nutrients for healthy maternal adaptation to pregnancy and optimum foetal growth and development. Indicate three food/fluid sources for each of the nutrients.

Nutrient	Importance for Pregnancy	Major Food Sources
Protein		
Iron		
Calcium		
Sodium		
Zinc		
Fat-soluble vitamins		
Water-soluble vitamins		

2. When assessing pregnant patients, it is critical that nurses are alert for factors that could place patients at nutritional risk so that early intervention can be implemented. Name five such indicators or risk factors of which the nurse should be aware.

3. Cite the pregnancy-related risks associated with the following nutritional problems.

   a. Underweight patients

   b. Inappropriate weight gain during pregnancy (inadequate; excessive)

   c. Patients with obesity

4. At her first prenatal visit, Marie, a 20-year-old primigravida, reports that she has been a strict vegetarian for the past 3 years. Identify two major guidelines that the nurse should follow when planning menus with Marie.

5. Evaluation of nutritional status is an essential part of a thorough physical assessment of pregnant patients. Cite four signs of good nutrition and four signs of inadequate nutrition that the nurse should observe for during the assessment of a pregnant patient.

6. Calculate the BMI for each of the following patients, and then determine the recommended weight gain and pattern for each patient based on their BMI.

Woman	BMI Meaning	Weight Gain (total; pattern)
a. Nicole: 1.6 m, 54 kg		
b. Alice: 1.68 m, 82 kg		
c. Annie: 1.65 m, 43 kg		

7. A nurse teaching a pregnant patient about the importance of iron in their diet would teach the patient to avoid consuming which of the following foods at the same time as an iron supplement because they will decrease iron absorption? (Select all that apply.)
   a. Tomatoes
   b. Spinach
   c. Meat
   d. Eggs
   e. Milk
   f. Bran

8. A 30-year-old pregnant patient with a BMI of 31 asks the nurse about recommendations for diet and weight gain during pregnancy. Which of the following would the nurse teach this patient?
   a. Counsel them to begin a lifestyle change for weight reduction
   b. Recommend a total weight gain goal of 4 kg during pregnancy
   c. Set a weight gain goal of 0.3 kg per week during the second and third trimesters
   d. Limit third trimester calorie increase to no more than 600 kcal more than prepregnant needs

9. A 25-year-old pregnant patient is at 10 weeks of gestation. Their BMI is calculated to be 24. Which one of the following is recommended in terms of weight gain during pregnancy?
   a. Total weight gain of 18 kg
   b. First trimester weight gain of 1 to 2 kg
   c. Weight gain of 0.4 kg each week for 40 weeks
   d. Weight gain of 3 kg per month during the second and third trimesters

10. A pregnant patient at 6 weeks of gestation tells the midwife that they have been experiencing nausea with occasional vomiting every day. The nurse could recommend which of the following as an effective relief measure?
   a. Eat starchy foods such as buttered popcorn or peanut butter with crackers in the morning before getting out of bed.
   b. Avoid eating before going to bed at night.
   c. Alter eating patterns to a schedule of small meals every 2 to 3 hours.
   d. Skip a meal if nausea is experienced.

11. A pregnant patient demonstrates an understanding of the importance of increasing her intake of foods high in folic acid (100 mcg or more) when includes which of the following foods into the diet? (Select all that apply.)
   a. Seafood
   b. Legumes
   c. Eggs
   d. Liver (beef)
   e. Asparagus
   f. Oranges

III. THINKING CRITICALLY

1. Nutrition and weight gain are important areas of consideration for nurses who care for pregnant patients. In addition, weight gain is often a source of stress and body image alteration for the pregnant patient. Discuss the approach you would use in each of the following situations.

   a. Kelly (1.7 m and 54 kg) states that her primary health care provider recommended a weight gain of approximately 14 kg during her pregnancy. She states, "Babies only weigh about 3.5 kg when they are born. Why do I have to gain much more than that?"

   b. Kate (1.63 m and 57 kg) has just found out that she is pregnant. She states, "I am so glad to be pregnant. I love to eat, and now I can start eating for two. It will be great not to have to watch the scale or what I eat."

   c. June tells you that she does not have to worry about her nutrient intake during her pregnancy. "I take plenty of vitamins—everything from A to Z."

   d. Cora, a primigravida beginning her second month of pregnancy, asks you why she needs to increase her intake of so many nutrients during pregnancy and states, "I work every weekday and rely on fast foods to get through the week, though I try to eat better over the weekends."

   e. Sara (BMI = 28.7) is 1 month pregnant. She asks you for dietary guidance, including a weight reduction diet because she does not want to gain too much weight with this pregnancy.

   f. Beth is 2 months pregnant. She states, "I have cut down on my water intake. I do get a little thirsty, but it's worth it since I don't have to urinate so often."

   g. Hedy is 2 months pregnant and has come for her second prenatal visit. During a discussion about nutritional needs during pregnancy she states, "I know I will never get enough calcium because I get sick when I drink milk."

2. Yvonne's hemoglobin is 130 g/L and her hematocrit is 0.37 at the onset of her pregnancy. She asks the nurse if she will have to take iron during her pregnancy if she tries to follow a good diet. "My friend took iron when she was pregnant and it made her sick to her stomach." Discuss the appropriate response by the nurse.

3. Identify three nursing measures appropriate for each of the following nursing diagnoses:

   a. Imbalanced nutrition related to inadequate intake associated with moderate nausea and vomiting of pregnancy

   b. Constipation associated with increased progesterone levels during pregnancy

   c. Pain related to reflux of gastric contents into oesophagus following dinner

4. Gloria is an 18-year-old woman (1.7 m and 44 kg) who is 8 weeks pregnant. In her discussions with you at her first prenatal visit, she expresses a lack of knowledge regarding the nutritional requirements of pregnancy and an interest in learning about what to eat because she wants to have a healthy baby.

   a. Outline the approach that you would use to help Gloria learn about and meet the nutritional requirements of her pregnancy.

   b. Gloria says her friends have told her she cannot drink coffee. What would you teach her regarding this?

   c. Gloria also states that she has heard something about listeriosis and wonders what this is and how this could impact a pregnancy. What should you teach her regarding this?

13 Pregnancy Risk Factors and Assessment

I. LEARNING KEY TERMS

FILL IN THE BLANKS: Insert the term that corresponds to each of the following descriptions.

1. _____ A pregnancy in which the life or health of the mother or the foetus is jeopardised by a disorder or medical, social, or environmental factors coincident with or unique to pregnancy.

2. _____ Assessment of foetal activity by the mother is a simple yet valuable method for monitoring the condition of the foetus.

3. _____ Diagnostic test that involves the use of sound having a frequency higher than that detectable by humans to examine structures inside the body. During pregnancy, it can be done by using either the _____ or _____ approach.

4. _____ Noninvasive study of blood flow in the foetus and placenta with ultrasound.

5. _____ Noninvasive dynamic assessment of the foetus and its environment that is based on acute and chronic markers of foetal disease. It uses real-time _____. This test includes assessment of five variables, namely _____, _____, _____, _____, and _____.

6. _____ Prenatal diagnostic test that is performed to obtain amniotic fluid to examine the foetal cells it contains.

7. _____ Prenatal diagnostic test that provides direct access to the foetal circulation during the second and third trimesters.

8. _____ Procedure that involves the removal of a small tissue specimen from the foetal portion of the placenta. Because this tissue originates from the zygote, it reflects the genetic makeup of the foetus and is performed between 10 and 13 weeks of gestation.

9. _____ What is tested for in a first trimester screening test, performed between 11 and 14 weeks of gestation. Assesses for foetal aneuploidy.

10. _____ Non-invasive prenatal testing that screens for foetal aneuploidy by obtaining maternal blood.

11. _____ Screening test for Rh incompatibility by examining the serum of Rh-negative patients for Rh antibodies.

12. _____ Test based on the fact that the heart rate of a healthy foetus with an intact central nervous system will usually accelerate in response to its own movement.

13. _____ Test used to identify the jeopardised foetus that is stable at rest but shows evidence of compromise when exposed to the stress of uterine contractions. If the resultant hypoxia of the foetus is sufficient, a deceleration of the FHR will result. Two methods used for this test are the _____ test and the _____ test.

II. REVIEWING KEY CONCEPTS

1. Identify social determinants of health that would place the pregnant patient and foetus/newborn at risk, including each of the following categories:

   Biology and genetic factors

   Demographic characteristics

   Personal health factors and coping strategies

2. Discuss the role of the nurse when caring for high risk pregnant patients who are required to undergo antepartal assessment testing to determine foetal well-being.

3. State two risk factors for each of the following pregnancy-related problems:

   Polyhydramnios

   Intrauterine growth restriction

   Oligohydramnios

   Chromosomal abnormalities

4. A 34-year-old patient at 36 weeks of gestation has been scheduled for an amniocentesis. The patient asks the nurse why the test needs to be performed. The nurse would tell them that the test:
   a. determines how well the baby will breathe after it is born.
   b. evaluates the response of the baby's heart to uterine contractions.
   c. measures the baby's head size and length.
   d. observes the foetus' activities in utero to predict fetal well-being.

5. As part of preparing a 24-year-old patient at 42 weeks of gestation for a nonstress test, the nurse would:
   a. instruct the patient to fast for 8 hours before the test.
   b. explain that the test will evaluate how well their baby is moving inside the uterus.
   c. show the patient how to indicate when the fetus moves.
   d. attach a spiral electrode to the presenting part to determine FHR patterns.

6. A pregnant patient at 13 weeks of gestation is having a first trimester screening test performed. The patient has obesity and is Rh negative. The primary purpose of this test is to screen for:
   a. spina bifida.
   b. Down syndrome.
   c. gestational diabetes.
   d. Rh antibodies.

7. During a contraction stress test, four contractions lasting 45 to 55 seconds were recorded in a 10-minute period. A late deceleration was noted during the third contraction. The nurse conducting the test would document that the result is:
   a. negative.
   b. positive.
   c. atypical.
   d. unsatisfactory.

8. A pregnant patient is scheduled for a transvaginal ultrasound test to establish gestational age. In preparing this patient for the test, the nurse would:
   a. place the patient in a supine position with her hips elevated on a folded pillow.
   b. instruct the patient to come for the test with a full bladder.
   c. administer an analgesic 30 minutes before the test.
   d. lubricate the vaginal probe with transmission gel.

73

III. THINKING CRITICALLY

1. Annie is a primigravida who is at 10 weeks of gestation. Her prenatal history reveals that she was treated for pelvic inflammatory disease 2 years ago. She describes irregular menstrual cycles and is therefore unsure about the first day of her last menstrual period. Annie is scheduled for a transvaginal ultrasound.

   a. Cite the likely reasons for the performance of this test.

   b. Describe how the nurse should prepare Annie for this test.

2. Latisha, a pregnant woman at 20 weeks of gestation, is scheduled for a series of transabdominal ultrasounds to monitor the growth of her fetus. Describe the nursing role as it applies to Latisha and transabdominal ultrasound examinations.

3. Mary is at 42 weeks of gestation. Her health care provider has ordered a biophysical profile (BPP). She is very upset and tells the nurse, "All my doctor told me is that this test will see if my baby is okay. I do not know what is going to happen and if it will be painful to me or harmful for my baby."

   a. Describe how the nurse should respond to Mary's concerns.

   b. Mary receives a score of 8 for the BPP. List the factors that were evaluated to obtain this score and specify the meaning of Mary's test result of 8.

4. Jan, is 18 weeks pregnant and is having an amniocentesis due to positive first trimester screening result. Jan's blood type is A negative and her partner's, the father of her baby, is B positive. Her primary health care provider has suggested an amniocentesis. Describe the nurse's role in terms of each of the following:

   a. Preparing Jan for the amniocentesis

   b. Supporting Jan during the procedure

74

c. Providing Jan with postprocedure care and instructions

5. Susan, who has diabetes and is in week 36 of pregnancy, has been scheduled for a nonstress test.

a. Discuss what you would tell Susan about the purpose of this test and what will be learned about her baby's well-being.

b. Describe how you would prepare Susan for this test.

c. Discuss how you would conduct the test.

d. Indicate the criteria you would use to determine whether the result of the test was:

Normal

Atypical

Abnormal

6. Beth is scheduled for a contraction stress test following an atypical result on a nonstress test. Nipple stimulation will be used to stimulate the required contractions.

a. Discuss what you would tell Beth about the purpose of this test and what will be learned about the well-being of her fetus.

b. Describe how you would prepare Beth for the test.

c. Indicate how you would conduct the test.

d. State how you would conduct the test differently if exogenous oxytocin is used instead of nipple stimulation.

e. Indicate the criteria you would use to determine whether the result of the test was:

Negative

Positive

Unsatisfactory

Equivocal-tachysystole

Atypical

14 Pregnancy at Risk: Gestational Conditions

I. LEARNING KEY TERMS

FILL IN THE BLANKS: Insert the term that corresponds to each of the following descriptions related to foetal assessment.

1. _____ A systolic BP greater than 140 mm Hg or a diastolic BP greater than 90 mm Hg recorded on two separate occasions at least 15 minutes apart.

2. _____ An obstetrical emergency in which there is a systolic BP of 160 mm Hg or greater or a diastolic BP of 110 mm Hg, based on at least two measurements taken at least 15 minutes apart.

3. _____ Development of hypertension after week 20 of pregnancy in a previously normotensive patient without proteinuria.

4. _____ A vasospastic pregnancy-specific syndrome in which gestational or chronic hypertension and new-onset proteinuria are criteria.

5. _____ Onset of seizure activity in the patient with preeclampsia, with no history of preexisting pathology, which can result in seizure activity.

6. _____ Hypertension present before pregnancy or diagnosed prior to 20 weeks gestation.

7. _____ Process which results in poor tissue perfusion in organ systems, increased peripheral resistance, and blood pressure, and increased cellular permeability.

8. _____ Laboratory diagnosis for a variant of severe preeclampsia that involves hepatic dysfunction; it is characterised by

_____, _____, and

_____.

9. _____ Protein concentration of ≥0.03 g/L in at least two random urine specimens collected at least 6 hours apart or a concentration of greater than 0.3 g/L per 24 hours for a 24-hour urine specimen.

10. Clinical signs that indicate resolution of preeclampsia include _____, and _____.

11. _____ Excessive vomiting during pregnancy that leads to significant weight loss along with dehydration, electrolyte imbalance, nutritional deficiency, and ketonuria.

12. _____ Pregnancy that ends as a result of natural causes before 20 weeks of gestation or less than 500 g birthweight. It is termed

_____ if it occurs before 12 weeks of

gestation and _____ if it occurs between 12 and 20 weeks of gestation.

13. _____ Pregnancy in which the foetus has died but the products of conception are retained in utero for up to several weeks.

14. _____ Three or more consecutive pregnancy losses before 20 weeks of gestation.

15. _____ Passive and painless dilation of the cervix during the second trimester leading to recurrent preterm births during the second trimester in the absence of other causes.

16. _____ Procedure that involves placement of a suture around the cervix beneath the mucosa to constrict the internal os of the cervix.

17. _____ Pregnancy in which the fertilised ovum is implanted outside the uterine cavity, most often in the uterine tube.

18. _____ Group of pregnancy-related trophoblastic proliferative disorders without a viable foetus that are caused by abnormal fertilisation. It includes _____,

_____, and _____.

77

19. _____ Disorder that results when an egg without an active nucleus has been fertilised.

20. _____ Disorder that results when two sperm fertilise an apparently normal ovum.

21. _____ Implantation of the placenta in the lower uterine segment totally covering the internal cervical os.

22. _____ Implantation of the placenta in the lower uterine segment without reaching the os.

23. _____ Detachment of part or all of the placenta from its implantation site.

24. _____ Condition in which the foetal vessels are implanted into the foetal membranes rather than the placenta. They often lie over the cervical os. _____ Variation of vasa previa in which the cord vessels begin to branch at the membranes and then course into the placenta. _____ A second variation of vasa previa in which the placenta is divided into two or more lobes rather than remaining as a single mass. Foetal vessels run between the lobes and collect at the periphery, eventually uniting to form the vessels of the umbilical cord.

25. _____ Marginal insertion of the cord into the placenta, which also increases the risk for foetal haemorrhage.

26. _____ Pathological form of clotting that is diffuse and consumes large amounts of clotting factors, causing widespread external or internal bleeding or both.

27. _____ The most common congenital clotting defect in North American persons of child-bearing age.

28. _____ Persistent presence of bacteria within the urinary tract of patients who have no symptoms.

29. _____ Bladder infection characterised by dysuria, urgency, and frequency, along with lower abdominal or suprapubic pain.

30. _____ Renal infection that is a common serious medical complication of pregnancy and the second most common nonbirth reason for hospitalization.

31. _____ The most common nonobstetrical surgical emergency during pregnancy.

32. _____ Presence of gallstones in the gallbladder.

33. _____ Inflammation of the gallbladder.

II. REVIEWING KEY CONCEPTS

1. State the principles you would follow to ensure the accuracy of BP measurement during pregnancy.

2. Describe the assessment technique used to determine whether the following findings are present in pregnant patients with preeclampsia. (Note: You may wish to review this information in a physical assessment textbook for a complete explanation of each technique.)

   a. Hyperreflexia and ankle clonus

   b. Proteinuria

MATCHING: Match the patient description with the appropriate diagnosis.

3. _____ At 30 weeks of gestation, a patient's BP is consistently above 140/90; her latest urinalysis indicated a protein level of 2+ on dipstick; biceps and patellar reflexes are 2 + .

4. _____ At 24 weeks of gestation, a normotensive patient's BP rose from a pre-pregnant baseline of 118/70 to 148/92. No other problematic signs and symptoms including proteinuria were noted.

5. _____ A 34-year-old pregnant patient has had a consistently high BP ranging from 148/92 to 160/98 since the age of 28. Their weight gain has followed normal patterns, and urinalysis remains normal as well.

6. _____ At 32 weeks of gestation, a patient, with hypertension since 28 weeks, hyperactive DTRs with clonus, and proteinuria of 4 + , has a convulsion.

7. _____ A pregnant patient has been hypertensive since their 24th week of pregnancy. Urinalysis indicates a protein content of 3 + . Further testing reveals a platelet count of 50 and elevated AST and ALT levels; they have begun to experience nausea with some vomiting and epigastric pain.

a. Eclampsia

b. Chronic hypertension

c. Gestational hypertension

d. HELLP syndrome

e. Preeclampsia

MATCHING: Match the medication description with the appropriate medication.

8. _____ Medication of choice in the prevention and treatment of seizure activity (eclampsia) caused by severe preeclampsia.

9. _____ Intravenous antihypertensive agent for the treatment of hypertension that occurs with severe preeclampsia.

10. _____ Antiemetic medication that is recommended to treat hyperemesis gravidarum.

11. _____ Synthetic prostaglandin E_1 analog administered orally or vaginally as part of the medical management of a miscarriage.

12. _____ Antimetabolite and folic acid antagonist that is used to destroy rapidly dividing cells; it is used for the medical management of an unruptured ectopic pregnancy.

13. _____ Prostaglandin derivative that can be administered intramuscularly to contract the uterus and treat excessive bleeding following evacuating the products of conception when a miscarriage has occurred.

a. pyridoxine

b. methotrexate

c. magnesium sulphate

d. misoprostol

e. labetolol

f. carboprost tromethamine

14. When measuring the BP to ensure consistency and to facilitate early detection of BP changes consistent with gestational hypertension, the nurse should:
   a. place the patient in a supine position.
   b. allow the patient to rest for at least 15 minutes before measuring her BP.
   c. use the same arm for each BP measurement.
   d. use a proper sized cuff that covers at least 50% of the upper arm.

15. A patient's preeclampsia has advanced to the severe stage. They are admitted to the hospital and the primary health care provider has ordered an infusion of magnesium sulphate be started. In fulfilling this order the nurse would implement which of the following? (Select all that apply.)

   a. Prepare a loading dose of 2 g of magnesium sulphate in 200 mL of 5% glucose in water to be given over 15 minutes.
   b. Prepare the maintenance solution by mixing 4 g of magnesium sulphate in at least 100 mL of IV fluid.
   c. Monitor maternal vital signs, foetal heart rate (FHR) patterns, and uterine contractions every 2 hours.
   d. Expect the maintenance dose to be approximately 1 to 2 g/hour.
   e. Report a respiratory rate of 14 breaths or less per minute to the primary health care provider immediately.
   f. Recognise that urinary output should be at least 25 to 30 mL per hour.

16. The primary expected outcome for care associated with the administration of magnesium sulphate would be met if the pregnant patient exhibits which of the following?
    a. Exhibits a decrease in both systolic and diastolic BP
    b. Experiences no seizures
    c. States that she feels more relaxed and calm
    d. Urinates more frequently, resulting in a decrease in pathological oedema

17. A pregnant patient has been diagnosed with mild hypertension and will be treated at home. The nurse, in teaching this patient about the treatment regimen for mild hypertension, would teach the patient to do which of the following? (Select all that apply.)
    a. Check respirations before and after taking an oral dose of magnesium sulphate.
    b. Place a dipstick into a clean-catch sample of urine to test for protein.
    c. Reduce fluid intake to four to five 240 mL glasses each day.
    d. Do gentle exercises such as hand and feet circles and gently tensing and relaxing arm and leg muscles.
    e. Avoid excessively salty foods.
    f. Maintain strict bed rest in a quiet dimly lighted room with minimal stimuli.

18. A pregnant patient has just been admitted with a diagnosis of hyperemesis gravidarum. They have been unable to retain any oral intake and as a result have lost weight and is exhibiting signs of dehydration with electrolyte imbalance and acetonuria. The care management of this patient would include which of the following?
    a. Administering labetalol to control nausea and vomiting
    b. Assessing the patient's urine for ketones
    c. Avoiding oral hygiene until the patient is able to tolerate oral fluids
    d. Providing small frequent meals consisting of bland foods and warm fluids together once the patient begins to respond to treatment

19. A primigravida at 10 weeks of gestation reports slight vaginal spotting without passage of tissue and mild uterine cramping. When examined, no cervical dilation is noted. The nurse caring for this patient would:
    a. anticipate that the patient will be sent home and with instructions to avoid stress and orgasm.
    b. prepare the patient for a dilation and curettage.
    c. inform the patient that frequent blood tests will be required to check the level of estrogen.
    d. tell the patient that the doctor will most likely perform a cerclage to help maintain the pregnancy.

20. A patient is admitted through the emergency department with a medical diagnosis of ruptured ectopic pregnancy. The priority nursing concern would be:
    a. acute pain.
    b. risk for infection.
    c. deficient fluid volume.
    d. anticipatory grieving related to unexpected pregnancy outcome.

21. A patient diagnosed with an ectopic pregnancy is given an intramuscular injection of methotrexate. The nurse would teach the patient which of the following?
    a. Methotrexate is an analgesic that will relieve the dull abdominal pain they are experiencing.
    b. Gastric distress, nausea and vomiting, stomatitis, and dizziness are common. Rare side effects include severe neutropenia, reversible hair loss, and pneumonitis.
    c. Follow-up blood tests will be required every other month for 6 months after the injection of the methotrexate.
    d. They should continue to take prenatal vitamin and folic acid to enhance healing.

22. A pregnant patient at 32 weeks of gestation comes to the emergency department due to experiencing bright red vaginal bleeding. They reports no pain. The admission nurse suspects:
    a. placental abruption.
    b. disseminated intravascular coagulation.
    c. placenta previa.
    d. preterm labour.

23. A pregnant patient, at 38 weeks of gestation diagnosed with marginal placenta previa, has just given birth to a healthy newborn. The nurse recognises that the immediate focus for the care of this patient would be:
    a. preventing haemorrhage.
    b. relieving pain.
    c. preventing infection.
    d. fostering attachment of the mother with their newborn.

24. Explain the current recommendations for screening for and diagnosing of gestational diabetes mellitus developed by Diabetes Canada Clinical Practice Guidelines Expert Committee.

III. THINKING CRITICALLY

1. Jean (G1-T0-P0-A0-L0) is at 30 weeks of gestation and has been diagnosed with mild gestational hypertension. The treatment plan includes home care with reduced activity and stress reduction. She and her partner are very anxious about the diagnosis and are also concerned about how they will manage the care of their active 3-year-old adopted daughter, Anne.

   a. What factors could be present in Jean's history that would increase her risk for developing preeclampsia?

   b. Indicate the clinical manifestations that would be present to indicate this diagnosis.

   c. Describe how you would help this couple organise their home care routine.

   d. Specify what you would teach them with regard to assessment of Jean's status in terms of each of the following:

   BP

   Protein in urine

   Foetal well-being

   Signs of a worsening condition

   e. Describe the instructions you would give Jean regarding her nutrient and fluid intake.

   f. Reduced activity can lead to a concern of constipation related to changes in bowel function associated with pregnancy and reduced activity. Cite two measures that Jean can use to enhance bowel elimination and prevent constipation.

2. Ellen, a pregnant patient at 37 weeks of gestation, is admitted to the hospital with a diagnosis of severe preeclampsia.

   a. Indicate the signs and symptoms that would be present to indicate this diagnosis.

b. Specify the precautionary measures that should be taken to protect Ellen and her foetus from injury.

c. Ellen's health care provider orders magnesium sulphate to be infused at 4 g in 20 minutes as a loading dose, and then a maintenance intravenous infusion of 2 g/hr.

- Identify the guidelines that must be followed when preparing and administering the magnesium sulphate infusion.

- Explain the expected therapeutic effect of magnesium sulphate to Ellen and her family.

d. List the maternal-fetal assessments that should be accomplished on a regular basis during the infusion of magnesium sulphate.

- Identify the progressive signs of magnesium sulphate toxicity.

- State the interventions that must be instituted immediately if magnesium sulphate toxicity occurs.

e. Despite all prevention efforts, Ellen has a seizure.

- Specify the nursing measures that should be implemented at the onset of the seizure and immediately afterward.

- List the problems that can occur as a result of the convulsion that Ellen experienced.

f. Ellen successfully gave birth vaginally despite her high risk status. Describe Ellen's care management during the first 48 hours of her postpartum recovery period.

3. Marie, an 18-year-old primigravida with obesity, is diagnosed with hyperemesis gravidarum at 9 weeks gestation. She is single and lives at home with her parents. Marie is admitted to the high risk antepartal unit. During the admission interview, Marie confides to the nurse that her parents have been very unhappy about her pregnancy. She now is worried that she may have made the wrong decision to continue with her pregnancy and raise her baby as a lone parent.

a. Identify the etiological factors that may have contributed to Marie's current health problem.

b. List the physiological and psychological factors that the nurse should be alert for when assessing Marie upon her admission.

c. Outline the nursing care measures appropriate for Marie while hospitalised.

d. Once stabilised, Marie is discharged to home care. She is able to tolerate oral food and fluid intake. Explain the important care measures that the nurse should discuss with Marie and her family before she goes home.

4. Lucia is admitted to the hospital, where a diagnosis of acute unruptured ectopic pregnancy in her fallopian tube is made.

   a. State the risk factors associated with ectopic pregnancy.

   b. Describe the findings that were most likely experienced and exhibited by Lucia as her ectopic pregnancy progressed and then ruptured.

   c. Identify the other health care problems that share the same or similar clinical manifestations as ectopic pregnancy.

   d. State the major care management problem at this time. Support your answer.

   e. Outline the nursing measures Lucia will require during the preoperative and postoperative period.

5. Kaycee is 10 weeks pregnant. She comes to the clinic and states that she has been experiencing slight bleeding with mild cramping for about 4 hours. No tissue has been passed and pelvic examination reveals that the cervical os is closed.

   a. Indicate the most likely basis for Kaycee's signs and symptoms.

   b. Outline the expected care management of Kaycee's problem.

83

6. Denise, a primigravida, calls the clinic. She is crying while she tells the nurse that she has noted "a lot of bleeding" and that she is sure she is losing her baby.

    a. Write several questions the nurse should ask Denise to obtain a more definitive picture of the bleeding she is experiencing.

    b. Based on the data collected, Denise is admitted to the hospital for further evaluation. A medical diagnosis of incomplete abortion is made. Describe the assessment findings that would indicate the diagnosis of incomplete abortion.

    c. What nursing priority would be most important at this time.

    d. Outline the nursing measures that would be appropriate for the priority nursing concern you identified and for the expected medical management of Denise's health problem.

    e. Specify the instructions that Denise should receive before her discharge from the hospital.

    f. List the nursing measures appropriate for the following nursing diagnosis: Anticipatory grieving related to unexpected outcome of pregnancy.

7. Maryam has been diagnosed with hydatidiform mole (complete).

    a. Identify the typical signs and symptoms Maryam would most likely exhibit to establish this diagnosis.

    b. Specify the posttreatment instructions that the nurse must stress when discussing follow-up management with Maryam.

    c. Name the major concern associated with complete hydatidiform mole and indicate the signs that would indicate that it is occurring.

8. Two pregnant patients are admitted to the labour unit with vaginal bleeding. Sonia is at 29 weeks of gestation and is diagnosed with marginal placenta previa. Diane is at 34 weeks of gestation and is diagnosed with a moderate (class II) premature separation of the placenta (placental abruption).

   a. Compare the clinical picture each of these women is likely to exhibit during assessment.

   Sonia   Diane

   b. Identify one priority nursing diagnosis for both Sonia and Diane.

   c. Contrast the nursing care required by each of the women as it relates to their diagnosis and the typical medical management.

   Sonia   Diane

   d. Indicate the considerations that must be given top priority following birth for each of these women.

   Sonia   Diane

9. Trauma continues to be a common complication during pregnancy that may require obstetrical critical care.

   a. Discuss the significance of this complication using statistical data to describe the scope of the problem in terms of incidence, timing during pregnancy, and forms of trauma.

   b. Indicate the effects trauma can have on pregnancy.

   c. Describe the potential impact of trauma on the foetus.

   d. Identify the priorities of care for the pregnant patient following trauma.

   e. Outline the major components of the assessment and care of a pregnant patient who has experienced trauma.

   Primary survey

   Secondary survey

   f. Explain how cardiopulmonary resuscitation (CPR) should be adapted for a pregnant patient.

10. Elena (G2-T1-P0-A0-L1) is a 32-year-old woman in week 28 of her pregnancy. Elena's BMI is 27. Her mother, who is 59, was recently diagnosed with type 2 diabetes. Elena's first pregnancy resulted in the birth of a 4.8 kg daughter who is now 2 years old. A 1-hour, 50-g glucose tolerance test last week revealed a glucose level of 8.3 mmol/L. A 3-hour glucose tolerance test was done yesterday with the following results: Fasting—6.0 mmol/L, 1 hr—10.7 mmol/L, 2 hr—9.4 mmol/L, 3 hr—7.8 mmol/L.

   a. Identify the complication of pregnancy Elena is exhibiting. State the rationale for your answer.

   b. List the risk factors for this health problem that are present in Elena's assessment data.

   c. Describe the pathophysiology involved in creating Elena's issue.

   d. Identify the maternal and foetal/neonatal risks and complications that are possible in this situation.

   e. Outline the ongoing assessment measures necessitated by Elena's health issue.

   f. Describe how Elena should be taught to maintain euglycemia for the remainder of her pregnancy. Explain to her why euglycemia is so important.

   g. Before discharge after the birth of her second daughter, Elena asks the nurse whether the health problem she experienced during this pregnancy will continue now that she has had her baby. She also wonders if it will happen with her next pregnancy because she wants to get pregnant again soon so she can "try for a son." Discuss the response the nurse should give to Elena's concerns.

15 Pregnancy at Risk: Pre existing Conditions

I. LEARNING KEY TERMS

FILL IN THE BLANKS: Insert the term that corresponds to each of the following descriptions related to diabetes mellitus.

1. _____ A group of metabolic diseases characterised by hyperglycemia resulting from defects in insulin secretion, insulin action, or both.

2. _____ Accumulation of excessive glucose in the blood.

3. _____ A normal blood glucose level.

4. _____ Blood glucose level that is too low.

5. _____ Excretion of large volumes of urine.

6. _____ Excessive thirst.

7. _____ Excessive eating.

8. _____ Excretion of unusable glucose into the urine.

9. _____ Accumulation of ketones in the blood resulting from hyperglycemia and leading to metabolic acidosis.

10. _____ Classification of diabetes mellitus primarily caused by pancreatic islet betacell destruction and prone to ketoacidosis; persons with this form of diabetes usually have an absolute insulin deficiency.

11. _____ Most prevalent classification of diabetes mellitus; persons with this form of diabetes have insulin resistance and usually relative (rather than absolute) insulin deficiency.

12. _____ Label given to diabetes mellitus that existed before pregnancy.

13. _____ Diabetes diagnosed during pregnancy. Related to carbohydrate intolerance.

14. _____ Blood test that provides a measurement of glycemic control over time, specifically over the previous 2 to 6 weeks.

15. _____ Excessive foetal growth; birth weight greater than 4000 to 4500 g or greater than the 90th percentile.

16. _____ Excessive amniotic fluid.

17. _____ Device persons with diabetes mellitus can use to measure blood glucose levels.

FILL IN THE BLANKS: Insert the term that corresponds to each of the following descriptions related to selected preexisting medical disorders during pregnancy.

18. _____ Inability of the heart to maintain a sufficient cardiac output. Physiological stress on the heart is greatest between week _____ and _____ of gestation because the cardiac output is at its peak. Risk for this complication is also higher during _____ and the first _____ to _____ hours after birth.

19. _____ Classification system for cardiovascular disorders developed by the New York Heart Association. Class I implies _____. Class II implies _____. Class III implies _____. Class IV implies _____.

20. _____ Cardiac disorder characterised by the development of heart failure in the last month of pregnancy or within 6 postpartum months, lack of another cause for heart failure, and the absence of heart disease before the last month of pregnancy.

21. _____ Damage of the heart valves and the chordae tendineae cordis as a result of an infection originating from an inadequately treated group A beta-haemolytic streptococcal infection of the throat.

22. _____ Narrowing of the valve between the left atrium and the left ventricle of the heart by stiffening of the valve leaflets, which obstructs blood flow from the atrium to the ventricles. _____ Narrowing of the opening of the aortic valve.

23. _____ Acute ischaemic event involving cardiac muscle.

24. _____ Inflammation of the innermost lining of the heart caused by invasion of bacteria.

25. _____ Common, usually benign, cardiac condition that involves the protrusion of the leaflets of the mitral valve back into the left atrium during ventricular systole, allowing some backflow of blood.

26. _____ A hemoglobin level of less than 110 g/L or a haematocrit of less than or equal to 0.32; it is mainly a result of an _____ deficiency.

27. _____ Disease caused by the presence of abnormal haemoglobin in the blood. It is a recessive, hereditary, familial hemolytic anemia that affects those of African or Mediterranean ancestry.

28. _____ Relatively common anemia in which an insufficient amount of hemoglobin is produced to fill red blood cells.

29. _____ Acute respiratory illness caused by allergens, irritants, marked changes in ambient temperature, certain medications, or exercise. In response to stimuli, there is widespread but reversible narrowing of the hyperactive airways making it difficult to breathe.

30. _____ Common autosomal recessive genetic disorder in which the exocrine glands produce excessive viscous secretions, causing problems with both respiratory and digestive functions.

31. _____ Generalised itching during pregnancy without the presence of a rash.

32. _____ Integumentary condition during pregnancy characterised by itching and urticarial papules and plaques most often appearing during the mid to late third trimester.

33. _____ Liver disorder unique to pregnancy that is characterised by generalised pruritus, usually beginning during the third trimester, most severely affecting the palms and soles, and is worse at night.

34. _____ Disorder of the brain causing recurrent seizures; it is the most common neurological disorder accompanying pregnancy.

35. _____ Patchy demyelinization of the spinal cord and CNS; may be viral in origin.

36. _____ Acute idiopathic facial paralysis that can occur during pregnancy.

37. _____ Chronic, multisystem, inflammatory disease characterised by autoimmune antibody production that affects the skin, joints, kidneys, lungs, central nervous system (CNS), liver, and other body organs.

II. REVIEWING KEY CONCEPTS

1. Identify the major maternal and foetal/newborn risks and complications associated with diabetic pregnancies. Indicate the underlying pathophysiological basis for each of the complications you identify.

2. State how hyperthyroidism and hypothyroidism can affect reproductive well-being and pregnancy.

3. Identify the maternal and foetal complications that are more common among pregnant patients who have cardiac problems.

4. A pregestational diabetic patient at 20 weeks of gestation exhibits the following: thirst, nausea and vomiting, abdominal pain, drowsiness, and increased urination. The skin is flushed and dry and their breathing is rapid with a fruity odour. A priority nursing action when caring for this patient would be to:
   a. provide the patient with a simple carbohydrate immediately.
   b. request an order for an antiemetic.
   c. assist the patient into a lateral position to rest.
   d. administer insulin according to the patient's blood glucose level.

5. During pregnancy, a patient with pregestational diabetes has been monitoring their blood glucose level several times a day. Which of the following levels would require further assessment?
   a. 4.1 mmol/L—before breakfast
   b. 5.0 mmol/L—before lunch
   c. 7.5 mmol/L—2 hours after supper
   d. 6.4 mmol/L—1 hour after breakfast

6. A nurse is working with a patient with pregestational diabetes to plan the diet they will follow during pregnancy. Which of the following nutritional guidelines should be used to ensure a euglycemic state and appropriate weight gain? (Select all that apply.)
   a. Substantial bedtime snack composed of complex carbohydrates with some protein and fat
   b. Average calories per day of 2200 during the first trimester and 2500 during the second and third trimesters
   c. Caloric distribution among three meals and one or two snacks
   d. Eat simple carbohydrates to maintain carbohydrate intake
   e. Increase fat intake to 50% of the daily caloric intake

7. When assessing a pregnant patient at 28 weeks of gestation who is diagnosed with mitral valve stenosis, the nurse must be alert for signs indicating cardiac decompensation. Signs of cardiac decompensation would include which of the following? (Select all that apply.)
   a. Dry, hacking cough
   b. Increasing fatigue
   c. Wheezing with inspiration and expiration
   d. Bradycardia
   e. Progressive generalised edema
   f. Orthopnea with increasing dyspnea

8. A patient at 30 weeks of gestation with a class II cardiac disorder calls the primary health care provider's office and speaks to the nurse practitioner. The patient tells the nurse that they have been experiencing a frequent, moist cough for the past few days. In addition, they have been feeling more tired and are having difficulty completing routine activities as a result of some difficulty with breathing. The nurse's best response would be:
   a. "Have someone bring you to the office so we can assess your cardiac status."
   b. "Try to get more rest during the day because this is a difficult time for your heart."
   c. "Take an extra diuretic tonight before you go to bed, since you may be developing some fluid in your lungs."
   d. "Ask your family to come over and do your housework for the next few days so you can rest."

9. A pregnant patient with a cardiac disorder will begin anticoagulant therapy to prevent clot formation. In preparing this patient for this treatment measure, the nurse would expect to teach the patient about self-administration of which of the following medications?
   a. Furosemide
   b. Propranolol
   c. Heparin
   d. Warfarin

10. At a previous antepartal visit, the nurse taught a pregnant patient diagnosed with a class II cardiac disorder about measures to use to lower the risk for cardiac decompensation. This patient would demonstrate need for further instruction if they tell the nurse they will use which of the following measures?
    a. Increase roughage in her diet
    b. Remain on bed rest, getting out of bed only to go to the bathroom
    c. Sleep 10 hours every night and take a short nap after meals
    d. Will call the nurse immediately if she experiences any pain or swelling in her legs

1. Fatima is a 24-year-old woman with Type I diabetes. When Fatima informed her primary health care provider that she and her partner are trying to get pregnant, she was referred to her endocrinologist for preconception counselling. Fatima tells the nurse that she just cannot understand why this is necessary. "I have had diabetes since I was 12 years old, and I have not had many problems. All I want to do is get pregnant!" Discuss how the nurse should respond to Fatima's comments.

2. Luann is a 25-year-old nulliparous woman in her first trimester of pregnancy (6th week of gestation). She has had type 1 diabetes since she was 15 years old. Recently, she has been experiencing some nausea and is eating less as a result. She took her usual dose of regular and NPH insulin before eating a very light breakfast of tea and a piece of toast. Just before her midmorning snack at work, she began to experience nervousness and weakness. She felt dizzy and became diaphoretic and pale.

    a. Identify the problem that Luann is experiencing. Indicate the basis for her symptoms.

    b. State the action that Luann should take.

3. Judy's first pregnancy has just been confirmed. She also has type 1 diabetes.

    a. As a result of her high risk status, a variety of additional assessment measures are emphasised during her prenatal period to evaluate her status and that of her foetus. Identify these additional assessment measures and their relevance in a diabetic pregnancy.

    b. Discuss the stressors that might confront Judy and her family as a result of her status as a pregnant patient with diabetes.

    c. Indicate the activity and exercise recommendations that Judy should be given.

d. Outline the nursing interventions and health teaching for self-management in terms of nutrition, blood glucose monitoring, and insulin requirements at each stage of Judy's pregnancy.

Antepartum

Intrapartum

Postpartum

e. Judy expresses a desire to breastfeed her baby and wonders if this is a good idea for her and her baby. What should the nurse tell Judy about breastfeeding?

f. Discuss the birth control options that would be best for Judy and her partner.

4. Linda, age 26, had rheumatic fever as a child and subsequently developed mitral valve stenosis. She is presently 6 weeks pregnant. She is classified as class II according to the New York Heart Association functional classification of heart disease. This is the first pregnancy for Linda and her partner.

a. Discuss a recommended therapeutic plan for Linda that will reduce her risk for cardiac decompensation in terms of each of the following:

Rest/sleep/activity patterns

Prevention of infection

Nutrition

Bowel elimination

91

b. Identify physiological and psychosocial factors that could increase the stress placed on Linda's heart during her pregnancy.

Physiological factors   Psychosocial factors

c. List the subjective symptoms that the nurse should teach Linda and her family to look for as indicators of possible cardiac decompensation.

d. List the objective signs that could indicate that Linda is experiencing signs of cardiac decompensation and heart failure.

e. Linda is admitted to the labour unit. Her cardiac condition is still classified as class II. Outline the nursing measures designed to assess Linda and promote optimum cardiac function during labour and birth.

f. Linda should be observed carefully during the postpartum period because cardiac risk continues. Indicate the physiological events after birth that place Linda at risk for cardiac decompensation.

g. Discuss the measures the nurse can use to reduce the stress placed on Linda's heart during the postpartum period.

h. Linda indicates that she wishes to breastfeed her infant. Describe the nurse's response.

i. Identify the important factors to be considered when preparing Linda's discharge plan.

5. Jean is a primigravida at 4 weeks of gestation. She has been an epileptic for several years and her seizures have been controlled with phenytoin (Dilantin). Jean expresses concern regarding how her medication use will affect her pregnancy and her baby. She wants to stop taking the Dilantin. Describe the approach you would take in addressing Jean's concern and the course of action she is contemplating.

6. Imagine that you are an advanced practice nurse who specialises in the treatment of men and women who are alcohol and drug dependent. You have been asked to establish a treatment program specifically designed for pregnant patients. Outline the approach you would take to ensure that the program you establish takes into consideration the unique characteristics and needs of persons in general and pregnant patients in particular who use alcohol and drugs.

7. Olivia is a 24-year-old pregnant patient, who has had a spinal cord injury at T-10 since she was 16.

   a. Discuss the risk factors that can occur during pregnancy and the appropriate nursing care.

   b. Describe the priorities for nursing care during labour.

   c. Olivia plans to breastfeed her newborn. Develop a plan for postpartum care for Olivia.

16 Labour and Birth Processes

I. LEARNING KEY TERMS

FILL IN THE BLANKS: Insert the term that corresponds to each of the following descriptions.

1. _____, _____, _____, _____, and _____ The five factors or "Ps" of labour and birth.

2. _____ Membrane-filled spaces that are located where the membranous sutures that unite the bones in the foetal/newborn skull intersect.

3. _____ Slight overlapping of the bones of the foetal skull that occurs during childbirth; it permits the skull to adapt to the various pelvic diameters.

4. _____ Part of the foetus that enters the pelvic inlet first. The three main types are _____ (head first), _____ (buttocks first), and _____.

5. _____ Part of the foetal body first felt by the examining finger during a vaginal examination. The three types are _____, _____, and _____.

6. _____ Relationship of the long axis (spine) of the foetus to the long axis (spine) of the mother. There are two types: _____, when the spines are parallel to each other, and _____, when the spines are at right angles or diagonal to each other.

7. _____ Relationship of the foetal body parts to one another. The most common type is one of general _____.

8. _____ Largest transverse diameter of the foetal skull. _____ Smallest anteroposterior diameter of the fetal skull to enter the maternal pelvis when the foetal head is in complete flexion.

9. _____ Relationship of a reference point on the fetal presenting part to the four quadrants of the maternal pelvis.

10. _____ Term that indicates that the largest transverse diameter of the presenting part has passed through the maternal pelvic brim or inlet into the true pelvis, reaching the level of the ischial spines.

11. _____ Relationship of the presenting part of the fetus to an imaginary line drawn between the maternal ischial spines; this is a measure of the degree of fetal descent through the birth canal.

12. _____ and _____ The two components of the maternal passageway or birth canal.

13. _____ Shortening and thinning of the cervix during the first stage of labour; it is expressed as a percentage or length in centimetres.

14. _____ Enlargement or widening of the cervical opening (os) and the cervical canal, which occurs once labour has begun; degree of progress is expressed in centimetres (cm) from less than 1 cm to 10 cm.

15. _____ Descent of the fetal presenting part into the true pelvis approximately 2 to 4 weeks before term for the primigravida and after uterine contractions are established and true labour is in progress for the multipara.

16. _____ Primary powers of labour.

17. _____ Secondary powers of labour.

18. _____ Brownish or blood-tinged cervical mucus representing the passage of the mucus plug as the cervix ripens in preparation for labour.

19. _____ The seven turns and adjustments of the fetal head, to facilitate passage through the birth canal. In a vertex presentation these turns and adjustments include _____, _____, _____, _____, _____, _____, and finally birth by _____.

20. _____ Pushing method discouraged during the second stage of labour characterized by a closed glottis with prolonged bearing down.

21. _____ The second stage of labour is composed of two phases: _____ and _____.

22. _____ Process of moving the fetus, placenta, and membranes out of the uterus and through the birth canal.

23. _____ Maternal urge to bear down that occurs when the fetal presenting part reaches the perineal floor and stretching of the cervix and vagina occur; oxytocin is released.

24. The first stage of labour is considered to last from the onset of _____ to full _____ and _____ of the cervix. It is traditionally divided into two phases, namely _____ and _____.

25. The second stage of labour lasts from the time the cervix is fully _____ to the _____.

26. The third stage of labour lasts from the _____ until the _____ is delivered.

27. The fourth stage of labour is the period of time immediately after the _____ and includes at least _____ after birth.

28. _____, _____, _____, and _____ The four factors that affect fetal circulation during labour.

29. _____ Morphine-like chemicals produced naturally in the body, which raise the pain threshold and produce sedation.

II. REVIEWING KEY CONCEPTS

1. Describe how the five factors (the five Ps) affect the process of labour and birth.

2. A vaginal examination during labour reveals the following information: LOA, −1, 75%, 3 cm. An accurate interpretation of this data would include which of the following? (Select all that apply.)
   a. Attitude: flexed
   b. Station: 3 cm below the ischial spines
   c. Presentation: cephalic
   d. Lie: longitudinal
   e. Effacement: 75% complete
   f. Dilation: 9 cm more to reach full dilation

3. Changes occur as a patient progresses through labour. Which of the following maternal adaptations would be expected during labour? (Select all that apply.)
   a. Increase in both systolic and diastolic blood pressure during uterine contractions in the first stage of labour
   b. Decrease in white blood cell count
   c. Slight increase in heart rate during the first and second stages of labour
   d. Decrease in gastric motility leading to nausea and vomiting during the first stage of labour
   e. Hypoglycemia
   f. Proteinuria up to 1+

4. A nurse is instructing a group of primigravid patients about the onset of labour. Which of the following signs could the patients observe preceding the onset of their labours? (Select all that apply.)
   a. Urinary frequency
   b. Weight gain of 2 kg
   c. Quickening
   d. Energy surge
   e. Bloody show
   f. Shortness of breath

95

III. THINKING CRITICALLY

1. As part of their care of the labouring patient, nurses perform vaginal examinations and interpret the results. State the meaning of each of the following vaginal examination findings.

Exam I	Exam II	Exam III	Exam IV
ROP	RMA	LST	OA
−1	0	+1	+3
50%	25%	75%	100%
3 cm	2 cm	6 cm	10 cm

2. Brooke is a primigravida at 34 weeks of gestation. During a prenatal visit she asks you the following questions regarding her approaching labour. Describe how you would respond.

   a. "What gets labour to start?"

   b. "Are there things I should watch for that would tell me my labour is getting closer to starting?"

   c. "My friend just had a baby and she told me the nurses kept helping her change her position and even encouraged her to walk! Isn't that dangerous for the baby and painful for the mom?"

   d. "How will my baby know to start breathing after it is born?"

17 Nursing Care of the Family During Labour and Birth

I. LEARNING KEY TERMS

FILL IN THE BLANKS: Insert the term that corresponds to each of the following descriptions associated with stages of labour.

1. The first stage of labour begins with the onset of _____ and ends with complete cervical _____ and _____. A blood-tinged mucus discharge (bloody show) from the vagina usually indicates the passage of the _____.

2. During the latent phase of the first stage of labour, in a primiparous patient, the cervix dilates up to ___ cm. Cervical dilation progresses from ___ to ____ cm during the active phase of the first stage of labour.

3. The second stage of labour begins with _____ and ends with the _____.

4. The third stage of labour lasts from the _____ until the _____. Detachment of the placenta from the wall of the uterus or separation is indicated by a firmly contracted _____; change in the shape of the uterus from _____ to _____; a sudden _____ from the introitus; apparent _____; and the finding of _____ and appearance of _____ at the introitus.

5. The fourth stage of labour is considered to be the first _____ after birth. During this stage, the mother and newborn recover from the physical process of childbirth and get to know each other.

MATCHING: Match the description with the appropriate term.

6. _____ Prolonged breath holding while bearing down (closed glottis pushing).

7. _____ Burning sensation of acute pain as vagina stretches and crowning occurs.

8. _____ Artificial rupture of membranes (AROM).

9. _____ Occurs when widest part of the head (parietal diameter) distends the vulva just before birth.

10. _____ Incision into perineum to enlarge the vaginal outlet.

11. _____ Test to determine whether membranes have ruptured by assessing pH of the fluid.

12. _____ Technique used to control birth of foetal head in order to prevent foetal intracranial injury, protect maternal tissues, and reduce postpartum perineal pain.

13. _____ Method of breathing during bearing-down efforts helping to maintain adequate oxygen levels for the mother and foetus.

14. _____ Cord encircles the foetal neck.

15. _____ Method used to palpate foetus through abdomen.

16. _____ Occurs when pressure of presenting part against pelvic floor stretch receptors results in a labouring patient's perception of an urge to bear down.

a. Ritgen maneuver (modified)

b. Episiotomy

c. Oxytocic

d. Ferguson reflex

e. Valsalva maneuver

f. Ring of fire

g. Crowning

h. Amniotomy

i. Nuchal cord

j. Prolapse of umbilical cord

k. Nitrazine test

l. Leopold manoeuvers

m. Ferning

n. Meconium staining

o. Open glottis pushing

17. _____ Frondlike crystalline pattern created by amniotic fluid when it is placed on a glass slide.

18. _____ Classification of medication that stimulates the uterus to contract (a uterotonic).

19. _____ Protrusion of umbilical cord in advance of the presenting part.

FILL IN THE BLANKS: Insert the term that corresponds to each of the following descriptions related to the characteristics of the powers of labour.

20. _____ The primary powers of labour that act involuntarily to expel the fetus and the placenta from the uterus.

21. _____ "Building up" of a contraction from its onset.

22. _____ The peak of a contraction.

23. _____ "Letting down" of a contraction.

24. _____ How often uterine contractions occur; the time that elapses from the beginning of one contraction to the beginning of the next contraction.

25. _____ The strength of a contraction at its peak.

26. _____ The time that elapses between the onset and the end of a contraction.

27. _____ The tension of the uterine muscle between contractions.

28. _____ An involuntary urge to push in response to the Ferguson reflex.

II. REVIEWING KEY CONCEPTS

1. Laura (G3-T1-P1-A0-L2) has just been admitted in the latent phase of the first stage of labour. As part of the admission procedure, you review her prenatal record and interview her regarding what has been happening during labour up until now and discuss her current health status.
   a. List the essential data you would need to obtain from her prenatal record to plan appropriate care for Laura.

   b. Identify the information required regarding the status of Laura's labour.

   c. State the information required regarding Laura's current health status.

2. A nurse caring for a labouring patient needs to be alert for signs indicative of obstetrical emergencies during labour. State the signs reflecting each of the following emergencies:

   Abnormal or atypical foetal heart rate and pattern

   Inadequate uterine relaxation

   Vaginal bleeding

   Infection

3. Identify two advantages for each of the following labour positions:

Semirecumbent

Lateral

Upright

Hands and knees

4. Outline the critical factors to be included in the physical assessment of both maternal and foetal status during labour.

5. Indicate the laboratory and diagnostic tests that are recommended during labour. State the purpose for each.

6. Identify the factors that can influence the duration of the second stage of labour.

7. Describe the maternal positions recommended to enhance the effectiveness of a patient's bearing-down efforts during the second stage of labour. State the basis for each position's effectiveness in facilitating the descent and birth of the foetus.

8. Explain why the nurse should encourage a patient planning to breastfeed to begin breastfeeding during the fourth stage of labour.

9. Identify signs of the second stage of labour that the nurse would see in the patient.

    a. Describe what physical assessment would be appropriate.

10. A primigravida calls the hospital and tells a nurse on the labour unit that they know that they are in labour. The nurse's initial response would be which of the following?
    a. "Tell me what is happening to indicate to you that you are in labour."
    b. "How far do you live from the hospital?"
    c. "When is your expected date of birth?"
    d. "Have your membranes ruptured?"

11. A pregnant patient's amniotic membranes have apparently ruptured. The nurse assesses the fluid to determine its characteristics and confirm membrane rupture. Which of the following would be an expected assessment finding?
    a. pH 5.5
    b. Absence of ferning
    c. Pale straw-coloured fluid with white flecks
    d. Strong odour

12. When admitting a primigravida to the labour unit, the nurse observes for signs that indicate the patient is in true labour and should be admitted. The nurse would recognise which of the following as signs indicative of true labour? (Select all that apply.)
    a. Patient reports that contractions seem stronger since walking from the car to the room on the labour unit.
    b. Progressive change in the cervix.
    c. Patient perceives pain to be in the back or abdomen above the level of the navel.
    d. Progressive descent of the foetus that is engaged in the pelvis at zero station.
    e. Cervix is in the posterior position.
    f. Patient continues to feel the contractions intensify following a backrub and with use of effleurage.

13. A vaginal examination is performed on a multiparous patient who is in labour. The results of the examination were documented as 6 cm, 75%, +2, LOT. Which of the following would be an accurate interpretation of this data?
    a. Patient is in the latent phase of the first stage of labour.
    b. Station is 2 cm above the ischial spines.
    c. Presentation is cephalic.
    d. Lie is transverse.

14. A physical care measure for a labouring patient that has been identified as unlikely to be beneficial and may even be harmful would be:
    a. allowing the labouring patient to drink fluids and eat light solids as tolerated.
    b. administering a Fleet enema at admission.
    c. ambulating periodically throughout labour as tolerated.
    d. using a whirlpool bath once active labour is established.

III. THINKING CRITICALLY

1. Alice, a primigravida, calls the labour unit. She tells the nurse that she thinks she is in labour. "I have had some pains for about 2 hours. Should my partner bring me to the hospital now?"

   a. Describe how the nurse should approach this situation.

   b. Write several questions the nurse could use to elicit the appropriate information required to determine the course of action required.

   c. Based on the data collected during the telephone interview, the nurse determines that Alice is in very early labour. Because she lives fairly close to the hospital, she is instructed to stay home until her labour progresses. Outline the instructions and recommendations for care Alice and her partner should be given.

2. Analyse the assessment findings documented for each of the following women.

	Denise (G2-T0-P0-A1-L0)	Teresa (G4-T3-P0-A0-L3)	Danielle (G2-T1-P0-A0-L1)
Dilation	6 cm	9 cm	2 cm
Contraction strength	moderate	very strong	mild
Contraction frequency	q4min	q2-3min	q6-8min
Contraction Length	40–55 sec	65–75 sec	30–35 sec
Pelvic station	0	+2	−1

   a. Identify the phase of labour being experienced by each woman.

b. Describe the behaviour and appearance you would expect to be exhibited by each patient.

c. Specify the physical care and emotional support measures you would implement if you were caring for each of these patients.

d. Denise's partner, Sam, is her major support person during labour. The nurse observes that he is beginning to appear fatigued and "stressed" after being with Denise since her admission 5 hours ago. Describe the actions this nurse can take to support Sam and his efforts to care for Denise.

3. Describe the procedure that should be followed before auscultating the FHR or applying an ultrasound transducer to the abdomen of a labouring patient. Explain the rationale for utilizing this procedure.

4. Tonya, a woman in active labour, begins to cry during a vaginal examination to assess her status. "Why not watch the monitor to see how I am progressing instead of doing these vaginal exams? They really hurt and they are embarrassing!"

a. Describe the response the nurse should make in regard to Tonya's concern.

b. Discuss the measures the nurse could use to meet Tonya's safety and comfort needs during a vaginal examination.

5. Tasha is dilated 6 cm. Her partner comes to tell you that her "water just broke with a gush!" Identify each action you would take in this situation, in order of priority. State the rationale for the actions you have identified.

Chapter **17** **Nursing Care of the Family During Labour and Birth**

6. Sara, a 17-year-old primigravida, is admitted in the latent phase of stage 1 labour. Her boyfriend, Dan, is with her as her only support. During the admission interview, Sara tells you that they did not go to any classes because she was embarrassed about not being married. Both Sara and Dan appear very nervous and assessment indicates they know little about what is happening, what to expect, and how to work together with the process of labour. Identify the labour support Sara and Dan should expect. State one expected outcome and list nursing measures appropriate for their care.

7. Identifying a labouring couple's cultural and religious beliefs and practices regarding childbirth is a critical factor in providing culturally sensitive care that enhances the couple's sense of control and eventual satisfaction with their childbirth experience.

   a. List the questions you would ask when assessing a couple's cultural and religious preferences for childbirth.

   b. Discuss the problems that can occur if the nurse does not consider the couple's cultural and religious preferences when planning and implementing care.

8. Cori (G4-T3-P0-A0-L3) is in the latent phase of stage 1 labour. She and her partner are being oriented to the birthing room. Their last birth occurred in a delivery room 15 years ago. Both Cori and her partner are amazed by the birthing room and the birthing bed that will allow her to give birth in an upright position. They are also informed that changes in bearing-down efforts in the active phase of stage 2 labour now allow a patient to follow her own body feelings and even to vocalise with pushing. Both Cori and her partner state that with every other birth they put her legs in stirrups; she held her breath for as long as she could, and pushed quietly. "Everything turned out okay, so why should we change?" Describe the response the primary nurse caring for this couple should make to their concerns.

9. A nurse living in a rural area is called to her neighbour's home to assist his partner who is in labour. "Everything is happening so fast. She says she is ready to give birth!"

   a. Identify the measures the nurse can use to reassure and comfort the patient.

   b. Shortly after the nurse arrives, crowning begins. State what the nurse should do.

c. Describe the action the nurse should take after the birth of the head.

d. List the measures the nurse should use to prevent excessive newborn heat loss after the birth.

e. Identify the infection control measures that should be implemented during a home birth.

f. Specify the measures the nurse should use to prevent excessive maternal blood loss or haemorrhage until the ambulance arrives.

g. Outline the information the nurse should document regarding the childbirth.

10. Beth is in the active phase of the second stage of labour. She is actively pushing to facilitate birth. Indicate the criteria a nurse would use to evaluate the effectiveness of Beth's technique.

11. Imagine that you are participating in a panel discussion on childbirth practices. Your topic is "Episiotomy—is it needed to ensure the safety and well-being of the labouring patient and their foetus?" Outline the information you would include in your presentation.

12. Imagine that you are a staff nurse on a childbirth unit. Your hospital is instituting a change in policy that would allow the participation of children in the labour and birth process of their parent. You are asked to be a part of the committee that will formulate the guidelines regarding sibling participation during childbirth. Discuss the suggestions you would make to help ensure a positive outcome for parents, children, and health care providers.

Chapter **17** **Nursing Care of the Family During Labour and Birth**

13. Annie is a primipara in the fourth stage of labour following a long and difficult childbirth process.

   a. Identify the essential nursing assessment and care measures required to ensure Annie's safety and recovery during this stage of her labour.

   b. As she performs the first assessment, the nurse notes that Annie seems disinterested in her baby. She looks him over quickly and then asks the nurse to put him in the isolette. Identify the factors that could be accounting for Annie's behaviour.

   c. Discuss the nursing measures you would use to encourage future maternal-newborn interactions and facilitate the attachment process.

18 Maximizing Comfort During Labour and Birth

I. LEARNING KEY TERMS

FILL IN THE BLANKS: Insert the term that corresponds to each of the following descriptions related to childbirth discomfort and its management.

1. _____ Decreased blood flow to the uterus during a contraction leading to an oxygen deficit.

2. _____ Pain that predominates during the first stage of labour; it results from cervical changes, distention of the lower uterine segment, and uterine ischemia.

3. _____ Pain that predominates during the second stage of labour; it results from stretching and distention of perineal tissues and the pelvic floor to allow passage of the fetus, from distention and traction on the peritoneum and uterocervical supports during contractions, and from lacerations of soft tissues.

4. _____ Pain in labour and birth that originates in the uterus and radiates to the abdominal wall, lumbosacral area of the back, iliac crests, gluteal area, and down the thighs.

5. _____ Level of pain a person is willing to endure.

6. _____ Theory of pain based on the premise that pain sensations travel along sensory nerve pathways to the brain, but only a limited number of sensations or messages can travel through these nerve pathways at one time; by using distraction techniques (e.g., massage, music, focal points, imagery) the capacity of nerve pathways are diminished

7. _____ Endogenous opioids secreted by the pituitary gland that act on the central and peripheral nervous systems to reduce pain; their level increases during pregnancy and birth, thereby enhancing a patient's ability to tolerate acute pain and reducing anxiety.

8. _____ Relaxed deep breath in through the nose and out through the mouth that begins each breathing pattern and ends each contraction.

9. _____ Paced breathing technique during which a labouring patient breathes at approximately 8 to 10 breaths per minute (half the normal breathing rate).

10. _____ Paced breathing technique during which a labouring patient breathes at approximately 32 to 40 breaths per minute (twice the normal breathing rate).

11. _____ Paced breathing technique during which a labouring patient breathes adt approximately 32 to 40 breaths per minute interspersed with blowing out of air in a ratio of 3:1 or 4:1; this technique enhances concentration.

12. _____ Undesirable reaction to a rapid-paced breathing pattern characterised by rapid deep respirations that lead to signs of respiratory alkalosis such as lightheadedness, dizziness, tingling of the fingers, or circumoral numbness. Breathing into a paper bag held tightly around the mouth will help to reestablish normal breathing.

13. _____ Light massage (stroking) of the abdomen or other body part in rhythm with breathing during contractions.

14. _____ Steady pressure against the sacrum using the fist or heel of the hand or a firm object to help the labouring patient cope with the sensations of internal pressure and pain in the lower back.

15. _____ Bathing, showering, or whirlpool baths using warm water to promote comfort and relaxation during labour, stimulate the release of endorphin, close the gate on pain, promote circulation and oxygenation, and help to soften the perineum.

16. _____ Method that involves placement of two pairs of electrodes on either side of the labouring patient's thoracic and sacral spine to provide continuous low-intensity electrical impulses that can be increased during a contraction, thereby stimulating the release of endorphins that make the pain less disturbing

17. _____ Application of pressure, heat, or cold over the skin of specific points on the body termed tsubos, which have increased density of neuroreceptors and increased electrical conductivity.

18. _____ Insertion of fine needles into specific areas of the body to restore the flow of qi (energy) and decrease pain, which is thought to be obstructing the flow of energy.

19. _____ Relaxation technique that can be used for labour that is based on the theory that, if a person can recognise physical signals, certain internal physiologic events can be changed (i.e., whatever signs the patient has that are associated with their pain).

20. _____ Use of oils distilled from plants, flowers, herbs, and trees to promote health and to treat and balance the mind, body, and spirit.

21. _____ Injection of small amounts of sterile water by using a fine-gauge needle into four locations on the lower back to relieve back pain; effectiveness of this method may be related to the mechanism of counterirritation, gate control, or an increase in the level of endorphins.

22. _____ Technique based on the concept of energy fields within the body called prana; it involves the laying-on of hands by a specially trained person to redirect energy fields associated with pain.

II. REVIEWING KEY CONCEPTS

1. Describe the factors that could influence the following nursing diagnosis identified for a patient in labour: Acute pain related to the processes involved in labour and birth.

2. Explain the theoretical basis for using techniques such as massage, stroking, music, and imagery to reduce the sensation of pain during childbirth.

MATCHING: Match the description with the appropriate pharmacological method for discomfort management during childbirth.

3. _____ Abolition of pain perception by interrupting nerve impulses going to the brain. Loss of sensation (partial or complete) and sometimes loss of consciousness occurs.

4. _____ Method used to repair a tear or hole in the dura mater around the spinal cord as a result of spinal anesthesia; the goal is to prevent or treat postdural puncture headaches (PDPH).

5. _____ Single-injection, subarachnoid anaesthesia useful for pain control during birth but not for labour; it is often used for Caesarean birth.

6. _____ Systemic analgesic such as nalbuphine that relieves pain without causing significant maternal or newborn respiratory depression and is less likely to cause nausea and vomiting.

7. _____ Provides rapid perineal anesthesia for performing and repairing an episiotomy or lacerations.

8. _____ Gas mixed with oxygen to provide analgesia during all stages of labour.

9. _____ Medication such as benzodiazepines that can be used to relieve anxiety, to induce sleep, to augment the effectiveness of analgesics, and to reduce nausea and vomiting.

10. _____ Technique that can be used to block pain transmission without compromising motor ability because an opioid with or without a local anesthetic is injected intrathecally and into the peridural space; with this technique labouring patients are able to walk if they choose to do so.

11. _____ Medication that promptly reverses the effects of opioids, including maternal and neonatal CNS depression, especially respiratory depression.

12. _____ Use of a medication such as an opioid analgesic that is administered IM or IV for pain relief during labour.

13. _____ Alleviation of pain sensation or raising of the pain threshold without loss of consciousness.

14. _____ Relief from pain of uterine contractions and birth by injecting a local anesthetic agent, an opioid, or both into the peridural space.

15. _____ Anaesthetic that relieves pain in the lower vagina, vulva, and perineum, making it useful if an episiotomy is to be performed or forceps or vacuum assistance is required to facilitate birth.

16. _____ Systemic analgesic such as meperidine or fentanyl that relieves pain and creates a feeling of well-being but can also result in respiratory depression (maternal and newborn), nausea, and vomiting.

a. Opioid agonist-antagonist analgesic

b. Anaesthesia

c. Analgesia

d. Combined spinal-epidural analgesic

e. Epidural analgesia/anesthesia (block)

f. Autologous epidural blood patch

g. Local infiltration anesthesia

h. Spinal anaesthesia (block)

i. Opioid antagonist

j. Nitrous oxide

k. Pudendal nerve block

l. Systemic analgesic

m. Sedative

n. Opioid agonist analgesic

17. Compare each of the following commonly used methods for nerve block analgesia and anesthesia. Indicate the effects, timing of administration, advantages and disadvantages, and nursing care management for each method in your comparison.

Local perineal infiltration anesthesia

Spinal anesthesia (block)

Epidural anesthesia/analgesia (block)

Combined spinal-epidural analgesia

Epidural and intrathecal opioids

18. Systemic analgesics cross the placenta and affect the foetus.

    a. List three factors that influence the effect systemic analgesics have on the foetus.

    b. Identify the foetal effects of systemic analgesics.

19. Explain why the intravenous route is preferred to the intramuscular route for the administration of systemic analgesics during labour.

20. In their birth plan, a patient requests the use the whirlpool bath during labour. When implementing this patient's request the nurse would do which of the following?
    a. Assist the patient to maintain a reclining position when in the tub.
    b. Tell the patient they will need to leave the tub as soon as their membranes rupture.
    c. Limit the patient to no longer than 1 hour in the tub.
    d. Maintain the water temperature between 35° C/95° F and 37.8° C/100° F.

21. The use of benzodiazepines can potentiate the action of analgesics and reduce nausea. When preparing to administer a benzodiazepine to a labouring patient, the nurse could expect to give which one of the following medications?
    a. Diazepam (Valium)
    b. Promethazine (Phenergan)
    c. Nalbuphine (Nubain)
    d. Fentanyl (Sublimaze)

22. The nurse has just administered ranitidine (Zantac) to a patient in labour. Which of the following would be an expected effect of this medication?
    a. Neutralization of stomach acid
    b. Nausea and vomiting
    c. Potentiation of opioid analgesics
    d. Respiratory depression

23. Following administration of fentanyl (Sublimaze) IV for labour pain, a patient's labour progresses more rapidly than expected. The health care provider orders that a stat dose of naloxone (Narcan) 1 mg be administered intravenously to the patient to reverse respiratory depression in the newborn after the birth. In fulfilling this order the nurse would:
    a. question the route because this medication should be administered orally.
    b. recognize that the dose is too low.
    c. monitor maternal condition for possible side effects.
    d. observe the patient for bradycardia and lethargy.

24. An anesthesiologist is preparing to begin a continuous epidural block using a combination local anesthetic and opioid analgesic as a pain relief measure for a labouring patient. Nursing care related to this type of nerve block would include which of the following? (Select all that apply.)
    a. Assist the patient into a modified lateral position or upright position with back curved for administration of the block.
    b. Alternate the patient's position from side to side every hour.
    c. Assess the patient for headaches because they commonly occur in the postpartum period if an epidural is used for labour.

d. Assist the patient to urinate every 2 hours during labour to prevent bladder distention.
e. Prepare the patient for use of forceps- or vacuum-assisted birth because they will be unable to bear down.
f. Assess blood pressure frequently because hypotension can occur.

25. Administering an opioid antagonist to a patient who is opioid dependent will result in the opioid abstinence syndrome. The nurse would recognize which of the following clinical manifestations as evidence that this syndrome is occurring? (Select all that apply.)
a. Yawning
b. Piloerection
c. Anorexia
d. Coughing
e. Dry skin, eyes, and nose
f. Tachypnea

26. After induction of a spinal block in preparation for an elective caesarean birth, a patient's blood pressure decreases from 124/76 to 96/60. The nurse's initial action would be to do which of the following?
a. Administer a vasopressor intravenously to raise the blood pressure.
b. Change the patient's position from supine to lateral.
c. Begin to administer oxygen by mask at 10 to 12 L/min.
d. Notify the patient's health care provider.

III. THINKING CRITICALLY

1. A nurse working with a group of expectant partners is asked if there really is "a physical reason for all the pain people say they feel when they are in labour." Describe the response that this nurse should give.

2. On admission to the labour unit in the latent phase of labour, a couple having their first baby tell you that they are so glad they took Lamaze classes and did so much reading about childbirth. "We will not need any medication now that we know what to do. But most importantly our baby will be safe." Describe how you would respond if you were their primary nurse for childbirth.

3. Imagine you are the nurse manager of a labour and birth unit. Major renovations are being planned for your unit and your input is required. You and your staff nurses believe that water therapy, including the use of showers and whirlpool baths, is a beneficial nonpharmacological method to relieve pain and discomfort and to enhance the progress of labour. Discuss the rationale you would use to convince planners that installation of a shower and a whirlpool bath into each birthing room is cost effective.

4. Tara has been in labour for 4 hours. Her blood pressure had been stable, averaging 130/80 when assessed between contractions, and the FHR pattern consistently exhibited criteria of a normal pattern. A lumbar epidural block was initiated. Shortly afterward, during assessment of maternal vital signs and FHR, Tara's blood pressure decreased to 102/60 and the FHR pattern began to exhibit some atypical features.

   a. State what Tara is experiencing. Support your answer and explain the physiological basis for what is happening to Tara.

   b. List the immediate nursing actions.

5. Moira, a primigravida, has decided to use a continuous epidural block as her pharmacological method of choice during childbirth.

   a. Identify the assessment procedures that should be used to determine Moira's readiness for the initiation of the epidural block.

   b. Describe the preparation methods that should be implemented.

   c. Describe two positions you could help Moira to assume for the induction of the epidural block.

   d. Outline the nursing care recommended while Moira is receiving the anaesthesia to ensure her well-being and that of her fetus.

19 Fetal Health Surveillance During Labour

I. LEARNING KEY TERMS

FILL IN THE BLANKS: Insert the term that corresponds to each of the following descriptions related to foetal assessment.

1. _____ Listening to foetal heart sounds at periodic intervals to assess foetal heart rate.

2. _____ Instrument used to assess the foetal heart rate through the transmission of ultrahigh-frequency sound waves reflecting movement of the foetal heart and the conversion of these sounds into an electronic signal that can be counted.

3. _____ Method used to continuously assess the FHR pattern.

_____ and _____ are the two modes used to accomplish this method of assessment.

4. _____ Device used in external monitoring to measure uterine activity transabdominally; it can determine the frequency, regularity, and approximate duration of uterine contractions but not their intensity.

5. _____ Device used in internal monitoring to obtain a continuous assessment of the foetal heart rate and pattern.

6. _____ Device used in internal monitoring to measure the frequency, duration, and intensity of uterine contractions as well as uterine resting tone.

7. _____ The interventions initiated when an abnormal FHR pattern is detected; these interventions involve instituting maternal position changes, increasing intravenous fluid administration, and providing supplemental oxygen if required.

8. _____ Assessment method that uses digital pressure to elicit an acceleration of the FHR.

9. _____ Abnormally small amount of amniotic fluid.

10. _____ Absence of amniotic fluid.

11. _____ Instillation of room temperature isotonic fluid into the uterine cavity when the volume of amniotic fluid is low for the purpose of adding fluid around the umbilical cord and thus preventing its compression during uterine contractions or foetal movement.

12. _____ Relaxation of the uterus achieved through the administration of medications that inhibit uterine contractions.

MATCHING: Match the definition with the appropriate term related to FHR pattern.

1. _____ Average of FHR during a 10-minute tracing segment that excludes accelerations, decelerations, and periods of marked variability.

2. _____ Amplitude range of the FHR fluctuations undetectable.

3. _____ Amplitude range detectable by the unaided eye, but is <5 beats/min.

4. _____ Persistent (≥10 minutes) baseline FHR <110 beats/min.

5. _____ Visually apparent decrease in the FHR of 15 beats/min or more below the baseline, which lasts between 2 and 10 minutes.

6. _____ Changes from baseline patterns in FHR that occur with uterine contractions.

7. _____ Persistent (≥10 minutes) baseline FHR >160 beats/min.

8. _____ Fluctuations in the baseline FHR that are irregular in amplitude and frequency and are visually quantified as the amplitude of the peak to trough in bpm.

9. _____ Visually apparent gradual decrease in and return to baseline FHR in response to transient foetal head compression during a uterine contraction; it is considered a normal and benign finding.

10. _____ Visually apparent gradual decrease in and return to baseline FHR in response to uteroplacental insufficiency resulting in a transient disruption of oxygen transfer to the foetus; lowest point occurs after the peak of the contraction and baseline rate is not usually regained until the uterine contraction is over.

11. _____ Visually abrupt decrease in FHR below baseline of 15 beats or more, lasting 15 seconds and returning to baseline in less than 2 minutes from the time of onset, which can occur at any time during a contraction as a result of umbilical cord compression.

12. _____ Visually apparent abrupt increase in the FHR of 15 beats/min or greater above the baseline, which lasts 15 seconds or more with return to baseline less than 2 minutes from the beginning of the increase.

13. _____ Changes from baseline patterns in FHR that are not associated with uterine contraction.

a. Acceleration

b. Early deceleration

c. Variability

d. Late deceleration

e. Variable deceleration

f. Tachycardia

g. Prolonged deceleration

h. Bradycardia

i. Baseline FHR

j. Absent variability

k. Periodic changes

l. Episodic changes

m. Minimal variability

14. Describe the factors associated with a reduction in foetal oxygen supply.

15. It is critical that a nurse working on a labour unit be knowledgeable concerning the characteristics of normal, atypical, and abnormal FHR patterns, and characteristics of normal and tachysystolic uterine activity. List the required information for each of the following:

    a. Characteristics of a normal FHR pattern

    b. Characteristics of an atypical FHR pattern

    c. Characteristics of abnormal FHR patterns

    d. Characteristics of normal uterine activity

    e. Characteristics of tachysystole

16. Nurses caring for patients in labour must review FHR tracings on a regular basis. Name several essential components that the nurse must evaluate each time the monitor tracing is observed.

17. Nurses caring for labouring patients use a variety of methods to assess foetal health and well-being during labour. State the advantages and disadvantages of each of the following methods to assess FHR and pattern as well as uterine activity. Outline the nursing care measures required for each of the monitoring methods.

    a. External fetal monitoring

    b. Internal fetal monitoring

    c. Portable telemetry

18. State the legal responsibilities related to foetal monitoring for nurses who care for patients during childbirth.

19. A labouring patient's uterine contractions are being internally monitored. When evaluating the monitor tracing, which of the following findings would be a source of concern and require further assessment?
    a. Frequency every 2.5 to 3 minutes
    b. Duration of 80 to 85 seconds
    c. Intensity during a uterine contraction of 55 to 80 mm Hg
    d. Average resting pressure of 25 to 30 mm Hg

20. External electronic foetal monitoring will be used for a high-risk patient just admitted to the labour unit in active labour. Guidelines the nurse should follow when implementing this form of monitoring would be which of the following? (Select all that apply.)
    a. Use Leopold manoeuvers to determine correct placement of the ultrasound transducer.
    b. Assist patient to maintain a dorsal recumbent position to ensure accurate monitor tracings for evaluation.
    c. Reposition the tocotransducer every hour.
    d. Teach the patient they can change positions as needed for comfort.
    e. Palpate the fundus to estimate the intensity of uterine contractions.

113

21. When evaluating the external foetal monitor tracing of a patient whose labour is being induced, the nurse identifies signs of persistent late deceleration patterns and begins intrauterine resuscitation interventions. Which of the following reflects that the appropriate interventions were implemented in the recommended order of priority?
    1. Increase rate of maintenance intravenous solution.
    2. Palpate uterus for tachysystole.
    3. Discontinue Oxytocin infusion.
    4. Change maternal position to a lateral position; then elevate her legs if patient is hypotensive.
        a. 2, 1, 4, 3
        b. 4, 1, 2, 3
        c. 3, 4, 1, 2
        d. 4, 1, 2, 3

22. The nurse caring for patients in labour should be aware of signs characterising normal, atypical, and abnormal FHR patterns. Which of the following would be abnormal signs? (Select all that apply.)
    a. Moderate baseline variability
    b. Average baseline FHR of 95 beats/min
    c. Acceleration with fetal movement
    d. Late deceleration patterns approximately every 2 contractions
    e. FHR of 155 beats/min between contractions
    f. Early deceleration patterns

23. A labouring patient's temperature is elevated as a result of an upper respiratory infection. The FHR pattern that reflects maternal fever would be:
    a. diminished variability.
    b. variable decelerations.
    c. tachycardia.
    d. early decelerations.

24. A nulliparous patient is in the active phase of labour and their cervix has progressed to 6 cm dilation. The nurse caring for this patient evaluates the external monitor tracing and notes the following: decrease in FHR shortly after onset of several uterine contractions returning to baseline rate by the end of the contraction; shape is uniform. Based on these findings the nurse should do which of the following?
    a. Change the patient's position to her left side.
    b. Document the finding on the patient's chart.
    c. Notify the health care provider.
    d. Perform a vaginal examination to check for cord prolapse.

III. THINKING CRITICALLY

1. Darlene, a primigravida with no risk factors is in active labour and has just been admitted to the labour unit. She asks about foetal monitoring and if it will be required for her labour. Describe the nurse's expected response.

2. Terry is a primigravida at 43 weeks of gestation. Her labour is being stimulated with oxytocin administered IV. Her contractions have been increasing in intensity with a frequency of every 2 to 2.5 minutes and a duration of 80 to 85 seconds. She is currently in a supine position with a 30-degree elevation of her head. On observation of the monitor tracing, you note that during the last two contractions the FHR decreased after the contraction peaked and did not return to baseline until about 10 seconds into the rest period. A slight decrease in variability and baseline rate was observed.

    a. Identify the pattern described and the possible factors responsible for it.

    b. Describe the actions you would take. State the rationale for each action.

3. Taisha is a multiparous woman in active labour. Her membranes rupture and the nurse caring for her immediately evaluates the EFM tracing.

    a. What type of periodic FHR pattern would the nurse be alert for when evaluating the tracing? Explain the rationale for your answer.

    b. State the actions the nurse should take in order of priority if the pattern is noted.

20 Labour and Birth at Risk

I. LEARNING KEY TERMS

FILL IN THE BLANKS: Insert the term that corresponds to each of the following descriptions.

1. _____ Regular uterine contractions and cervical change occurring between 20 and 36 6/7 weeks of pregnancy.

2. _____ Any birth that occurs after 20 weeks and before the completion of 37 weeks of pregnancy regardless of birth weight.

3. _____ Weight at the time of birth of 2500 g or less.

4. _____ Glycoproteins found in plasma and produced during foetal life; their reappearance in the cervical canal between 24 and 34 weeks of gestation could predict preterm labour.

5. _____ Characteristic of the cervix that could be a predictor for preterm labour.

6. _____ Spontaneous rupture of the amniotic sac and leakage of amniotic fluid beginning before the onset of labour at any gestational age.

7. _____ Spontaneous rupture of the amniotic sac and leakage of fluid before the completion of 37 weeks of gestation often associated with weakening of the membranes caused by inflammation, stress from uterine contractions, or other factors that cause increased intrauterine pressure.

8. _____ A bacterial infection of the amniotic cavity that is potentially life threatening for the foetus and the pregnant patient.

9. _____ Long, difficult, or abnormal labour caused by various conditions associated with the lack of labour progress.

10. _____ Abnormal uterine activity often experienced by an anxious first-time mother who is having painful and frequent contractions that are ineffective in causing cervical dilation and effacement to progress. It usually occurs in the latent phase of the first stage of labour.

11. _____ Abnormal uterine activity that usually occurs when a labouring patient initially makes normal progress into the active phase of the first stage of labour and then uterine contractions become weak and inefficient or stop altogether.

12. _____ Abnormal labour caused by contractures of the pelvic diameters that reduce the capacity of the bony pelvis, including the inlet, midpelvis, outlet, or any combination of these planes.

13. _____ Abnormal labour caused by obstruction of the birth passage by an anatomical abnormality other than that involving the bony pelvis; the obstruction may result from placenta previa, leiomyomas (uterine fibroid tumours), ovarian tumours, or a full bladder or rectum.

14. _____ Abnormal labour caused by foetal anomalies, excessive foetal size, malpresentation, malposition, or multifoetal pregnancy.

15. _____ Abnormal labour caused by disproportion between the size of the foetus and the size of the pelvis of the labouring patient

16. _____ The most common foetal malposition.

17. _____ The most common form of malpresentation.

18. _____ Gestation of twins, triplets, quadruplets, or more newborns.

19. _____,

    _____, _____,

    _____, _____,

    _____ Six abnormal labour patterns identified according to the nature of the cervical dilation and foetal descent

20. _____ Labour pattern that lasts, 3 hours from the onset of contractions to the time of birth, often resulting from hypertonic uterine contractions that are tetanic in intensity.

21. _____ Attempt to turn the foetus from a breech or shoulder presentation to a vertex presentation for birth by exerting gentle, constant pressure on the abdomen.

22. _____ Observance of a labouring patient and their foetus for a reasonable period of spontaneous active labour to assess the safety of a vaginal birth for both.

23. _____ Chemical or mechanical initiation of uterine contractions before their spontaneous onset for the purpose of bringing about the birth.

24. _____ Rating system used to evaluate the inducibility of the cervix.

25. _____ Artificial rupture of the membranes often used to induce labour when the cervix is ripe or to augment labour if the progress begins to slow.

26. _____ Stimulation of uterine contractions after labour has started spontaneously but progress is unsatisfactory. Common methods include infusion of oxytocin and rupture of membranes.

27. _____ Chemical, mechanical, and physical methods used to prepare the cervix for stimulation of labour by making it more inducible by making it softer and thinner.

28. _____ Term applied to the occurrence of more than ten or more contractions in 20 minutes; it can occur in both spontaneous and stimulated labours.

29. _____ Birth method in which an instrument with two curved blades is used to assist the birth of the foetal head.

30. _____ Birth method involving the attachment of a vacuum cup to the foetal head, using negative pressure.

31. _____ Birth of the foetus through a transabdominal incision of the uterus.

32. _____ Pregnancy that extends beyond the end of week 42 of gestation.

33. _____ Uncommon obstetrical emergency in which the head of the fetus is born but the anterior shoulder cannot pass under the pubic arch. Two major causes are _____ or _____ maternal.

34. _____ Obstetrical emergency in which the umbilical cord lies below the presenting part of the fetus; it may be occult (hidden) or more commonly frank (visible).

35. _____ Obstetrical emergency in which a foreign substance present in the amniotic fluid enters the maternal circulation triggering a rapid, complex series of pathophysiological events that lead to life-threatening maternal symptoms including acute hypoxia, hypotension, cardiovascular collapse, and coagulopathies.

II. REVIEWING KEY CONCEPTS

1. Compare and contrast spontaneous and indicated preterm birth.

2. Explain why bed rest may be more harmful than helpful as a component of preterm labour care management.

MATCHING: Match the description of medications used as part of the management of preterm labour with the appropriate medication.

3. _____ An antenatal glucocorticoid used to accelerate fetal lung maturity when there is risk for preterm birth.

4. _____ A prostaglandin synthesis inhibitor that relaxes uterine smooth muscle; it is administered orally.

5. _____ A calcium channel blocker that relaxes smooth muscles including those of the contracting uterus; maternal hypotension is a major concern.

a. Tocolytic

b. Betamethasone

c. Indomethacin (Indocin)

d. Magnesium sulphate

e. Nifedipine (Adalat)

117

6. _____ Classification of medications used to arrest labour after uterine contractions and cervical changes have occurred.

7. _____ A central nervous system (CNS) depressant that inhibits uterine contractions; it is administered intravenously.

Match the description of medications used during the process of stimulating uterine contractions and cervical ripening with the medication listed.

8. _____ Classification of medications that can be used to ripen the cervix, stimulate uterine contractions, or both.

9. _____ Cervical ripening agent in the form of a vaginal insert that is placed in the posterior fornix of the vagina.

10. _____ Cervical ripening agent in the form of a gel that is inserted into the cervical canal just below the internal os or into the posterior fornix.

11. _____ Pituitary hormone used to stimulate uterine contractions in the augmentation or induction of labour.

12. _____ Natural cervical dilator made from seaweed.

13. _____ Synthetic cervical dilator containing magnesium sulphate.

14. _____ Cervical ripening agent, used in the form of a tablet that is most commonly inserted intravaginally into the posterior fornix.

a. Oxytocin (Syntocinon)

b. Misoprostol (Cytotec)

c. Dinoprostone (Cervidil)

d. Dinoprostone (Prepidil)

e. Prostaglandin

f. Laminaria tent

g. Lamicel

15. Describe factors that cause labour to be long, difficult, or abnormal. Explain how they interrelate.

16. Explain the treatment approach of therapeutic rest.

17. A primigravida is experiencing hypertonic uterine dysfunction and a multigravida is experiencing hypotonic uterine dysfunction. Compare and contrast each patient's labour in terms of causes/precipitating factors, maternal-foetal effects, change in pattern of progress, and care management.

   a. Primigravida—hypertonic uterine dysfunction

   b. Multigravida—hypotonic uterine dysfunction

18. Identify four indications for oxytocin induction and four contraindications to the use of oxytocin to stimulate the onset of labour.

   Indications

   Contraindications

19. When assessing a pregnant patient, the nurse is alert for factors associated with spontaneous preterm labour. Which of the following factors, if exhibited by this pregnant patient, would increase their risk for spontaneous preterm labour? (Select all that apply.)
   a. BMI of 22
   b. Obstetrical history: G2-T0-P2-A0-L1
   c. Periodontal disease
   d. Singleton gestation
   e. Personal history of being born prematurely

20. A patient is receiving intravenous magnesium sulphate for foetal neuroprotection. Which of the following measures should be implemented during the infusion?
    a. Limit fluid intake to 2500 to 3000 mL per day.
    b. Discontinue infusion if maternal respirations are 12 breaths per minute.
    c. Ensure that calcium gluconate is available should toxicity occur.
    d. Assist patient to maintain a comfortable semirecumbent position when in bed.

21. The health care provider has ordered that dinoprostone (Cervidil) be administered to ripen a pregnant patient's cervix in preparation for an induction of their labour. In fulfilling this order, the nurse would do which of the following? Select all that apply
    a. Assist the health care provider to insert the Cervidil into the posterior fornix of the cervical canal just below the internal os.
    b. Instruct the patient to remain in bed for at least 2 hours.
    c. Observe the patient for signs of tachysystole.
    d. Begin induction using oxytocin 30 to 60 minutes after removal of the insert.

22. A nulliparous patient experiencing a postterm pregnancy is admitted for labour induction. Assessment reveals a Bishop score of 9. The nurse would:
    a. call the woman's primary health care provider to order a cervical ripening agent.
    b. mix 20 units of oxytocin in 500 mL of 5% glucose in water.
    c. piggyback the oxytocin solution into the port nearest the drip chamber of the primary IV tubing.
    d. begin the oxytocin infusion at a rate between 0.5 to 2 milliunits/min as determined by the induction protocol.

23. A patient's labour is being induced. The nurse assesses the patient's status and that of their foetus and the labour process just before an oxytocin infusion increment of 2 milliunits/min. The nurse would discontinue the infusion and notify the patient's primary health care provider if which of the following had been noted during the assessment?
    a. Frequency of uterine contractions: every 1.5 minutes
    b. Variability of FHR: present
    c. Deceleration patterns: early decelerations noted with several contractions
    d. Strong uterine contractions lasting 80 to 90 seconds each.

24. A labouring patient's vaginal examination reveals the following: 3 cm, 50%, LSA, 0. The nurse caring for this patient would:
    a. place the ultrasound transducer in the left lower quadrant of the patient's abdomen.
    b. recognise that passage of meconium would be a definitive sign of fetal distress.
    c. expect the progress of foetal descent to be slower than usual.
    d. assist the patient into a knee-chest position for each contraction.

25. A nurse is caring for a pregnant patient at 30 weeks of gestation in preterm labour. The primary health care provider orders Betamethasone 12 mg for two doses with the first dose to be given at 1100. In implementing this order, the nurse would do which of the following?
    a. Consult with the health care provider because the dose is too high.
    b. Administer the medication orally.
    c. Schedule the second dose for 2300.
    d. Assess the patient for signs of hyperglycemia.

26. A nurse caring for a pregnant patient suspected of being in preterm labour would recognise which of the following as diagnostic of preterm labour?
    a. Cervical dilation of at least 2 cm
    b. Uterine contractions occurring every 15 minutes
    c. Spontaneous rupture of the membranes
    d. Presence of foetal fibronectin in cervical secretions

III. THINKING CRITICALLY

1. Imagine that you are a nurse working at an inner-city women's health clinic. You are concerned about the rate of preterm labour and birth among the pregnant patients who come to your clinic for care. Outline a preterm labour and birth prevention program that you would implement at your clinic to reduce the rate of preterm labours and birth.

2. Sara, a multiparous woman (G2-T0-LP1-A0-1) at 22 weeks of gestation, comes to the clinic for her scheduled prenatal visit. She is anxious because her last labour began at 26 weeks and she is worried that this will happen again. "I had no warning the last time. Is there anything I can do this time to have my baby later or at least know that labour is starting so I can let you know?"

a. Identify the signs of preterm labour that the nurse should teach Sara.

b. Explain how the nurse could help Sara implement a plan to reduce her risk for preterm labour.

c. Sara calls the clinic 3 weeks later and tells the nurse that she has been having uterine contractions about every 8 minutes or so for the last hour. She is admitted for possible tocolytic therapy. Specify the criteria that Sara must meet before tocolysis can be safely initiated.

d. Sara is started on a tocolysis regimen that involves the oral administration of nifedipine. Outline the nursing care measures that must be implemented during the administration of this medication to ensure the safety of Sara and her foetus.

e. The nurse is preparing to give Sara a dose of betamethasone as prescribed by the primary health care provider.

   1. State the purpose of this medication.

   2. Explain the protocol that the nurse should follow in fulfilling this order.

3. Denise, a primigravida, has reached the second stage of labour with the foetus at zero station and positioned LOP. She is experiencing intense low back pain. Denise did not attend any childbirth classes and is having difficulty pushing effectively. No anesthesia has been used.

a. Identify the factors that can have a negative effect on the secondary powers of labour (bearing-down efforts).

b. Describe how you would help Denise use her expulsive forces to facilitate the descent and birth of her baby.

c. Specify the positions that would be recommended based on the position of the presenting part of Denise's foetus.

4. Anne, a primigravida, attended childbirth classes with her partner, Mark. They were looking forward to working together during the labour and birth of their baby. Because of an atypical fetal heart rate tracing, an emergency low-segment Caesarean section with a transverse incision was performed after 18 hours of labour. Even though Anne and her son are in stable condition and she is glad that "everything turned out okay" for her son, she expresses a sense of failure, stating, "I could not manage to give birth to my son in the normal way and now I never will!"

   a. List the preoperative nursing measures that should have been implemented to prepare Anne physically and emotionally for the unexpected Caesarean birth.

   b. Describe the major focus of care for Anne's care immediately after unplanned Caesarean section.

   c. Specify the assessment measures that are critical when Anne is in the recovery room following the birth of her son.

   d. Identify the nursing diagnosis reflected in Anne's statement, "I could not manage to give birth to my son in the normal way and now I never will!" Specify the support measures the nurse could use to put her Caesarean birth into perspective.

5. A vaginal examination reveals that Marie's fetus is RSA. Specify the considerations that the nurse should keep in mind when providing care for Marie.

6. Angela (G2-T0-P0-A1-L0) is at 42 weeks of gestation and has been admitted for induction of her labour.

   a. Assessment of Angela at admission included determination of her Bishop score. State the purpose of the Bishop score and identify the factors that are evaluated.

   b. Angela's score was 5. Interpret this result in terms of the planned induction of her labour.

   c. Angela's primary health care provider ordered that dinoprostone (Cervidil) be inserted. State the purpose of the Cervidil, method of application, and potential side effects that can occur.

   d. Before induction of her labour, Angela's primary health provider performs an amniotomy. State the rationale for performing an amniotomy at this time. Specify the nursing responsibilities before, during, and after this procedure.

e. Indicate which of the following actions reflect appropriate care (A) for Angela during the induction of her labour with intravenous oxytocin. If the action is not appropriate (NA), state what the correct action would be.

1. _____ Assist Angela into a lateral or upright position.

2. _____ Apply an external electronic fetal monitor and evaluate the tracing every 30 minutes throughout labour.

3. _____ Explain to Angela what to expect and techniques used.

4. _____ Add oxytocin into intravenous bag of an isotonic electrolyte solution (as per hospital protocol).

5. _____ Piggyback the oxytocin solution to the proximal port (port nearest the venous insertion site) of the primary IV.

6. _____ Begin infusion at 4 milliunits/min (if using high-dose protocol).

7. _____ Increase oxytocin by 1 to 2 milliunits/min at 5- to 10-minute intervals after the initial dose until the desired pattern of contractions is achieved.

8. _____ Stop increasing the dosage and maintain level of oxytocin when strong contractions occur every 2 to 3 minutes, and last 80 to 90 seconds each.

9. _____ Monitor maternal blood pressure and pulse every 15 minutes and after every increment.

10. _____ Limit IV intake to 1500 mL/8 hours.

f. State the reportable conditions associated with oxytocin induction for which the nurse must be alert when managing Angela's labour.

g. The nurse notes a uterine hyperstimulation pattern when evaluating Angela's monitor tracing. List the actions the nurse should take in order of priority.

7. Julia is in latent labour. Her BMI prior to pregnancy was 35 and she gained 36 kg during her pregnancy. If you were the nurse caring for Julia, what considerations related to her BMI would you keep in mind as you manage her care?

21 Physiological Changes in the Postpartum Patient

I. LEARNING KEY TERMS

FILL IN THE BLANKS: Insert the term that corresponds to each of the following descriptions.

1. _____ Increased sweating that occurs after birth, especially at night for the first 2 to 3 days, to rid the body of fluid retained during pregnancy.

2. _____ Uncomfortable uterine cramping that occurs during the early postpartum period as a result of periodic relaxation and vigorous contractions.

3. _____ Lactogenic hormone secreted by the pituitary gland of lactating patients. _____ Pituitary hormone that is responsible for uterine contraction and suppression of ovulation.

4. _____ Surgical incision of the perineum at birth.

5. _____ Result of the failure of the uterine muscle to contract firmly.

6. _____ Anal varicosity.

7. _____ Return of the uterus to a nonpregnant state.

8. _____ Self-destruction of excess hypertrophied uterine tissue as a result of the decrease in oestrogen and progesterone level following birth.

9. _____ Terms used interchangeably with postpartum to refer to the period of recovery after childbirth when reproductive organs return to their nonpregnant state; it lasts approximately 6 to 12 weeks though the time can vary from person to person.

10. _____ Separation of the abdominal wall muscles related to the effect of the enlargement of the uterus on the abdominal musculature.

11. _____ Postbirth uterine discharge or flow.

12. _____ Dark red, bloody uterine discharge that occurs for the first few days following birth; it consists primarily of blood, decidual tissue, trophoblastic debris, and sometimes small clots.

13. _____ Pink to brownish uterine discharge that begins about 3 to 4 days after birth; it consists of old blood, serum, leukocytes, and tissue debris.

14. _____ Yellowish white flow that begins about 10 days after birth and continues for 4 to 6 weeks; it consists of leukocytes, decidua, epithelial cells, mucus, serum, and bacteria.

15. _____ Term that describes distended, firm, tender, and warm breasts during the postpartum period.

16. _____ Failure of the uterus to return to a nonpregnant state. The most common causes for this failure are _____ and

_____.

17. _____ Medication most commonly administered intravenously or intramuscularly immediately after expulsion of the placenta to ensure that the uterus remains firm and well contracted.

18. _____ Coital discomfort or pain with intercourse.

19. _____ Exercises that help to strengthen perineal muscles and encourage healing.

20. _____ Yellowish fluid produced in the breasts before lactation.

21. _____ Increased production of urine that occurs in the postpartum period to rid the body of fluid retained during pregnancy.

22. _____ Stretch marks that appear during pregnancy on the breasts, abdomen, and thighs.

II. REVIEWING KEY CONCEPTS

1. When caring for a patient following vaginal birth, it is of critical importance for the nurse to assess the patient's bladder for distention.

   a. Explain why bladder distention is more likely to occur during the immediate postpartum period.

   b. Identify the problems that can occur if the bladder is allowed to become distended.

2. Cite the factors that can interfere with bowel elimination in the postpartum period.

3. Indicate the factors that place a postpartum patient at increased risk for the development of thrombophlebitis.

4. Compare and contrast the characteristics of lochial bleeding and nonlochial bleeding.

5. A nurse has assessed a patient who gave birth vaginally 12 hours ago. Which of the following findings would require further assessment?
   a. Bright to dark red uterine discharge
   b. Midline episiotomy—approximated, moderate oedema, slight erythema, absence of ecchymosis
   c. Protrusion of abdomen with sight separation of abdominal wall muscles
   d. Fundus firm at 1 cm above the umbilicus and to the right of midline

6. A patient, 24 hours after giving birth, tells the nurse that their sleep was interrupted the night before because of sweating and the need to have their gown and bed linen changed. The nurse's first action would be to:
   a. assess this patient for additional clinical manifestations of infection.
   b. explain to the patient that the sweating represents her body's attempt to eliminate the fluid that was accumulated during pregnancy.
   c. notify her primary health care provider of the finding.
   d. document the finding as postpartum diaphoresis.

7. Which of the following patients at 24 hours after giving birth is least likely to experience afterpains?
   a. Primipara who is breastfeeding twins that were born at 38 weeks of gestation
   b. Multipara who is breastfeeding their 4.5 kg full-term baby
   c. Multipara who is bottle-feeding her 3.6 kg baby
   d. Primipara who is breastfeeding her 3.5 kg baby

III. THINKING CRITICALLY

1. Describe how you would respond to each of the following typical questions/concerns of postpartum patients.

   a. Mary is a primipara who is breastfeeding. "Why am I experiencing so many painful cramps in my uterus? I thought this happens only in women who have had babies before."

   b. Susan is being discharged after giving birth 20 hours ago. "For how many days should I be able to palpate my uterus to make sure it is firm?"

   c. Gheeta is a primipara. "My friend, who had a baby last year, said she had a bleeding for 6 weeks. Isn't that a long time to bleed after having a baby?"

   d. Jean is at 24 hours postpartum. "I cannot believe it—I look as if I am still pregnant! How can this be?"

   e. Marion is 1 day postpartum. "It seems like I am urinating all the time; do you think that I have a bladder infection?"

   f. Mila is a primipara who is breastfeeding her baby. "My friend told me that I cannot get pregnant as long as I continue to breastfeed. This is great because I do not like to use birth control."

   g. Stella, a primiparous, bottle-feeding woman, is concerned. She states, "My mother told me that I should be getting a drug to dry up my breasts like she got after she gave birth. How will my breasts ever stop making milk and get back to normal?"

   h. Andrea, a primipara, is 1 day postpartum. While breastfeeding her baby she confides to the nurse that she does not know how long she will continue to breastfeed. "My partner and I have always had a satisfying sex life, but my friend told me that as long as I breastfeed, intercourse is painful."

22 Nursing Care of the Family During the Postpartum Period

I. LEARNING KEY TERMS

FILL IN THE BLANKS: Insert the term that corresponds to each of the following descriptions regarding the postpartum period.

1. _____ Classification of medications that stimulate contraction of the uterine smooth muscle.

2. _____ Failure of the uterine muscle to contract firmly. It is the most frequent cause for excessive bleeding following childbirth.

3. _____ Perineal treatment that involves sitting in warm water for approximately 20 minutes to soothe and cleanse the site and to increase blood flow, thereby enhancing healing.

4. _____ Menstrual-like cramps experienced by many women as the uterus contracts after childbirth.

5. _____ Dilation of the blood vessels supplying the intestines as a result of the rapid decrease in intraabdominal pressure after birth. It causes blood to pool in the viscera and thereby contributes to the development of

   _____ when the patient who has recently given birth sits or stands, first ambulates, or takes a warm shower.

6. _____ Exercises that can assist postpartum patients to regain muscle tone that is often lost when pelvic tissues are stretched and torn during pregnancy and birth.

7. _____ Swelling of breast tissue caused by increased blood and lymph supply to the breasts as the body begins the process of lactation.

8. _____ Vaccine that can be given to postpartum patients whose antibody titre is less than 1:8 or whose enzyme immunoassay level is less than 0.8. It is used to prevent nonimmune patients from contracting this infection during a subsequent pregnancy.

9. _____ Blood product that is administered to Rh-negative, antibody (Coombs)-negative patients who give birth to Rh-positive newborns. It is administered at 28 weeks of gestation and again within 72 hours after birth.

10. _____ Telephone-based postpartum consultation service that can provide information and support; it is not a crisis intervention line to be used for emergencies.

II. REVIEWING KEY CONCEPTS

1. Explain to a patient who has just given birth why breastfeeding their newborn during the fourth stage of labour is beneficial to both themselves and the newborn.

2. A postpartum patient at 6 hours after a vaginal birth is having difficulty voiding. List the measures that you would try to help this patient void spontaneously.

3. Identify the measures the nurse should teach a postpartum patient in an effort to prevent the development of venous thromboembolism (VTE).

4. Identify the measures you would teach a bottle-feeding mother to suppress lactation naturally and to relieve discomfort during breast engorgement.

5. State the two most important interventions that can be used to prevent excessive postpartum bleeding in the early postpartum period. Indicate the rationale for the effectiveness of each intervention you identified.

6. Identify the signs of potential psychosocial complications that may occur during the postpartum period.

7. The nurse is preparing to assess a postpartum patient's fundus. The nurse would assist the patient to:
   a. elevate the head of the bed.
   b. place hands under the head.
   c. empty the bladder.
   d. lie flat with legs extended and toes pointed.

8. A nurse is preparing to administer Rh Immune Globulin to a postpartum patient. Before implementing this care measure the nurse should:
   a. ensure that medication is given at least 24 hours after the birth.
   b. verify that the Coombs test results are negative.
   c. make sure that the newborn is Rh negative.
   d. cancel the administration of the Rh Immune Globulin if it was given to the patient during pregnancy at 28 weeks of gestation.

9. When teaching a postpartum patient with an episiotomy about using a sitz bath, the nurse should emphasize:
   a. using sterile equipment.
   b. filling the sitz bath basin with hot water (at least 42 °C).
   c. taking a sitz bath once a day for 10 minutes.
   d. squeezing the buttocks together before sitting down, then relaxing them.

10. Prior to discharge at 1 day postpartum, a nurse evaluates a patient's level of knowledge regarding the care of a second degree perineal laceration. Which of the following statements if made by the patient would indicate the need for further instruction before being discharged? (Select all that apply.)
    a. "I will wash my stitches at least once a day with mild soap and warm water."
    b. "I will change my pad every time I go to the bathroom—at least 4 times each day."
    c. "I will use my squeeze bottle filled with warm water to cleanse my stitches after I urinate."
    d. "I will take a sitz bath once a day before bed for about 10 minutes."
    e. "I will apply the anaesthetic cream to my stitches at least 6 times per day."

11. When assessing postpartum patients during the first 24 hours after birth, the nurse must be alert for signs that could indicate the development of postpartum physiological complications. Which of the following signs would be of concern to the nurse? (Select all that apply.)
    a. Temperature—38 °C
    b. Fundus—midline, boggy
    c. Lochia—75% of pad saturated in 3 hours
    d. Anorexia
    e. Voids approximately 150 to 200 mL of urine for each of the first three voidings after birth.

12. Before discharge, a postpartum patient and their partner ask the nurse about the baby blues. "Our friend said she felt so let down after she had her baby, and we have heard that some people actually become very depressed. Is there anything we can do to prevent this from happening to us or at least to cope with the blues if they occur?" The nurse should teach this couple:
    a. "Postpartum blues usually happen in pregnancies that are high risk or unplanned, so there is no need for you to worry."
    b. "Try to become skillful in breastfeeding and caring for your baby as quickly as you can."
    c. "Get as much rest as you can and sleep when the baby sleeps, because fatigue can precipitate the blues or make them worse."
    d. "I will call your primary health care provider before you leave to get you a prescription for an antidepressant to prevent the blues from happening."

III. THINKING CRITICALLY

1. Tara is a breastfeeding patient at 12 hours postpartum. She requests medication for pain. Describe the approach that you would take when fulfilling Tara's request.

2. When caring for a woman who gave birth 4 hours earlier, the nurse notes an excessive rubra flow and early signs of hypovolemic shock.

   a. State the criteria that the nurse should have used to determine that the flow is rubra and excessive and that the early signs of hypovolemic shock are being exhibited.

   b. Identify the nurse's priority action in response to these assessment findings.

   c. Identify additional interventions that a nurse may need to implement to ensure this patient's safety and to prevent the development of further complications.

3. Carrie is a postpartum woman awaiting discharge. Because her rubella titre indicates that she is not immune, a rubella vaccination has been ordered before discharge. State what you would teach Carrie with regard to this vaccination.

4. A primary health care provider has written the following order for a postpartum patient: "Administer Rh immune globulin, if indicated." Describe the actions the nurse should take in fulfilling this order.

5. Sindy, a postpartum breastfeeding woman, confides to the nurse, "My partner and I have always had a very satisfying sex life, even when I was pregnant. My sister told me that this will definitely change now that I have had a baby." Describe what the nurse should tell Sindy regarding sexual changes and activity after birth.

6. Identify the priority nursing diagnosis as well as one expected outcome and appropriate nursing care for each of the following situations.

   a. Tina is 2 days postpartum. During a home visit the nurse notes that Tina's laceration is oedematous and slightly reddened, with approximated wound edges and no drainage. A distinct odour is noted. During the interview, Tina reveals that she is afraid to wash the area. "I rinse with a little water in my peri bottle in the morning and again at night. I also apply plenty of my topical anaesthetic gel."

   Nursing Diagnosis   Expected Outcome   Nursing Care

   b. Erin, who gave birth 3 days ago, has not had a bowel movement since a day or two before labour. She tells the visiting nurse during the interview that she has been avoiding "fibre" foods for fear that the baby will get diarrhea. Her activity level is low. "My family is taking good care of me. I do not have to lift a finger! Besides I would prefer to wait until my "bottom" is less sore before trying to have a bowel movement."

   Nursing Diagnosis   Expected Outcome   Nursing Care

   c. Mary gave birth 24 hours ago. She states she has perineal discomfort. "My haemorrhoids and stitches are killing me, but I do not want to take any medication because it will get into my breast milk and hurt my baby."

   Nursing Diagnosis   Expected Outcome   Nursing Care

   d. Jane is 2 days postpartum. When the nurse makes a home visit, Jane is found crying. Jane states, "I have such a let-down feeling. I cannot understand why I feel this way when I should be so happy about the healthy outcome for myself and my baby." Jane's husband confirms her behaviour and expresses confusion as well, stating, "I wish I knew what to do to help her."

   Nursing Diagnosis   Expected Outcome   Nursing Care

7. Dawn gave birth 8 hours ago. Upon palpation, her fundus was found to be 2 fingerbreadths above the umbilicus and deviated to the right of midline. It was also assessed to be less firm than previously noted.

   a. State the most likely basis for these findings.

   b. Describe the action that the nurse should take based on these assessment findings.

8. Jill gave birth 3 hours ago. During labour, epidural anaesthesia was used for pain relief. Jill's primary health care provider has written the following order: "Out of bed and ambulating when able." Discuss the approach the nurse should take in safely fulfilling this order.

9. Cultural beliefs and practises must be considered when planning and implementing care in the postpartum period.

   a. Discuss the importance of using a culturally sensitive approach when providing care to postpartum patients and their families.

   b. A patient who has recently immigrated from Korea, has just given birth. Assessment reveals that she and her family are guided by beliefs and practises based on a balance of heat and cold. Describe how the nurse would adjust typical postpartum care in order to respect and accommodate the patient's cultural beliefs and practices.

   c. An Indigenous woman has been admitted to the postpartum unit following the birth of her second son. Describe the approach you would use in managing this woman's care in a culturally sensitive manner.

10. Tamara gave birth vaginally 2 hours ago. She has a second-degree laceration.

   a. Describe the position that Tamara should assume in order to facilitate palpation of her fundus.

   b. Identify the characteristics of Tamara's fundus that should be assessed.

   c. Describe the position Tamara should assume in order to facilitate the examination of her laceration.

   d. Identify the characteristics that should be assessed to determine progress of healing and adequacy of Tamara's perineal self-care measures.

   e. State the characteristics of Tamara's uterine blood flow that should be assessed.

11. Imagine that you are the nurse who cared for a patient during labour and birth and recovery during the fourth stage of labour. Outline the information that you would report to the mother-baby nurse when you transfer the new mother and baby to a room on the postpartum unit.

12. Infection control measures should guide the practise of nurses working on a postpartum unit.

    a. Discuss the measures designed to prevent transmission of infection from person to person.

    b. Discuss measures a postpartum patient should be taught to reduce the risk of infection.

23 Transition to Parenthood

I. LEARNING KEY TERMS

FILL IN THE BLANKS: Insert the appropriate term for each of the following descriptions regarding parent-infant interaction and parenting.

1. _____ Process by which a parent comes to love and accept a child and a child comes to love and accept a parent. The term _____ is often used to refer to this process.

2. _____ Process that occurs as parents interact with their newborn and maintain close proximity as they identify the infant as an individual and claim them as a member of the family; parents will touch, talk to, make eye contact with, and explore their newborn.

3. _____ Infant behaviours and characteristics call forth a corresponding set of caregiver behaviours and characteristics.

4. _____ Infant behaviours such as crying, smiling, and cooing that initiate the contact and bring the caregiver to the child.

5. _____ Process in which parents identify the new baby, first in terms of likeness to other family members, second in terms of differences, and third in terms of uniqueness.

6. _____ Position used for mutual gazing in which the parent's face and the infant's face are approximately 20 cm apart and are on the same plane.

7. _____ Newborns move in time with the structure of adult speech by waving their arms, lifting their heads, and kicking their legs, seemingly "dancing in tune" to a parent's voice.

8. _____ Personal biorhythm developed by the infant; parents facilitate this process by giving consistent loving care and using their infant's alert state to develop responsive behaviour and thereby increase social interaction and opportunities for learning.

9. _____ Type of body movement or behaviour that provides the observer with cues. The observer or receiver interprets those cues and responds to them.

10. _____ The "fit" between the infant's cues and the parents' response.

11. _____ Period from the decision to conceive through the first months of having a child.

12. _____ Parents action of looking at their baby demonstrating interest in them, which often makes them feel closer to them.

13. _____ Involves a stabilisation of tasks and coming to terms with commitments to the parental role.

14. _____ Process of transformation and growth of the mother identity during which the person learns new skills and increases their confidence in themselves as they meet new challenges in caring for their child(ren).

15. _____ Father's absorption, preoccupation, and interest in his infant.

16. _____ Contingent responses that occur within a specific time and are similar in form to a stimulus behaviour.

II. REVIEWING KEY CONCEPTS

1. Attachment of the newborn to parents and family is critical for optimum growth and development.

   a. List conditions that must be present for the parent-newborn attachment process to begin favourably.

   b. Discuss how you would assess the progress of attachment between parents and their new baby.

c. Indentify what nurses can do to facilitate the process of attachment in the immediate postbirth period.

2. Describe three parental tasks and responsibilities that are part of parental adjustment to a new baby.

3. Discuss how each of the following forms of parent-infant contact can facilitate attachment and promote the family as a focus of care.

   a. Early contact

   b. Extended contact

4. Describe how a parent's touching of their newborn progresses during the immediate postbirth period.

5. Describe how each of the following factors influences the manner in which parents respond to the birth of their child. State two nursing implications/actions related to each factor.

   Adolescent parents

   Parental age older than 35

   LBGTQ2 couple

Indigencus family

Social support

Culture

Socioeconomic conditions

Personal aspirations

Sensory impairment

6. During maternal attachment and bonding with the newborn, which of the following might a mother say?
   a. "She has her grandfather's nose."
   b. "His ears lay nice and flat against his head, not like mine and his sister's, which stick out."
   c. "She gave me nothing but trouble during pregnancy, and now she is so stubborn she won't wake up to breastfeed."
   d. "He has such a sweet disposition and pleasant expression. I have never seen a baby quite like him before."

7. Which of the following nursing actions would be least effective in facilitating parent attachment to their newborn?
   a. Referring the couple to a lactation consultant to ensure continuing success with breastfeeding
   b. Keeping the baby in the nursery as much as possible for the first 24 hours after birth so the mother can rest
   c. Extending visiting hours for the postpartum patient's partner as desired
   d. Providing guidance and support as the parents care for their baby's nutrition and hygiene needs

8. Which of the following behaviours illustrates engrossment?
   a. A father is sitting in a rocking chair, holding his new baby boy, touching his toes, and making eye contact.
   b. A mother tells her friends that her baby's eyes and nose are just like hers.
   c. A mother picks up and cuddles her baby when she begins to cry.
   d. A grandmother gazes into her new grandchild's face, which she holds about 20 cm away from her own; she and the baby make eye-to-eye contact.

9. Which of the following infant behaviours affect parental attachment? (Select all that apply.)
   a. Grasp reflex
   b. Unpredictable feeding and sleeping schedule
   c. Seeks attention from any adult in room
   d. Differential crying, smiling and vocalising
   e. Approaches through locomotion

III. THINKING CRITICALLY

1. Describe what you would teach a couple who have just had a baby regarding the communication process as it relates to their newborn.

   a. Techniques they can use to communicate effectively with their newborn.

   b. The manner in which the baby is able to communicate with them.

2. Allison had a difficult labour that resulted in an emergency Cesarean birth under general anaesthesia. She did not see her baby until 4 hours after her birth. Allison tells the nurse who brings the baby to her room, "I am so disappointed. I had planned to breastfeed my baby and hold her close, skin to skin, right after her birth just like all the books say. I know that this is so important for our relationship." Describe how the nurse should respond to Allison's concern.

3. Angela is the mother of a 1-day-old boy and a 3-year-old girl. As you prepare Angela for discharge, she states, "My little girl just saw her brother. She says she loves him and cannot wait for him to come home. I am so glad that I do not have to worry about any of that sibling rivalry business!" Indicate how you would respond to Angela's comments.

4. A couple have just experienced the birth of their first baby. They are very happy with their newborn but appear very unsure of themselves and are obviously anxious about how to tell what their baby needs. Sara is trying very hard to breastfeed and is having some success but not as much as she had hoped. Both parents express self-doubt about their ability to succeed at the "most important role in our lives."

   a. State the nursing diagnosis that is most appropriate for this couple.

   b. Describe what the nurse caring for this family can do to facilitate the attachment process.

5. Mary and Jim are the parents of three sons. They very much wanted to have a girl this time, but after a long and difficult birth they had another son who weighed 4.5 kg. His appearance reflects the difficult birth process: occipital moulding, caput succedaneum, and forceps marks on each cheek. Mary and Jim express their disappointment not only in the appearance of their son but also in the fact that they had another boy. "This was supposed to be our last child—now we just do not know what we will do." Discuss how you would facilitate Mary and Jim's attachment to their son and reconcile their fantasy ("dream") child with the reality of their actual child.

6. A couple has just given birth to their first baby. This is the first grandchild for both sets of grandparents. The grandmothers approach the nurse to ask how they can help the new family, stating, "We want to help them but at the same time not interfere with what they want to do." Discuss the role of the nurse in helping these grandparents to recognise their importance to the new family and to develop a mutually satisfying relationship with the parents and the new baby.

7. Ali has just become a father with the birth of his first child.

   a. Describe the process Ali will follow as he adjusts to fatherhood.

   b. Identify several measures the nurse caring for Ali's partner and newborn can use to facilitate his adjustment to fatherhood and attachment to his baby.

24 Postpartum Complications

I. LEARNING KEY TERMS

FILL IN THE BLANKS: Insert the term that corresponds to each of the following descriptions of postpartum complications.

1. _____ Loss of 500 mL or more of blood after vaginal birth or 1 000 mL or more after Caesarean birth. _____ Excessive blood loss that occurs within 24 hours after birth; it is most often caused by marked uterine hypotonia. _____ Blood loss that occurs more than 24 hours after birth but less than 12 weeks after birth.

2. _____ Marked hypotonia of the uterus; the uterus fails to contract well or maintain contraction.

3. _____ Collection of blood in the connective tissue as a result of blood vessel damage. _____ are the most common type. _____ are usually associated with a forceps-assisted birth, an episiotomy, or primigravidity.

4. _____ Unusual placental adherence in which there is slight penetration of the myometrium by placental trophoblast.

5. _____ Unusual placental adherence in which there is deep penetration of the myometrium by the placenta.

6. _____ Unusual placental adherence in which there is perforation of the uterus by the placenta.

7. _____ Turning of the uterus inside out after birth.

8. _____ Delayed return of the enlarged uterus to normal size and function.

9. _____ Emergency situation in which profuse blood loss (haemorrhage) can result in severely compromised perfusion of body organs. Death may occur.

10. _____ Coagulopathy resulting from an autoimmune disorder in which antiplatelet antibodies decrease the life span of the platelets.

11. _____ Type of haemophilia; it is among the most common congenital clotting defects in North American women of childbearing age.

12. _____ Pathological form of clotting that is diffuse and consumes large amounts of clotting factors; it is also known as consumptive coagulopathy.

13. _____ Results from a formation of a blood clot or clots inside a blood vessel.

14. _____ Inflammation of a vein with clot formation.

15. _____ Clot involves the superficial saphenous venous system. _____ Clot involvement can extend from the foot to the iliofemoral region.

16. _____ Complication occurring when part of a blood clot dislodges and is carried to the pulmonary artery, where it occludes the vessel and obstructs blood flow to the lungs.

17. _____ or _____ Clinical infection of the genital canal that occurs within 42 days after miscarriage, induced abortion, or childbirth. Common symptoms include, pyrexia (presence of fever of greater than 38 °C), tachycardia and subjective feelings of localised pain

18. _____ Infection of the lining of the uterus; it is the most common postpartum infection and usually begins as a localised infection at the placental site.

19. _____ Infection of the breast affecting approximately 2% to 10% of postpartum patients, soon after childbirth, most of whom are first-time breastfeeding mothers; it almost always is unilateral and develops well after lactation has been established.

20. _____ Downward displacement of the uterus, with varying degrees of displacement from into the vagina to complete protrusion outside the introitus.

21. _____ Predominant classification of mental health disorders in the antepartum and postpartum period.

22. _____ characterised by tearfulness, agitation, mood swings, anxiety, sleep and appetite disturbances and feelings of being overwhelmed; however, resolves within a few days and does not need treatment.

23. _____ An intense and pervasive sadness with severe and labile mood swings; it is serious and persistent. Intense fears, anger, anxiety, and despondency that persist past the baby's first few weeks are not a normal part of postpartum blues.

24. _____ Syndrome most often characterised by rapid onset of bizarre behaviour, auditory or visual hallucinations, paranoid or grandiose delusions, and extreme deficits in judgement.

25. _____ Symptom of postpartum depression that may include not feeling love for the newborn.

26. _____ Treatment for moderate to severe postpartum depression.

27. _____ Mood disorder defined by the presence of one or more episodes of abnormally elevated energy levels, cognition, and mood and one or more depressive episodes.

28. _____ and _____ Screening scales to assess postpartum depression.

29. _____, _____, _____, and _____ Four criteria used to measure the seriousness of a suicidal plan.

30. _____ Pervasive feeling of anxiety most of the time and excessive worry about multiple concerns.

31. _____ Unpredictable, intermittent episodes of symptoms similar to those of generalised anxiety disorder.

32. _____ Prolonged grief in the form of depression.

II. REVIEWING KEY CONCEPTS

1. State the twofold focus of medical management of haemorrhagic shock.

2. Identify the priority nursing care for postpartum haemorrhage and hypovolemic shock. Include the rationale for each intervention identified.

3. State the standard of care for bleeding emergencies.

4. Identify measures found to be effective in preventing genital tract infections during the postpartum period.

5. Describe nursing care that should be provided to families prior to discharge regarding perinatal mood disorders.

6. Describe how you, as a nurse, would help family members with maternal death.

7. A woman has been diagnosed with severe perinatal depression. The nurse caring for this woman is concerned that she may harm herself, her baby, or both of them.

   a. What questions should the nurse ask to determine whether the patient is considering such a harmful action?

   b. The woman admits that she has been thinking that her family and even her baby might be better off without her. Identify the four criteria the nurse could use to determine how serious the woman might be.

8. Methylergonovine 0.2 mg is ordered to be administered intramuscularly to a patient who gave birth vaginally 1 hour ago for a profuse lochial flow with clots. The fundus is boggy and does not respond well to massage. The patient was treated for preeclampsia prior to the birth. The patient's blood pressure, measured 5 minutes ago, was 155/98. In fulfilling this order, the nurse would do which of the following?
   a. Measure the patient's blood pressure again 5 minutes after administering the medication.
   b. Question the order based on the patient's hypertensive status.
   c. Recognise that methylergonovie should be administered rectally.
   d. Teach the patient that the medication will lead to uterine cramping.

9. A postpartum patient in the fourth stage of labour received Carboprost tromethamine 100 mcg intramuscularly. The expected outcome of care for the administration of this medication would be which of the following?
   a. Relief from the pain of uterine cramping
   b. Prevention of intrauterine infection
   c. Reduction in the blood's ability to clot
   d. Limitation of excessive blood loss that is occurring after birth

10. The nurse responsible for the care of postpartum patients should recognise that the first sign of puerperal infection would most likely be which of the following?
    a. Fever with body temperature at 38° C or higher after the first 24 hours following birth
    b. Increased white blood cell count
    c. Foul-smelling profuse lochia
    d. Bradycardia

11. A breastfeeding patient's Caesarean birth occurred 2 days ago. Investigation of the pain, tenderness, and swelling in her left leg led to a medical diagnosis of venous thromboembolism (VTE). Care management for this patient during the acute stage of the VTE would involve which of the following actions? (Select all that apply.)
    a. Explaining that they will need to stop breastfeeding until anticoagulation therapy is completed
    b. Administering heparin via continuous intravenous drip
    c. Placing the patient on bed rest with the left leg elevated
    d. Encouraging the patient to change positions frequently when on bed rest
    e. Teaching the patient and family how to administer warfarin (Coumadin) subcutaneously after discharge
    f. Teaching the patient to use acetaminophen (Tylenol) for discomfort

12. Which of the following would be a priority question to ask a patient experiencing postpartum depression?
    a. Have you thought about hurting yourself?
    b. Does it seem like your mind is filled with cobwebs?
    c. Have you been feeling insecure, fragile, or vulnerable?
    d. Does the responsibility of motherhood seem overwhelming?

13. Which disorder is carboprost tromethamine contraindicated
    a. Hypertension
    b. von Willebrand disease
    c. Asthma
    d. Cardiac disease

14. Signs of pulmonary embolus include:
    a. decreased pulse.
    b. elevated blood pressure.
    c. skin warm to touch.
    d. tachypnea.

15. Which of the following are management techniques used in postpartum haemorrhage? (Select all that apply.)
    a. Bimanual compression
    b. Administration of uterotonic medications
    c. Call the haemorrhage team
    d. Start an IV with lactated Ringer with magnesium sulfate

16. A postpartum patient experiencing postpartum depression asks the nurse if there are any herbal remedies they can use as part of the treatment regimen. Which of the following would the nurse discuss with the woman?
    a. Blue cohosh
    b. Shepherd's purse
    c. St. John's wort
    d. Lavender tea
    e. Lady's mantle
    f. Red raspberry leaves

17. The expected outcome for care when methylergonovine (Methergine), an oxytocic, is administered to a postpartum patient during the fourth stage of labour would be which of the following? The patient will:
    a. demonstrate decreased lochial flow.
    b. achieve relief of pain associated with uterine cramping.
    c. remain free from infection.
    d. void spontaneously within 4 hours of birth.

III. THINKING CRITICALLY

1. Andrea is a multiparous woman (G6-T6-P1-A0-L7) who gave birth to full-term twins vaginally 1 hour ago. Oxytocin was used to augment her labour when hypotonic uterine contractions protracted the active stage of her labour. Special forceps were used to assist the birth of the second twin. Currently her vital signs are stable, her fundus is at the umbilicus, midline and firm, and her lochial flow is moderate to heavy without clots.

    a. Early postpartum haemorrhage is a major concern at this time. State the factors that have increased Andrea's risk for haemorrhage at this time.

    b. During the second hour after birth, the nurse notes that Andrea's perineal pad became saturated in 15 minutes and a large amount of blood had accumulated on the bed under her buttocks. Describe the nurse's initial response to this finding. State the rationale for the action you described.

    c. The nurse prepares to administer 10 units of oxytocin intravenously as ordered by Andrea's health care provider. Explain the guidelines the nurse should follow in fulfilling this order.

    d. During the assessment of Andrea, the nurse must be alert for signs of developing hypovolemic shock. Cite the signs the nurse would be watching for.

    e. Describe the measures that the nurse should use to support Andrea and her family in an effort to reduce their anxiety.

Chapter **24** **Postpartum Complications**

2. Nurses working on a postpartum unit must be constantly alert for signs and symptoms of postpartum infection in their patients.

   a. List the factors that can increase a postpartum patient's risk for postpartum infection.

   b. State the typical clinical manifestations of endometritis for which the nurse should be alert when assessing postpartum patients.

   c. Describe the critical nursing care measures that are essential related to postpartum infection.

3. Sara, a primiparous breastfeeding mother at 2 weeks postpartum, calls the breastfeeding clinic to say that her right breast is painful and she's not "feeling well."

   a. Explain the assessment findings the nurse would be alert for to indicate whether Sara is experiencing mastitis.

   b. A medical diagnosis of mastitis of Sara's right breast is made. State two nursing diagnoses appropriate for this situation.

   c. Describe the treatment measures and health teaching that Sara needs regarding her infection and breastfeeding, because she wishes to continue to breastfeed.

   d. Identify several behaviours that Sara should learn to prevent recurrence of mastitis.

4. Susan is a 36-year-old multiparous patient with obesity (G5-T4-P0-A1-L4) who experienced a Caesarean birth 2 days ago. During this pregnancy, she was able to reduce her smoking of 1 pack of cigarettes each day to 1/2 pack per day. Although she has never experienced a venous thrombophlebitis, she did develop varicose veins in both legs with her third pregnancy. A major complication of the postpartum period is the development of thromboembolic disease.

   a. State the risk factors for this complication that Susan presents.

140

b. When assessing Susan on the afternoon of her second postpartum day, the nurse notes signs indicative of VTE. List the signs the nurse most likely observed.

c. A medical diagnosis of VTE is confirmed. State one nursing diagnosis appropriate for this situation.

d. Outline the expected care management for Susan during the acute phase of the VTE.

e. Upon discharge Susan will be taking warfarin for at least 3 months. Specify the discharge instructions that Susan and her family should receive.

5. Denise (G1-T0-P0-A0-L0), is a postpartum patient who has been diagnosed with a pelvic haematoma.

a. Describe the signs and symptoms Denise most likely exhibited that lead to this diagnosis.

b. State the risk factors for this complication that Denise presents.

c. Outline the care approach recommended for Denise's diagnosis.

6. Miriam, a 35-year-old primiparous woman beginning her second week postpartum, is bottle-feeding her baby. She and her partner, Tom, moved from Red Deer Alberta, where they lived all their lives, to Toronto 2 months ago to take advantage of a career opportunity for Tom. They live in a community with many other young couples who are also starting families. Last month they joined the church near their home. Tom tries to help Miriam with the baby but he has to spend long hours at work to establish his position. Miriam's prenatal record reveals that she often exhibited anxiety about her well-being and that of her baby. During a home visit by a nurse, Mariam tells the nurse that she always wants to sleep and just cannot seem to get enough rest. Miriam is very concerned that she is not being a good mother and states, "Sometimes I just do not know what to do to care for my baby the right way, and I am not even breastfeeding my baby. It seems that Tom enjoys spending what little time he has at home with the baby and not with me. I even find myself yelling at him for the silliest things." The nurse recognises that Miriam is exhibiting behaviours strongly suggestive of perinatal depression.

a. Indicate the signs and symptoms that Miriam exhibited that led the nurse to suspect perinatal depression.

b. Specify the risk factors for perinatal depression that are present in Mary's situation.

c. Write several questions that the nurse could ask Mary to determine the depth of the perinatal depression that she is experiencing.

d. Describe the measures the nurse could use to help Mary and Tom cope with perinatal depression.

7. Angela gave birth vaginally to a newborn at 41 weeks of gestation. Her infant was 4.5 kg. After the birth, Anita experienced a postpartum haemorrhage. Explain the care for Angela involving an interprofessional health care team.

8. A patient gave birth to a baby by Caesarean section after a prolonged labour. Later the patient was diagnosed with a urinary tract infection.

a. Discuss risk factors that place the patient at risk for a urinary tract infection.

b. Review a possible management plan for patient after this diagnosis.

25 Physiological Adaptations of the Newborn

I. LEARNING KEY TERMS

FILL IN THE BLANKS: Insert the term that corresponds to each of the following descriptions related to newborn characteristics and care.

1. _____ Environment that allows the newborn to maintain a stable normal body temperature.

2. _____ Heat production or generation; for the newborn, it occurs as a result of increased muscle activity.

3. _____ Heat production process unique to the newborn accomplished primarily by metabolism of brown fat and secondarily by increased metabolic activity in the brain, heart, and liver.

4. _____ Flow of heat from the body surface to cooler ambient air. Two measures to reduce heat loss by this method would be to wrap the infant and place a cap on the head.

5. _____ Loss of heat from the body surface to a cooler, solid surface not in direct contact but in relative proximity. To prevent this type of heat loss, cribs and examining tables are placed away from outside windows and care is taken to avoid direct air draught.

6. _____ Loss of heat that occurs when a liquid is converted to vapour; in the newborn heat loss occurs when moisture from the skin is vapourized. This heat loss can be intensified by failure to dry the newborn directly after birth or by drying the newborn too slowly after a bath.

7. _____ Loss of heat from the body surface to cooler surfaces in direct contact. Placing a protective cover on the scale when weighing the newborn will minimise heat lost by this method.

8. _____ The newborn has a decreased ability to increase evaporative skin water losses because sweat glands do not function sufficiently to allow the newborn to sweat; serious overheating can cause cerebral damage from dehydration or heat stroke and death.

9. _____ Accelerates the depletion of brown fat and can lead to metabolic and respiratory complications.

10. _____ Small, flat pink areas, cn the upper eyelids, nose, upper lip, back of head, and nape of neck that easily blanch.

11. _____ Overlapping of cranial bones to facilitate movement of the foetal head through the maternal pelvis during the process of labour and birth.

12. _____ Generalised, easily identifiable edematous area of the scalp usually over the occiput.

13. _____ Collection of blood between a skull bone and its periosteum that does not cross cranial suture lines that results from pressure during the birthing process.

14. _____ Bluish-black pigmented areas [slate grey] usually found on back and buttocks but can occur anywhere on the exterior surface of the body including the extremities.

15. _____ Hands and feet appear slightly cyanotic, especially when chilled, as a result of vasomotor instability and capillary stasis; it may occur during the first 7 to 10 days of life.

16. _____ White, cheese-like substance that coats and protects the foetus's skin while in utero.

143

17. _____ Small white facial bumps caused by distended sebaceous glands.

18. _____ Yellow skin discolouration caused by increased levels of serum bilirubin.

19. _____ Thick, tarry, dark green-black stool usually passed within 24 hours of birth.

20. _____ Transient newborn rash characterised by erythematous macules, papules, and small vesicles; it may appear suddenly anywhere on the body.

21. _____ Substance present in the urine of newborns that cause a pink-tinged stain or "brick dust" on the diaper; it is a normal finding during the first week and not representative of bleeding.

22. _____ Contraction of the anal sphincter in response to touch; it is a sign of good sphincter tone.

23. _____ Accumulation of fluid in the scrotum, around the testes.

24. _____ Bruising.

25. _____ Heart sound heard when foetal shunts (foramen ovale, ductus arteriosus) remain fully or partially open after birth.

26. _____ Soft, downy hair on face, shoulders, and back.

27. _____ Bleeding into the space below the aponeurosis layer of the skull that contains loosely arranged connective tissue; it is located beneath the tendinous sheath that connects the frontal and occipital muscles and forms the inner surface of the scalp. The injury can be associated with deliveries assisted by vacuum extraction and may lead to hypovolemic shock.

28. _____ Peeling of the skin that occurs in the term infant a few days after birth; if present at birth, it may be an indication of postmaturity.

29. _____ Flat red to purple birthmark composed of a plexus of newly formed capillaries in the papillary layer of the corium; it varies in size, shape, and location but is usually found on the neck and face. It does not blanch under pressure or disappear.

30. _____ Birthmark consisting of dilated, newly formed capillaries occupying the entire dermal and subdermal layers with associated connective tissue hypertrophy; it is typically a raised, sharply demarcated bright or dark red, rough-surfaced swelling that appear at or around the time of birth; lesion will progress in size before beginning the slow process of involution.

31. _____ Slightly blood-tinged mucoid vaginal discharge associated with an oestrogen decrease after birth.

32. _____ Foreskin.

33. _____ Small, white areas found on the gum margins or palates.

34. _____ Extra digits, fingers or toes. _____ Missing digits.

35. _____ Fused fingers or toes.

36. _____ Variations in the state of consciousness of newborn infants.

37. _____ and _____ The two sleep states. The newborn sleeps about 17 hours a day, with periods of wakefulness _____ gradually.

38. _____, _____, _____, and _____ The four wake states.

39. _____ The optimum state of arousal in which the infant can be observed smiling, responding to voices, watching faces, vocalising, and moving in synchrony.

40. _____ Behaviour of the newborn to modulate its state of consciousness, develop predictable sleep and wake states, and react appropriately to stress.

41. _____ Protective mechanism that allows the infant to become accustomed to environmental stimuli. It is a psychologic and physiologic phenomenon in which the response to a constant or repetitive stimulus is decreased.

42. _____ Quality of alert states and ability to attend to visual and auditory stimuli while alert.

43. _____ Ability of the newborn to self-sooth and reduce stress; one behaviour a newborn uses is hand-to-mouth movements with or without sucking.

44. _____ Individual variations in a newborn's primary reaction pattern.

45. _____ A protective mechanism that allows the infant to become accustomed to environmental stimuli.

46. _____ The language an infant uses to signal hunger, discomfort, pain, desire for attention, or fussiness.

II. REVIEWING KEY CONCEPTS

1. The most critical adjustment that a newborn must make at birth is the establishment of respirations. List the factors that are responsible for the initiation of breathing after birth.

2. During the first 6 to 8 hours after birth, newborns experience a transitional period characterised by three phases of instability. Indicate the timing/duration and typical behaviours for each phase of this transitional period.

   First period of reactivity

   Period of decreased responsiveness

   Second period of reactivity

3. A newborn, at 5 hours old, wakes from a sound sleep and becomes very active and begins to cry. Which of the following signs if exhibited by this newborn would indicate expected adaptation to extrauterine life? (Select all that apply.)
   a. Increased mucus production
   b. Passage of meconium
   c. Heart rate of 160 beats per minute
   d. Respiratory rate of 24 breaths per minute and irregular
   e. Retraction of sternum with inspiration
   f. Expiratory grunting with nasal flaring

4. When assessing a newborn infant at 12 hours of age, the nurse notes a rash on the abdomen and thighs composed of erythematous macules, papules, and small vesicles. The nurse would:
   a. document the finding as erythema toxicum.
   b. isolate the newborn and parent until infection is ruled out.
   c. apply an antiseptic ointment to each lesion.
   d. request nonallergenic linen from the laundry.

5. A breastfed full-term newborn infant is 12 hours old and is being prepared for early discharge. Which of the following assessment findings, if present, could delay discharge?
   a. Dark green-black stool, tarry in consistency
   b. Yellow discolouration of sclera and face
   c. Swollen breasts with a scant amount of thin discharge
   d. Blood-tinged mucoid vaginal discharge

6. As part of a thorough assessment, the newborn should be checked for hip dislocation and dysplasia. Which of the following techniques would be used?
   a. Check for syndactyly bilaterally
   b. Stepping or walking reflex
   c. Magnet reflex
   d. Ortolani manoeuvre

7. When assessing a newborn after birth, the nurse notes flat, irregular, pink marks on the bridge of the nose, nape of neck, and over the eyelids. The areas blanch when pressed with a finger. The nurse would document this finding as:
   a. milia
   b. infantile haemangioma
   c. telangiectatic nevi
   d. nevus flammeus

III. THINKING CRITICALLY

1. When caring for newborns, especially during the transition period following birth, the nurse recognises that newborns are at increased risk for cold stress.

   a. Explain the basis for this risk.

   b. State the danger that cold stress poses for the newborn.

   c. Identify one nursing diagnosis and one expected outcome related to this danger.

   d. Describe care measures the nurse should implement to prevent cold stress from occurring.

2. After a long and difficult labour, baby James was born with a caput succedaneum and significant moulding over the occipital area. Low forceps were used for the birth, resulting in ecchymotic areas on both facial cheeks. James's parents tell the nurse that they are very concerned that James may have experienced brain damage. Describe what the nurse should tell the parents of James about these assessment findings.

3. During the first 24 hours of life, it is essential that the nurse monitor a newborn's breathing pattern for signs of distress. Create a checklist that could be used by a nurse to determine if a newborn is exhibiting eupnea (normal breathing pattern) or dyspnea (respiratory distress).

4. Roberto and Maria are first-time parents of their recently born infant. They ask the nurse about their baby's ability to see and hear things around her and to interact with them.

   a. Specify what the nurse should tell these parents about the sensory capabilities of their healthy full-term newborn.

   b. Name four stimuli Roberto and Maria could provide for their baby that would help foster development.

5. Shanice and Malik, a black couple, express concern that their new baby has several bruises on their back and buttocks. They ask if their baby was injured during birth or in the nursery. Describe the appropriate response of the nurse to this couple's concern.

6. Jaundice in the newborn can represent a normal physiologic response or indicate pathology. Compare and contrast each type of jaundice identified below in terms of causation, characteristics, and significance.

   a. Physiologic (nonpathologic) jaundice

   b. Pathologic (nonphysiologic) jaundice

   c. Breastfeeding-associated jaundice

   d. Breast-milk jaundice

26 Nursing Care of the Newborn and Family

I. LEARNING KEY TERMS

FILL IN THE BLANKS: Insert the term that corresponds to each of the following descriptions of newborns and their care.

1. _____ Assessment method used to rapidly assess the newborn's transition to extrauterine existence at 1 and 5 minutes after birth; it is based on five signs that indicate his or her physiologic state, namely: _____, _____, _____, _____, and _____.

2. _____ Automatic sensor usually placed on the upper quadrant of the abdomen immediately below the right or left costal margin; functions as a servo-control mechanism to maintain newborn skin temperature within preset range.

3. _____ Inflammation of the newborn's eyes from gonorrhoeal or chlamydial infection contracted by the newborn during passage through the mother's birth canal. _____ ointment may not be indicated in exposed asymptomatic newborns; Nurses should understand local policy and guidelines regarding administration.

4. _____ Single-dose medication administered intramuscularly to the newborn to prevent haemorrhagic disease of the newborn

5. _____ Evaluation tool used to assess and estimate gestational age at birth

6. _____ Term that describes an infant whose birthweight falls between the 10th and 90th percentiles reflecting appropriate growth during foetal life regardless of length of gestation.

7. _____ Infant born before the completion of 37 weeks of gestation, regardless of birth weight.

8. _____ Infant born after completion of week 42 of gestation.

9. _____ Infant born after completion of week 42 of gestation and showing the effects of progressive placental insufficiency.

10. _____ Infants born from 37 0/7 to 38 6/7 weeks of gestation.

11. _____ Pinpoint haemorrhagic areas acquired during birth that may extend over the upper trunk and face; they are benign if they disappear within 2 to 3 days of birth and no new lesions appear.

12. _____ Derived from the breakdown of red blood cells; its accumulation in the blood results in a yellow discolouration of the skin, sclera, and oral mucous membranes.

13. _____ Yellow discolouration of the integument and sclera that first appears after the first 24 hours of life, peaks at 3-5 days in term infants, and resolves after 1-2 weeks.

14. _____ Yellow staining of brain cells that may result in bilirubin encephalopathy.

15. _____ Device used for noninvasive monitoring of bilirubin via cutaneous reflectance measurements; is not accurate once phototherapy commences.

16. _____ Common method used to reduce the level of circulating unconjugated bilirubin or to keep it from increasing; it uses light energy to change the shape and structure of unconjugated bilirubin and convert it to molecules that can be excreted.

17. _____ Blood glucose concentration less than adequate to support neurologic, organ, and tissue function during the early newborn period; neurological injury can occur if severe or prolonged.

18. _____ Early onset usually occurs in first 24-48 hours; presenting symptoms similar to hypoglycemia although may also be asymptomatic.

19. _____ Newborn respiratory rate of 30 breaths per minute or lower.

20. _____ Newborn respiratory rate of 60 breaths per minute or higher.

21. _____ The most important single measure in the prevention of neonatal infection.

22. _____ An alternative device for phototherapy in the treatment of hyperbilirubinemia; flexible device may be placed under the newborn or around the torso.

23. _____ Surgical procedure that involves removing the prepuce (foreskin) of the glans penis.

II. REVIEWING KEY CONCEPTS

MATCHING: Match the description with the appropriate newborn reflex.

1. _____ Place infant supine, then partially flex both legs and apply light pressure with fingers to the soles of the feet—legs extend against examiner's pressure.

2. _____ Place infant supine on flat surface and make a loud abrupt noise (e.g., sharp hand clap)—symmetric abduction and extension of arms, fingers fan out, thumb and forefinger form a C; arms are then adducted into an embracing motion and return to relaxed flexion and movement.

3. _____ Place finger in palm of hand or at base of toes—infant's fingers curl around examiner's finger; toes curl downward.

4. _____ Place infant prone on flat surface, run finger down side of back first on one side and then down the other 4 to 5 cm lateral to spine—body flexes and pelvis swings toward stimulated side.

5. _____ Tap over forehead, bridge of nose, or maxilla when eyes are open—blinks for first four to five taps.

6. _____ Use finger to stroke sole of foot beginning at heel, upward along lateral aspect of sole, and then across ball of foot—all toes hyperextend, with dorsiflexion of big toe.

7. _____ Touch infant's lip, cheek, or corner of mouth with nipple or finger—turns head toward stimulus, opens mouth, takes hold, and sucks.

8. _____ Place infant in a supine neutral position, turn head quickly to one side—arm and leg extend on side to which head is turned while opposite arm and leg flex.

9. _____ Hold infant vertically under the arms or around the trunk allowing one foot to touch a flat surface—alternates flexion and extension of its feet; term infants will use soles of feet and preterm infants will use toes.

10. _____ Touch or depress tip of tongue—infant forces tongue outward.

11. _____ Place infant supine and then extend one leg, press knee downward, and stimulate the bottom of the foot—opposite leg flexes, adducts, and then extends as if the infant is attempting to push away the stimulation.

a. Rooting

b. Palmar grasp

c. Extrusion

d. Glabellar (Myerson)

e. Tonic neck

f. Moro

g. Stepping (walking)

h. Babinski

i. Truncal incurvation (Galant)

j. Magnet

k. Crossed extension

12. Outline the specific measures nurses should use when caring for newborns to ensure a safe and protective environment.

13. Describe the approach you would use to ensure accuracy when performing each of the following measurements of a newborn.

    a. Weight

    b. Length

    c. Head circumference

    d. Chest circumference

14. Preparing parents for the discharge of their newborn requires informing them about the essential aspects of newborn care. Identify three points that you would emphasise when teaching parents about each of the following aspects of newborn characteristics and care.

    a. Vital signs: temperature and respirations

    b. Feeding Patterns and Elimination

    c. Positioning and holding

    d. Safety

    e. Hygiene: bathing, cord care, skin care, and genital care

15. Maintaining a patent airway and supporting respirations to ensure an adequate oxygen supply in the newborn are essential focuses of nursing care management of the newborn, especially in the early postbirth period.

    a. State the four conditions that are essential for maintaining an adequate oxygen supply in the newborn.

    b. List four signs that the nurse who is assessing a newborn would recognise as indicative of abnormal breathing.

16. A newborn estimated to be 40 weeks gestation following an assessment using the New Ballard scale. Which of the following would be a Ballard scale finding consistent with this newborn's full-term status? (Select all that apply.)
    a. Apical pulse rate of 120 beats per minute, regular, and strong
    b. Popliteal angle of 160 degrees
    c. Weight of 3200 g, placing him at the 50th percentile
    d. Thinning of lanugo with some bald areas
    e. Testes descended into the scrotum
    f. Elbow does not pass midline when arm is pulled across the chest

17. A newborn has been designated as large for gestational age. The birth mother was diagnosed with gestational diabetes late in pregnancy. The nurse should be alert for signs of hypoglycemia in the infant. Which of the following assessment findings would be consistent with a diagnosis of hypoglycemia?
    a. Hyperthermia
    b. Jitteriness
    c. Loose, watery stools
    d. Laryngospasm

18. A newborn male has been scheduled for a circumcision using a Gomco device. Essential nursing care measures following this surgical procedure would include which one of the following?
    a. Administer oral acetaminophen every 6 hours for a maximum of 4 doses in 24 hours.

b. Apply petrolatum to the site with every diaper change.
c. Check the penis for bleeding every 15 minutes for the first 4 hours.
d. Teach parents to remove the yellowish exudate that forms over the glans using a diaper wipe.

19. The doctor has prescribed a hepatitis B vaccination for a newborn prior to discharge. In fulfilling this order, the nurse should do which of the following? (Select all that apply.)
a. Confirm that the mother is hepatitis B positive before the injection is given.
b. Obtain parental consent prior to administering the vaccination.
c. Inform the parents that the next vaccine in the series would need to be given in 1 to 2 months.
d. Administer the injection into the vastus lateralis muscle.

III. THINKING CRITICALLY

1. Apgar scoring is a method of newborn assessment used in the immediate postbirth period, at 1 and 5 minutes. Indicate the Apgar score for each of the following newborns.

   a. Baby Nunez at 1 minute after birth:
   Heart rate—160 beats/min
   Respiratory effort—good, crying vigorously
   Muscle tone—active movement, well flexed
   Reflex irritability—cries with stimulus to soles of feet
   Colour—body pink, feet and hands cyanotic
      Score:
      Interpretation:

   b. Baby Yoo at 5 minutes after birth:
   Heart rate—102 beats/min
   Respiratory effort—slow, irregular with weak cry
   Muscle tone—some flexion of extremities
   Reflex irritability—grimace with stimulus to soles of feet
   Colour—pale
      Score:
      Interpretation:

2. Baby Bogdan is 24 hours old. The nurse is preparing to perform a physical examination of this newborn before his discharge.

   a. List the actions the nurse should take in order to ensure safety and accuracy. Include the rationale for the actions identified.

   b. Identify the major points that should be assessed as part of this physical examination.

   c. Support the premise that Bogdan's parents should be present during this examination.

3. Ivan and James are taking their newly circumcised (6 hours postprocedure) baby home. This is their first baby and they express anxiety concerning care of both the circumcision and the umbilical cord.

   a. State one nursing diagnosis related to this situation.

   b. State one expected outcome related to the nursing diagnosis identified.

   c. Specify the instructions that the nurse should give to Ivan and James regarding assessment of both sites and the care measures required to facilitate healing.

4. Andrew and Marion are parents of a newborn, 30 hours old, who has developed hyperbilirubinemia. They are very concerned about the colour of their baby and the need to put the baby under special lights. "A relative was yellow just like our baby and later died of liver cancer!"

   a. Describe how the nurse should respond to Andrew and Marion's concern.

   b. Identify the expected assessment findings and physiologic effects related to hyperbilirubinemia.

   c. List the precautions and care measures required by the newborn undergoing phototherapy in order to prevent injury to the newborn yet maintain the effectiveness of the treatment. State the rationale for each action identified.

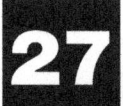 **Newborn Nutrition and Feeding**

I. LEARNING KEY TERMS

FILL IN THE BLANKS: Insert the term that corresponds to the following descriptions of breast structures and the breastfeeding process.

1. _____ Structures in the breast that are composed of alveoli, milk ducts, and myoepithelial cells.

2. _____ Milk-producing cells.

3. _____ Breast structure that transports milk from the alveoli to the nipple.

4. _____ Reflex that occurs when the infant cries, suckles, or rubs against the breast; facilitates effective latch. _____

_____ Nipple type that remains flat and soft and does not protrude even when stimulated.

5. _____ Cells surrounding alveoli; these cells contract in response to oxytocin, resulting in the milk ejection reflex or letdown.

6. _____ Rounded, pigmented section of tissue surrounding the nipple.

7. _____ The process of milk production.

8. _____ The lactogenic hormone secreted by the anterior pituitary gland in response to the infant's suck and emptying of the breast.

9. _____ Posterior pituitary hormone that triggers the let-down reflex.

10. _____ Reflex that aids in the propulsion of milk through the ducts to the nipple pores.

11. _____ Plastic device that can be placed over the nipple and areola to keep clothing off the nipple and put pressure around the base of the nipple to encourage nipple eversion.

12. _____ Herbal or pharmaceutical agent reported to increase breast milk production.

13. _____ Very concentrated, clear yellow fluid that is rich in protein and antibodies; it is present in the breasts before the formation of milk.

14. _____ The ideal food for human infants.

15. _____ Newborn behaviours that indicate hunger and a desire to eat such as hand-to-mouth movements, rooting, and sucking motions.

16. _____ or

_____ Reflex triggered by the contraction of myoepithelial cells. Colostrum, and later milk, is ejected toward the nipple.

17. _____ Reflex stimulated when a hungry baby's upper lip is touched which stimulates the mouth to open.

18. _____ Placing the baby onto the breast with the mouth open wide and the tongue down. The nipple and some of the areola should be in the baby's mouth, making a seal between the mouth and the breast to create adequate suction for milk removal.

19. _____ Breast response that occurs around the third to fifth day, when the "milk comes in" and blood supply to the breasts increases. The breasts become tender, swollen, hot and hard, and even shiny and red.

20. _____ Breastfeeding position in which the mother holds the baby's head and shoulders in her hand with the baby's back and body tucked under her arm.

21. _____ Breastfeeding position in which the baby is positioned across the lap.

153

22. _____ Certified health care provider with specialised training and experience to support breastfeeding families.

23. _____ Inflammation of the breast manifested by a swollen, erythematous, tender breast and sudden onset of flulike symptoms.

24. _____ Short frenulum, which interferes with tongue extrusion and effective sucking.

25. _____ Transition period from exclusive breastfeeding while incorporating other foods into infant's daily intake.

26. _____ Jaundice (hyperbilirubinemia) that occurs in breastfeeding infants as a result of insufficient feeding and infrequent stooling.

27. _____ Jaundice (hyperbilirubinemia) that occurs in breastfed newborns between 5 and 10 days of age; they are typically thriving, gaining weight, and stooling normally

II. REVIEWING KEY CONCEPTS

1. Consider the sociocultural values that may influence breastfeeding initiation and continuation amongst a multiethnic community. Outline strategies to support members of the LGBTQ2 community who want to breastfeed their infant.

2. Proper latch (latch-on) is essential for effective breastfeeding and preservation of nipple and areolar tissue integrity.

   a. Indicate the steps the nurse should teach a breastfeeding woman to follow to ensure a proper latch-on.

   b. When observing a woman breastfeeding, it is essential that the nurse determine the effectiveness of the latch-on. State the signs a nurse should look for that would indicate a proper latch-on.

   c. Describe the way a woman should remove her baby from her breast after feeding is completed.

3. During a home visit, the mother of a 1-week-old infant tells the nurse that she is very concerned about whether her baby is getting enough breast milk. The nurse would tell this mother that at 1 week of age a well-nourished newborn should exhibit which of the following?
   a. Weight gain sufficient to return to birthweight
   b. Passing meconium stools twice daily
   c. Frequent [>4] wet diapers each day with clear pale yellow urine
   d. Breastfeeding at a frequency of every 4 hours or about 6 times each day

4. The nurse teaches breastfeeding mothers about breast care measures to preserve the integrity of the nipples and areola. Which of the following should the nurse include in these instructions?
   a. Cleanse nipples and areola twice a day with mild soap and water.
   b. Apply vitamin E cream to nipples and areola at least four times each day before a feeding.
   c. Insert plastic-lined pads into the bra to absorb leakage and protect clothing.
   d. Place a breast shell into the bra if nipples are sore.

5. A breastfeeding woman asks the nurse about what birth control she should use during the postpartum period. Which is the best recommendation for a safe, yet effective method during the first 6 weeks after birth?
   a. Combination oral contraceptive that she used before she was pregnant
   b. Barrier method using a combination of a condom and spermicide foam
   c. Use injectable progesterone
   d. Exclusive breastfeeding—baby only receives breast milk for nourishment

6. A woman has determined that formula-feeding is the best feeding method for her baby. Instructions the woman should receive regarding this feeding method includes which of the following?
   a. Provide the infant with supplemental vitamins along with the iron-fortified formula.
   b. Sterilise water by boiling, then cool and mix with formula powder or concentrate.
   c. Expect a 2-week-old newborn to drink approximately 30 mL of formula at each feeding.
   d. Microwave refrigerated formula for about 2 minutes before feeding the newborn.

7. A nurse is evaluating a woman's breastfeeding technique. Which of the following actions would indicate that the woman needs further instruction regarding breastfeeding to ensure success? (Select all that apply.)
   a. Washes her breasts and nipples thoroughly with soap and water twice a day
   b. Massages a small amount of breast milk into her nipple and areola before and after each feeding
   c. Lines her bra with a thick plastic-lined pad to absorb leakage
   d. Positions baby supporting back and shoulders securely and then brings her breast toward the baby, putting the nipple in the baby's mouth
   e. Feeds her baby every 2 to 3 hours
   f. Inserts her finger into the corner of her baby's mouth between the gums before removing her baby from the breast

III. THINKING CRITICALLY

1. Shonda, as a first-time breastfeeding mother, has many questions. Describe how you would respond to the following questions and comments.

   a. "I am so afraid that I will not make enough milk for my baby. My breasts are not as large as some of my friends who breastfeed."

   b. "Everyone keeps talking about this let-down that is supposed to happen. What is it and how will I know I have it?"

   c. "How can I possibly know if breastfeeding is going well and my baby is getting enough if I cannot tell how many ounces they get with each feeding?"

   d. "It is only the first day that I am breastfeeding and my nipples already feel sore. What can I do to relieve this soreness and prevent it from getting worse?"

   e. "My friends all told me to watch out for the fourth day and engorgement. What can I do to keep it from being too bad and to take care of myself when it occurs?"

   f. "Every time I breastfeed, I get cramps and my flow seems to get heavier. Is there something wrong with me?"

   g. "I am so glad I do not have to worry about getting pregnant again as long as I am breastfeeding. I hate using birth control and my friend told me I do not have to as long as I am breastfeeding."

   h. "I would like to keep breastfeeding my baby for at least 6 months but I need to return to work in 6 weeks. What should I do when I am ready to stop breastfeeding my baby?"

2. Simone is 2 days old and last fed 5 hours ago. Her mother tells the nurse that Simone is so sleepy that she just does not have the heart to wake her.

   a. Identify one nursing diagnosis and one expected outcome appropriate for this newborn.

   b. Discuss the approach the nurse should take with regard to this situation.

3. Prior to discharge, a nurse is evaluating a woman's ability to breastfeed and her newborn's response to breastfeeding.

   a. Identify the factors that the nurse should assess before and during breastfeeding to ensure that this mother and newborn are ready to breastfeed at home.

   b. After determining that breastfeeding is progressing well, the woman is discharged. One week later the nurse calls the woman to discuss breastfeeding. Write several questions this nurse should ask to determine whether breastfeeding is continuing to progress normally.

28 Infants with Gestational Age-Related Conditions

I. LEARNING KEY TERMS

MATCHING: Match each term with its definition.

1. Oxygenation assessment of sick neonates includes _____ and _____

2. _____ has a strong analgesic effect during painful procedures.

3. _____ Infant whose birthweight is <2 500 g, regardless of gestational age.

4. _____ Infant whose birthweight is <1 500 g.

5. _____ Infant whose birthweight is <1 000 g.

6. _____ Infant born before completion of 37 weeks of gestation.

7. _____ Infants born between 34 0/7 and 36 6/7 weeks of gestation.

8. _____ Infant born between 39 0/7 weeks and 40 6/7 weeks of gestation.

9. _____ Infant whose birthweight falls above the 90th percentile as a result of growing at an accelerated rate during foetal life.

10. _____ Infant whose birthweight falls below the 10th percentile as a result of growing at a restricted rate during foetal life.

11. _____ inhibits surfactant function.

12. _____ Cessation of respirations of 20 seconds or more.

13. _____ Phospholipid protein that reduces alveolar surface tension and prevents alveolar collapse.

14. _____ The environmental temperature at which oxygen consumption and metabolic rate are minimal but adequate to maintain the body temperature.

15. _____ Death that occurs in the first 27 days of life; it is described as early if it occurs in the first week of life and late if it occurs at 7 to 27 days.

16. _____ Method incorporates skin-to-skin contact with the newborn that can reduce stress in the infant.

17. _____ Growth restriction in which the weight, length, and head circumference are all affected.

18. _____ is a structure in the foetus connecting the pulmonary artery to the aorta

19. _____ Common condition that occurs in infants of diabetic mothers (IDM) within minutes to hours after birth; signs and symptoms are variable and infant may be asymptomatic or may have tremors, poor feeding, or respiratory distress.

a. Late preterm infant

b. Kangaroo care

c. Surfactant

d. continuous pulse oximetry

e. Neutral thermal environment

f. Neonatal death

g. Apnea

h. blood gas analysis

i. Premature or preterm infant

j. Large for gestational age

k. Small for gestational age

l. Full-term infant

m. Skin-to-skin care

n. Meconium

o. Low birthweight (LBW)

p. Very low birthweight (VLBW)

q. Extremely low birthweight (ELBW)

r. Symmetric intrauterine growth restriction

s. Ductus arteriosus

t. Hypoglycemia

FILL IN THE BLANKS: Insert the term that corresponds to each of the following descriptions.

20. _____ remains the leading cause of neonatal deaths in Canada.

21. Determining who makes decisions related to the resuscitation of extremely-low-birth-weight infants is an example of an _____ in the care of ELBW infants.

22. Oxygen therapy may prevent _____ accumulation that results from hypoxia.

23. _____ provides positive pressure during both inspiratory and expiratory phases of a neonate's spontaneous breath.

24. _____ may be required for infants who exhibit severe hypoxemia or severe hypercapnia on blood gas analysis.

25. Extremely low birth weight infants may be placed in a _____ at birth to decrease heat and water loss.

26. The duration in hours that specific postnatal neuroprotective practises are recommended immediately after birth for LBW and ELBW infants is _____.

27. Coordination of sucking and swallowing mechanisms occurs at approximately _____ weeks of gestation.

28. Early introduction of small amounts of breast milk enteral feeds will stimulate the infant's gastrointestinal tract and prevent _____.

29. _____ feeding involves the surgical placement of a tube through the skin of the abdomen into the stomach.

30. _____ to help promote regular sleep for preterm infants in isolettes can be facilitated by covering the isolette with a blanket.

31. _____ Common type of neurological injury in preterm and term infants.

32. _____ A colourless gas administered through the ventilator circuit that promotes pulmonary vasodilation and improves oxygenation in neonates who experience persistent pulmonary hypertension.

33. _____ Acute inflammatory disease of the bowel that occurs with increased incidence in preterm infants.

34. _____ is a method of providing breast milk or formula through a nasogastric or orogastric tube.

35. _____ Lung disorder usually affecting preterm neonates and is caused by surfactant deficiency.

36. _____ Combined findings of pulmonary hypertension, right-to-left shunting, and a structurally normal heart; it is also called *persistent foetal circulation* because the syndrome includes reversion to foetal pathways for blood flow.

II. REVIEWING KEY CONCEPTS

1. Explain why maternal transfer prior to the delivery of a high-risk infant is preferred and describe what mechanisms need to be implemented for the critically ill newborn if maternal transfer is not possible.

2. Explain the relationship between neonatal hypoglycemia and intrauterine hyperinsulinism in the infant of a diabetic mother (IDM).

3. The preterm infant is vulnerable to a number of complications related to immaturity of body systems. Identify the potential problems and their physiologic basis for each of the areas listed:

Respiratory function

Thermoregulation

Nutritional status

Renal function

Haematological status

Immune status and infection prevention

4. Preterm infants are at increased risk for developing respiratory distress. The nurse regularly assesses for signs that would indicate that the newborn is having difficulty breathing. Which of the following are signs of respiratory distress? (Select all that apply.)
a. Use of abdominal muscles to breathe
b. Tachypnea
c. Periodic breathing pattern
d. Suprasternal retraction
e. Nasal flaring
f. Acrocyanosis

5. When caring for a preterm infant born at 30 weeks of gestation. the nurse should recognise which of the following as the newborn's primary nursing diagnosis?
a. Risk for infection related to decreased immune response
b. Ineffective breathing pattern related to surfactant deficiency and weak respiratory muscle effort
c. Ineffective thermoregulation related to immature thermoregulation centre
d. Imbalanced nutrition: less than body requirements related to ineffective suck and swallow

6. The nurse is caring for a newborn whose birth mother had gestational diabetes. The estimated gestational age is 41 weeks, and the birthweight is 4800 g. When assessing this newborn, the nurse should be alert for which of the following?
a. Fracture of the femur
b. Hypercalcemia
c. Blood glucose level less than 2.6mmol/L
d. Signs of a congenital heart defect

III. THINKING CRITICALLY

1. Navneet, a preterm newborn who weighs 1800g at 34 weeks of gestation, is admitted to the neonatal intensive care unit (NICU) after birth for observation and supportive care. Navneet's nutritional needs are an important aspect in overall care. Oral feedings are being considered.

a. State the assessment data that the nurse should document after each of Navneet's feedings to indicate feeding method effectiveness.

b. The nurse determines that Navneet's suck is weak and becomes too fatigued during oral feedings to obtain sufficient nutrients and fluid. The nurse consults with the practitioner and a decision is made to provide intermittent gavage feedings with occasional oral feedings. Describe the guidelines the nurse should follow when inserting the gavage tube.

c. State the priority nursing diagnosis for Navneet.

d. Discuss the principles the nurse should follow before, during, and after a gavage feeding to ensure safety and maximum effectiveness.

e. List the complications that may ensue with indwelling naso/oro gastric feeding tubes.

2. The nurse is preparing to insert a gavage tube and feed a preterm newborn. As part of the protocol for this procedure, the nurse should consider the determination of optimal feeding tube placement. Describe current evidence-informed guidelines for ensuring safety of feeding tube placement in infants.

3. The NICU is a stressful environment for preterm infants and their families.
   a. Identify the common sources of stress facing infants in an intensive care environment.

   b. Identify specific measures that can be used to protect infants from overstimulation and yet provide appropriate stimulation to meet the developmental and emotional needs of infants.

4. Nishiime is beginning their 43rd week of pregnancy.

   a. Support this statement: Perinatal mortality is significantly higher in the postterm neonate.

   b. State the assessment findings that are typical of a postterm infant.

   c. Discuss the two major complications that can be experienced by a postterm infant.

5. A medically stable 26 week gestation neonate is receiving intravenous total parenteral nutrition. Minimal enteral (trophic) feedings with maternal breast milk are being considered. Describe the concept of these trophic feedings in preterm infants and the reported advantages and disadvantages.

6. Anita and Juan are the parents of a 2-day-old preterm newborn. Their baby, who is 27 weeks' gestation and weighs 1 kg, is in the NICU and will be in the hospital for several weeks. The nurse caring for this baby recognises that they must also provide supportive care for Anita and Juan.

   a. Outline strategies to support Anita and Juan during their first encounter with their baby in NICU.

   b. Outline mechanisms that may enable a father-friendly culture within the NICU.

160

29 The Newborn at Risk: Acquired and Congenital Conditions

I. LEARNING KEY TERMS

MATCHING: Match each term with its definition.

1. _____ Birth injury in which the upper brachial nerve plexus is damaged as the head and neck are delivered at birth with additional traction applied.

2. _____ Birth injury in which the lower brachial plexus is injured during the birthing process resulting in wrist drop and relaxed fingers on the affected side.

3. _____ Form of brain injury stemming from perinatal complications.

4. _____ Leading infectious cause of hearing loss in infants and children.

5. _____ Important source of neonatal morbidity.

6. _____ Term used to describe the fibrinous material that holds newborn skull bones together.

7. _____ Ping-pong ball indentation on neonate's head noted shortly after birth.

8. _____ Abnormal neurological finding that occurs in VLBW infants in the neonatal period.

9. _____ Common cause of fractured clavicle.

10. _____ A type of sentinel event that may lead to moderate or severe hypoxic ischemic encephalopathy in the neonate.

11. _____ Type of maternal immunoglobulin that does not cross the placenta to protect the foetus.

12. _____ The presence of microorganisms or their toxins in the bloodstream.

13. _____ Predisposing factors of prolonged courses of antibiotics and altered skin integrity may contribute to the development of this form of invasive infection in the preterm infant.

14. _____ Indicated by maternal fever or foul-smelling amniotic fluid.

15. _____ A sequelae of septicemia.

16. _____ Death that occurs in the first 27 days of life; it is described as early if it occurs in the first week of life and late if it occurs at 7 to 27 days.

17. _____ Comprised of live microorganisms that may positively influence the gut flora.

a. Hypoxic ischemic encephalopathy

b. Birth trauma

c. Cytomegalovirus (CMV)

d. Early-onset sepsis-

e. Depressed skull fracture

f. Neonatal death

g. Shoulder dystocia

h. Sepsis

i. Sutures

j. Erb's palsy

k. Klumpke palsy

l. Intracranial haemorrhage

m. Uterine rupture

n. IgM

o. Fungal

p. Chorioamnionitis

q. Phototherapy

r. Hyperbilirubinemia

s. Disseminated intravascular coagulation (DIC)

t. Probiotics

18. _____ Presence of a bacterial infection in the newborn with symptoms usually manifesting within 72 hours of birth; infection is acquired in the perinatal period.

19. _____ Noninvasive method used to treat increased levels of circulating bilirubin in newborn infant.

20. _____ May occur as a result of haemolytic disease of the newborn (HDN).

FILL IN THE BLANKS: Insert the term that corresponds to each of the following descriptions.

21. _____ Acronym used to designate certain maternal infections during early pregnancy that are known to be associated with various congenital malformations or negative long-term sequelae.

22. _____ Neonatal infection typically acquired from the pregnant woman experiencing a primary genital infection.

23. The single most effective measure to reduce healthcare-associated infections in high-risk infants is

_____.

24. _____ Constellation of effects caused by foetal exposure to alcohol that include growth restriction, dysmorphic facial features, and cognitive/behavioural problems in children; may present as generalised irritability and poor feeding in the newborn period.

25. _____ Destruction of red blood cells that leads to anaemia; may cause elevated bilirubin levels.

26. _____ Condition in which the foetus produces large numbers of immature red blood cells in response to progressive haemolysis. The most severe form of this condition is called

_____ and is characterised by foetal hypoxia, cardiac decompensation, generalised oedema and fluid effusions in pericardial, pleural or peritoneal spaces.

27. Hemolytic disease can occur when the foetal blood group is type A or B and the pregnant woman's blood type is O blood group which is referred to as

_____.

28. _____ The term used to describe the set of behaviours exhibited by infants exposed to opioids or other substances in utero.

29. _____ Type of specimen collected from the newborn to screen for possible substance exposure in the last trimester of pregnancy.

30. _____ A group of disorders caused by a metabolic defect that results from the absence or deficiency of a substance essential to cellular metabolism, usually an enzyme; most commonly characterised by abnormal protein, carbohydrate or fat metabolism.

31. _____ In this disorder the infant is placed on a low phenylalanine diet and this diet is maintained throughout life to prevent severe cognitive impairment.

32. _____ Disorder in which the affected infant does not properly convert galactose into glucose resulting in hepatic dysfunction and jaundice developing in the newborn period. *E. coli* sepsis many be a presenting clinical sign.

33. _____ Treatment of this disorder involves the lifelong administration of thyroxine commencing upon confirmation of diagnosis to prevent severe cognitive developmental delay

34. Smoking and passive exposure to second-hand smoke during pregnancy increases the risk for

_____ weight and _____ birth.

35. _____ Main psychoactive component in cannabis that crosses the placenta and may contribute to increased risk of growth restriction and preterm birth.

36. _____ Use of this substance during pregnancy can cause maternal increased blood pressure, decreased uterine blood flow and increased vascular resistance leading to reduced blood flow and oxygenation to the foetus.

162

37. _____ Type of counselling that provides information about risk of occurrence of a genetic disorder within a family.

38. _____ The bone most often fractured at birth,

39. _____ Nerve injury occurring at birth in which the diaphragm does not expand adequately, often resulting in respiratory distress.

40. _____ Cooling of the infant's head or entire body to reduce severity of neurologic injury in hypoxic ischemic encephalopathy.

II. REVIEWING KEY CONCEPTS

1. The clinical manifestations of perinatal drug exposure may occur in any one or all of the following categories: CNS, gastrointestinal, and respiratory. List some common signs that nurses can observe in each category:

    Central nervous system

    Gastrointestinal

    Respiratory

    Outline non-pharmacological strategies that nurses can employ or encourage families to implement in caring for an infant experiencing Neonatal Abstinence Syndrome.

2. Explain the impact of ABO incompatibility and Rh isoimmunisation on the foetal red blood cell.

3. The nursing care management of a newborn whose biological mother is HIV positive would most likely include which of the following? (Select all that apply.)
    a. Isolating the newborn in a special nursery
    b. Implementing routine precautions immediately after birth
    c. Counselling family to provide formula feeds and avoid breastfeeding
    d. Initiating neonatal antiretroviral prophylaxis treatment within 72 hours

III. THINKING CRITICALLY

1. Clara and Miguel are parents of baby Luca, born at term gestation and who has developed severe unconjugated hyperbilirubinemia within the first 24 hours of life. Serum bilirubin levels have continued to increase, despite administration of intensive phototherapy and immunoglobulin therapy, and an exchange transfusion is required. Describe the nursing measures necessary to care for Luca throughout the procedure.

2. Baby Winnie was delivered vaginally, birthweight 4.2kg, after a difficult and prolonged labour. As the RN caring for Winnie, you note that they do not completely close their left eye. Describe the other aspects of your physical assessment that you would particularly monitor, and outline the principle nursing measures that may be required when caring for a newborn who has experienced a facial nerve palsy.

Pediatric Nursing

30 Pediatric Nursing in Canada

I. LEARNING KEY TERMS

MATCHING: Match each term with its corresponding definition.

1. _____ Actions by the nurse that include acknowledging parents' presence, listening, involving parents and child in care, showing interest and concern for parents' and the child's welfare.

2. _____ Interaction with patients in which boundaries are blurred and the nurse's personal needs may be served rather than the patient's.

3. _____ Refers to behavioural, social, and educational problems that can significantly alter a child's health.

4. _____ Deemed as one of the most important public health intervention provided to Canadians.

5. _____ Therapeutic care that minimises the psychological and physical distress experienced by children and their families in the health care system.

6. _____ The philosophy that recognises the family as the constant in a child's life.

7. _____ Meaningful interaction with caring, well-defined boundaries separating the nurse from the patient.

8. _____ An interaction of professionals with families that assists families to maintain or acquire a sense of control over their family lives and acknowledge positive changes through the fostering of their own strengths, abilities, and actions.

9. _____ A 5-step model of problem identification and problem solving that describes what the nurse actually does.

10. _____ An imbalance between demands on a person and the ability of a person to cope with those demands; disrupts the equilibrium of the person.

11. _____ Process of enabling people to increase control over and optimise the health of children and their families.

12. _____ Leading cause of death and disability in children, the majority of which are preventable.

13. _____ Accounts for the majority of all acute conditions.

14. _____ Involves ensuring that families are aware of all available health services, adequately informed of treatments and procedures, involved in the child's care, and encouraged to change or support existing health care practises.

15. _____ Symptoms severe enough to limit activity or require medical attention.

a. Morbidity
b. Vaccination
c. Family-centred care
d. Stress
e. Personable care
f. Atraumatic care
g. Nursing process
h. Therapeutic relationship
i. Nontherapeutic relationships
j. Health promotion
k. Empowerment
l. Advocacy
m. Injuries
n. Respiratory illness
o. Acute illness

II. REVIEWING KEY CONCEPTS

1. Risk factors impacting infant mortality in Canada include the following except:
   a. inadequate housing
   b. global warming
   c. food insecurity
   d. lack of access to health care

2. The decline in congenital anomalies present at birth for Canadian infants can be attributed to:
   a. increased prenatal diagnosis and pregnancy termination
   b. changes in maternal health behaviours (e.g., smoking cessation)
   c. reduced prematurity
   d. a and b only
   e. all of the above

3. LGBTQ2 children may experience:
   a. low self-rated mental health.
   b. internalised stress.
   c. higher potential for death by suicide.
   d. all of the above.

4. Antimicrobial stewardship includes the following except:
   a. testing to diagnose viral or bacterial etiologies.
   b. maintaining a questioning attitude for possible specimen contamination.
   c. confirming pneumonia through sputum culture
   d. cautious use of antimicrobials to reduce adverse outcomes from antimicrobials.

5. List three communication barriers that nurses can eliminate in their practise to optimise a patient-nurse therapeutic relationship.

6. Adverse childhood events can:
   a. include parental separation or divorce.
   b. include parental addiction.
   c. contribute to the development of toxic stress in children.
   d. all of the above.

7. While providing discharge instructions to the child and/or family member, the nurse may suspect information overload when observing the following behaviours except:
   a. long periods of silence.
   b. maintaining notes on all instructions provided.
   c. sudden disruptions such as asking to go the washroom.
   d. attempting to change the topic of discussion.

8. T F Upon first introduction, the nurse should inquire about the preferred name a child may use and record it on the medical record.

9. T F Patient interviews may occur wherever information can be shared quickly and efficiently.

10. T F Assuring patients and families that confidentiality will be maintained at all times is a primary nursing value as outlined by the Canadian Nurses Association.

11. T F Incorporating a child's special toy or doll into an interview rarely helps to ease the child into the conversation and facilitate communication with the nurse.

12. T F Paediatric patients require a family member to be with them at all times during an interview to verify the accuracy of information.

13. T F Providing the opportunity to touch or inspect physical examination tools prior to using them during a health assessment will help to gain the cooperation of pre-school aged children.

167

14. T F A unified interdisciplinary team approach facilitates holistic care for paediatric patients.

15. T F Nurses engaged in community organisations may influence government legislation.

III. THINKING CRITICALLY

1. Four-year-old Usman has been recently diagnosed with Type I Diabetes Mellitus. Usman lives with two other siblings and a single parent who has two part-time jobs. Please outline how family low-income may influence Usman's diabetes management.

2. Indigenous adolescents experience death by suicide at greater rates than non-Indigenous youth. While conducting a health assessment of 15-year-old Adlartok, what cultural factors should the nurse explore to help determine potential risk for a break in mental health?

31 Family, Social, and Cultural Influences on Children's Health

I. LEARNING KEY TERMS

MATCHING: Match each term with its corresponding definition.

1. _____ Prompts the nurse to understand what life is like for the child and family and assess their own history and contextual factors that have shaped their own life.

2. _____ Legal term recognising anyone who has decision-making authority over a child and assumes all the rights, duties, obligations, and responsibilities of the child.

3. _____ The pattern of assumptions, beliefs, and practises encompassing other products of human work and thoughts specific to members of an intergenerational group, community, or population.

4. _____ Common approach to understand and assess families as a whole, and the individuals that make up the whole.

5. _____ Family situation in which each parent is awarded custody of one or more of the children, thereby separating siblings.

6. _____ Family situation in which the children do not reside with both parents, but both parents share parenting responsibilities.

7. _____ What an individual considers it to be; an institution where individuals, related through biology or enduring commitments, and representing similar or different generations and genders, participate in roles involving mutual socialisation, nurturance, and emotional commitment.

8. _____ Made up of family, school, neighbourhood, youth organisations, and other members; may be source of opportunity and growth and support positive child and adolescent development.

9. _____ Seen widely in North America as a result of a biological cause; scientific methods and processes implemented to diagnose and address health issues

10. _____ The placement of a child in a stable and approved environment with a nonrelated family.

11. _____ Relates to a family's economic and education levels; may have a pronounced adverse influence on health

12. _____ A legal relationship between a child and parent who are not related by birth

a. Family

b. Family systems theory

c. Culture

d. Cultural humility

e. Parent

f. Divided, or split, custody

g. Joint custody

h. Adoption

i. Foster care

j. Socioeconomic status

k. Community

l. Illness

II. REVIEWING KEY CONCEPTS

1. The nurse provides individualised support that builds on family strengths that are evidenced by which of the following qualities:
   a. A balanced access of internal and external family resources to aid in coping with life events and planning for the future.
   b. A collection of coping strategies that promote positive functioning in dealing with life events.
   c. An ability to communicate with one another in a way that emphasises positive interactions.
   d. All of the above

2. Factors that affect parenting practises of infants and young children include
   a. the birth order of children.
   b. access to play-groups and daycare facilities.
   c. parental personality and mental well-being.
   d. all of the above

3. Government and adoption agency eligibility requirements to adopt in Canada include:
   a. Canadian citizenship
   b. lack of criminal record
   c. over 21 years of age
   d. a and b only
   e. All of the above.

4. When establishing a family that incorporates adoption, parents will engage in purposeful actions for which of the following?
   a. The initial attachment process.
   b. Disclosure of adoption to the child.
   c. Understanding the influence of adoption on identity formation during adolescence.
   d. Consistent limit-setting and discipline with all children in the family.
   e. all of the above

5. Which of the following is not an important consideration for parents when telling their children about the decision to divorce?
   a. Initial disclosure should include both parents and siblings.
   b. Time should be allowed for discussion with each child individually.
   c. Initial disclosure should be kept simple and reasons for divorce should not be included.
   d. Disclosure may include the expression of authentic parental sadness.

6. When considering the impact of culture on the paediatric patient, the nurse recognises that culture:
   a. is synonymous with race.
   b. affects the development of health beliefs.
   c. refers to a group of people with similar physical characteristics.
   d. refers to the universal manner and sequence of growth and development.

7. Cultural beliefs and practises are an important part of nursing assessment because, when analysed and incorporated into the nursing process, these beliefs:
   a. often assist in the plan of care.
   b. can be manipulated more easily if known.
   c. must be in unison with standard health practices.
   d. are very similar from one culture to another.

8. The health of Indigenous children under 16 years of health differs from other Canadian children because:
   a. infant mortality rates are lower in the Indigenous population.
   b. infectious diseases contribute significantly to morbidities for Indigenous children.
   c. injuries occur less frequently for Indigenous children.
   d. immunisation rates are higher among Indigenous children.

9. Cultural beliefs may attribute the cause of illness to:
   a. natural forces.
   b. supernatural forces.
   c. an imbalance between natural and supernatural forces.
   d. all of the above.

10. T F It is recommended that children be told they are adopted before entering school.

11. T F Research has shown that children of divorce suffer no lasting psychological or social difficulties.

12. T F The most common natural forces blamed for ill health are cold air entering the body and impurities in the air.

13. T F The 'evil eye' is recognised as a supernatural force that contributes to illness.

14. T F A neutral state of emotion can create weakness, and lead to a state of imbalance and illness.

15. T F Health equilibrium can be explained by applying the concept of hot and cold imbalances.

16. T F Home remedies for treatment of illness exist in some form in all cultures.

170

III. THINKING CRITICALLY

1. Twenty-six-year-old Noemi, a newcomer to Canada, has brought her three children Liseth, a 3-month-old infant, to the ambulatory clinic for a well-baby check-up along with Liseth's siblings who are 18-months and 3 years of age. One of your goals is to promote continuation of the immunisation schedule. List questions you would ask to determine whether there are social and cultural influences that affect Noemi's intent to have her children immunised.

32 Developmental Influences on Child Health Promotion

I. LEARNING KEY TERMS

MATCHING: Match each term with its corresponding definition.

1. _____ Processes by which early cells and structures are systematically modified and altered to achieve specific and characteristic physical and chemical properties.

2. _____ Rate of metabolism when the body is at rest.

3. _____ An increase in competence and adaptability; a change in the complexity of a structure; to function at a higher level.

4. _____ Cognitive component of how a person describes themselves; includes the beliefs and convictions that make up an individual's self-knowledge.

5. _____ A gradual change and expansion; advancement from lower to more advanced stages of complexity.

6. _____ Process by which developing individuals become acquainted with the world; ability to reason abstractly, think in a logical manner, organise intellectual functions into higher-order structures.

7. _____ A set of skills and competencies peculiar to each stage that children accomplish to deal effectively with their environment.

8. _____ Pattern of growth and development; near-to-far or midline-to-peripheral.

9. _____ An increase in the number and size of cells as they divide and synthesise new proteins; results in an increased size and weight.

10. _____ Subjective concepts and attitudes that individuals have toward their own body; evolves and changes during the process of growth and development.

11. _____ Regularity in timing of physiological functions such as hunger, sleep, and elimination.

12. _____ Pattern of growth and development; head-to-tail.

13. _____ Type of behaviour on social media or other internet sites that negatively impacts other users and leads to their potential experience of worry, sadness, depression, anxiety.

14. _____ Manner of thinking, behaving, or reacting; traits that stay relatively constant over time.

15. _____ Particular time during which an organism will interact with a particular environment in a specific manner.

a. Maturation

b. Developmental task

c. Cephalo-caudal

d. Growth

e. Proximodistal

f. BMR; basal metabolic rate

g. Temperament

h. Self-concept

i. Cyberbully

j. Development

k. Cognition

l. Sensitive period

m. Differentiation

n. Body image

o. Rhythmicity

172

II. REVIEWING KEY CONCEPTS

1. Categorising growth and behaviour into approximate age stages:
   a. helps to account for individual differences in children.
   b. can be applied to all children with some degree of precision.
   c. provides a convenient means to describe the majority of children.
   d. determines the speed of each child's growth.

2. Growth in children with Down syndrome differs from that in other children as noted in their
   a. shorter stature achievement after their pubertal growth spurt
   b. lower weight in infancy
   c. greater head circumference in childhood
   d. none of the above.

3. The average newborn will
   a. gain approximately 2-3 kg per year after the first year until the adolescent growth spurt
   b. triple their birthweight by 6 months
   c. double their birthweight by 4 to 7 months
   d. continue to grow in length/height at a consistent rate until adulthood.

4. Bone formation begins in utero when
   a. placental transfer of maternal calcium intake is optimised through maternal multivitamin supplements.
   b. calcium salts are deposited in the intercellular substance to form calcified cartilage.
   c. blood circulation commences and increased oxygen delivery occurs.
   d. at 7 months when foetal erythropoiesis develops.

5. The foetal nervous system grows proportionately more rapidly than the postnatal nervous system as noted by
   a. the dramatic increase in neurons between 15 and 20 weeks gestation
   b. a surge in number of neurons at approximately 30 weeks
   c. the postnatal increase in intricacy of communications between cells
   d. all of the above

6. Lymphoid tissue follows a growth pattern unlike other body tissues because
   a. they reach adult dimensions by 4 years of age
   b. children are regularly responding to new organisms and infections and the lymph tissues respond to these antigens
   c. they regress in size prior to the onset of puberty
   d. there is a size discordance in children with Down syndrome throughout the lifespan

7. The basal metabolic rate reflects body temperature and
   a. will decrease during prolonged of illness
   b. fluid requirements when temperature is elevated
   c. will continue to increase until a child fully matures
   d. all of the above

8. Erickson's theory of personality development outlines that the development of *identity*
   a. occurs during the period of 6 to 12 years of age.
   b. is characterised by the latent period of physical growth.
   c. represents an internal struggle youth experience when they try to integrate their own concepts and values with those of society.
   d. all of the above.

9. Language development, including oral speaking skills, requires
   a. intelligence
   b. stimulation
   c. intact physiological structure and function
   d. all of the above

10. An infant will achieve mastery of performing tasks when
    a. care-givers readily provide assistance during tasks
    b. care-givers redirect the infant's focus on the task at hand
    c. kinesthetic stimulation is provided after an infant has developed head control
    d. care-givers express enjoyment in the infant's accomplishments.

11. Hypothermia in the healthy infant can lead to
    a. hypoglycaemia, reduced bilirubin levels, metabolic acidosis
    b. hyperglycaemia, elevated bilirubin levels, metabolic alkalosis
    c. hypoglycaemia, elevated bilirubin levels, metabolic acidosis
    d. hyperglycaemia, reduced bilirubin levels, metabolic alkalosis

12. T   F   The most accurate measure of general development is bone age.

13. T   F   The rate of metabolism is inversely proportionate to the child's caloric requirement.

14. T   F   Nutrition is the single most important influence on growth.

15. T   F   A child may develop behavioural problems if there is dissonance between the child's temperament and the environment

173

16. T F The epiphyseal cartilage plate is resistant to interference caused by trauma or infections.

17. T F Females maintain a temperature slightly above males throughout life.

18. T F *Canada's Food Guide* identifies water as the drink of choice and recommends a diet that includes plenty of protein and whole grain foods (half a dinner plate each).

19. T F Easy-going children can display a mild to moderate intense mood that is usually positive and are regular and predictable in their habits.

20. T F As children grow, interaction with age-mates increases in importance and contributes to the socialisation process.

MATCHING: Match each type of play with the corresponding example of that type of play.

21. _____ Colouring a picture alone with other children in the same area engaged in other activities.

22. _____ Acting out events of daily life; predominant form of play in preschool children.

23. _____ Not playful but focusing their attention momentarily on anything that strikes their interest; daydreaming.

24. _____ Playing peek-a-boo/patty-cake.

25. _____ Children watch what other children are doing but make no attempt to enter into the play activity.

26. _____ Children who engage in group activities or play formal games.

27. _____ Play demonstrated by repeating an action over and over again.

28. _____ The work of children.

29. _____ Children play together but there is no organisation.

30. _____ Characteristic play of toddlers, each child plays beside but not with the other child.

a. Play

b. Skill play

c. Unoccupied behaviour

d. Dramatic play

e. Imitative games

f. Onlooker play

g. Solitary play

h. Parallel play

i. Associative play

j. Cooperative play

III. THINKING CRITICALLY

1. Svetlana, a 10-year-old child, presents at the clinic for an annual health checkup. Past anthropometric data consistently showed height and weight at 50th percentile and Svetlana is generally considered healthy. Svetlana reports watching television for about 4 to 5 hours daily. Past family history includes heart disease. Svetlana's mother is concerned about Svetlana's increase in physical aggressiveness lately. Measurements today show Svetlana's height to be at the 50th percentile, and weight is at the 95th percentile. A random serum cholesterol level is elevated.

   1. Outline the factors in Svetlana's current history that need to be addressed.

   2. Describe at least three strategies Svetlana's family can use to deal with the child's aggressiveness.

   3. Describe achievable outcomes Svetlana could work toward.

33 Pediatric Health Assessment

I. LEARNING KEY TERMS

MATCHING: Match each term with its corresponding description.

1. _____ An essential parameter of nutritional status; the measurement of height, weight, head circumference, proportions, skinfold thickness, and arm circumference.

2. _____ The capacity to understand what another person is experiencing from within that person's frame of reference.

3. _____ Specific reason for the child's visit to the clinic or hospital.

4. _____ Refers to all those individuals who are considered by the patient to be significant to the nuclear unit.

5. _____ Specific review of each body system.

6. _____ Small, distinct, pinpoint haemorrhages 2 mm or less in size; can denote a type of blood disorder such as leukemia.

7. _____ Appears translucent, light pearly pink, or gray.

8. _____ Lateral curvature of the spine.

9. _____ Redness that may be a result of increased blood flow from climatic conditions, local inflammation, infection, skin irritation, allergy, or other dermatoses or may be caused by increased numbers of red blood cells as a compensatory response to chronic hypoxia.

10. _____ Response of the testes to stimulation by cold, touch, emotional excitement, or exercise.

11. _____ Yellow staining of the skin usually caused by bile pigments.

12. _____ Bowel sounds.

13. _____ The amount of elasticity in the skin; determined by grasping the skin on the abdomen or arm between the thumb and index finger, pulling it taut, and quickly releasing it.

14. _____ Large diffuse area that is usually black and blue; caused by haemorrhage of blood into skin; typically a result of injuries.

15. _____ Placing the hands against the skin to feel for muscle tone, tenderness, and superficial lesions.

16. _____ Paleness may be a sign of anaemia, chronic disease, edema, or shock.

17. _____ Using the stethoscope to evaluate breath sounds

a. Empathy

b. presenting health concern

c. Family

d. Review of systems

e. Anthropometry

f. Recumbent length

g. Stature

h. Skin turgor

i. Cyanosis

j. Pallor

k. Erythema

l. Ecchymosis

m. Petechiae

n. Jaundice

o. Tympanic membrane

p. Binocularity

q. Strabismus

r. Auscultation

s. Palpation

t. Peristalsis

u. Cremasteric reflex

v. Scoliosis

18. _____ A person's standing height.

19. _____ Occurs when one eye deviates from the point of fixation; sometimes called "cross eye."

20. _____ A patient's length measured while the patient is lying down.

21. _____ The ability to visually fixate on one visual field with both eyes simultaneously.

22. _____ A bluish tone to the skin indicating reduced (deoxygenated) haemoglobin.

II. REVIEWING KEY CONCEPTS

1. Mrs. G. has brought Karen to the clinic as a new patient. Karen, age 12 years, requires a physical examination to play volleyball. Which of the following techniques used by the nurse to establish effective communication during the interview process is not correct?
   a. The nurse introduces themself and asks the names of all family members present.
   b. After the introduction, the nurse is careful to direct questions about Karen to Mrs. G. as the best source of information.
   c. After the introduction and explanation of the nursing role, they begin the interview by saying to Karen, "Tell me about your volleyball team."
   d. The nurse chooses to conduct the interview in a quiet area with few distractions.

2. While conducting an assessment of the child, the nurse communicates with the child's family. Which of the following does the nurse recognise as *not* productive in obtaining information?
   a. Obtaining input from the child, verbal, and nonverbal
   b. Observing the relationship between parents and child
   c. Using broad, open-ended questions
   d. Using leading questions to direct the focus of the interview

3. T F Children are alert to their surroundings and attach meaning to gestures.

4. T F Active attempts to make friends with children before they have had an opportunity to evaluate an unfamiliar person increases their anxiety.

5. T F When communicating with small children the nurse should assume a position that is at eye level with the child.

6. List eight components of a complete paediatric health history.

7. In eliciting the presenting health issue or concern, it would be inappropriate for the nurse to:
   a. isolate the presenting health issue to a brief statement restricted to one or two symptoms.
   b. use labeling-type questions such as "How are you? Are you sick?" to facilitate information exchange.
   c. record the presenting health issue in the child's or parent's own words.
   d. use open-ended neutral questions to elicit information.

8. Which component of the paediatric health history is illustrated by the following statement? "Nausea and vomiting for 3 days. Started with abdominal cramping after eating hamburger at home. No pain or cramping at present. Unable to keep any foods down but able to drink clear liquids without vomiting. No temperature elevation; no diarrhoea."
   a. Presenting health issue or concern
   b. Past history
   c. Present illness
   d. Review of systems

9. Which of the following components is *not* a part of the past history in a paediatric health history?
   a. Symptom analysis
   b. Allergies
   c. Birth history
   d. Current medications

10. The nurse knows that the best description of the reproductive health history for an adolescent's health assessment:
    a. includes a discussion of plans for future children.
    b. allows the patient to introduce sexual activity history.
    c. includes a discussion of contraception methods only when the patient discloses current sexual activity.
    d. alerts the nurse to the need for sexually transmitted infection screening or pregnancy testing.

11. When assessing respirations in a 3-month-old, the nurse would assess respirations by observing which muscle group?
    a. Thoracic muscles
    b. Abdominal muscles
    c. Intercostal muscles
    d. Accessory muscles

12. The dietary history of a paediatric patient includes:
    a. a 12-hour dietary intake recall.
    b. a more specific, detailed history for the older child.
    c. concern for food security.
    d. criticism of parents' allowance of nonessential foods.

13. Jin-Lee brings her 11-month-old child to the clinic because she is "sleeping poorly and tugging at her ear when she is awake." Based on the information provided, the nurse can correctly record which of the following?
    a. presenting health issue or concern
    b. Present illness
    c. Past medical history
    d. Symptom analysis

14. The nurse is measuring a 20-month-old child's length. The most accurate method to obtain this measurement is with the child:
    a. sitting on the mom's lap.
    b. laying on a recumbent measuring board.
    c. laying on the exam table paper.
    d. standing with head and shoulders against a tape measure on the wall.

15. In examining paediatric patients, the normal head-to-toe sequence is often altered to accommodate the patient's developmental needs. With this approach, the nurse will:
    a. increase the stress and anxiety associated with the assessment of body parts.
    b. record the findings according to the normal sequence.
    c. hinder the trusting nurse-child relationship.
    d. decrease the security of the parent-child relationship.

16. A father brings his 12-month-old son in for the child's regular well-infant examination. The nurse knows that the best approach to the physical examination for this patient will be to:
    a. have the infant sit on the parent's lap to complete as much of the examination as possible.
    b. place the infant on the examining table with parent out of view.
    c. perform examination in head-to-toe direction.
    d. completely undress the child and leave him undressed during the examination.

17. Of the following behaviours, the behaviour that indicates to the nurse that a child may be reluctant to participate and cooperate during a physical examination is:
    a. talking to the nurse.
    b. making eye contact with the nurse.
    c. allowing physical touching.
    d. sitting on parent's lap, focused on a toy.

18. Growth charts used in Canada to evaluate the 0 to 19 years of age population are adapted from World Health Organisation (WHO) Growth Standards and

    Growth References. However, the _____ growth chart is recommended for premature or very low-birth-weight infants who weigh less than 1 500g until 10 weeks postterm.

19. The assessment method that provides the best information about the physical growth pattern of a preschool-age child is to:
    a. record child's height and weight measurements on the standardised growth reference chart.
    b. keep a flow sheet for height, weight, and head circumference increases.
    c. obtain a history of sibling growth patterns.
    d. measure the height, weight, and head circumference of the child.

20. T F A wall-mounted unit is the most accurate measuring device to evaluate height.

21. T F Growth is a continuous but uneven process, and the most reliable evaluation lies in comparison of growth measurements over a given time period (e.g., over a year).

22. T F Growth measurements during the physical examination should be age-specific and include length, height, weight, skinfold thickness, and arm and head circumference.

23. Head circumference is:
    a. measured in all children up to the age of 24 months.
    b. equal to chest circumference at about 1 to 2 years of age.
    c. about 8 to 9 cm smaller than chest circumference during childhood.
    d. measured slightly below the eyebrows and pinna of the ears.

24. In infants and small children, the _____ pulse should be taken because it is the most reliable. This

    pulse should be counted for _____ because of the possibility of irregularities in rhythm.

25. Which of the following observations would not be recorded as part of the child's general appearance?
    a. Impression of child's nutritional status
    b. Behaviour, interactions with parents
    c. Hygiene, cleanliness
    d. Vital signs

26. When assessing a 7-year-old's lymph nodes, the nurse uses the distal portions of the fingers and gently but firmly presses in a circular motion along the

177

submandibular node area. The nurse records the findings as "tender, enlarged, warm lymph nodes." The nurse knows that the:
a. findings are within normal limits for the child's age.
b. assessment technique was incorrect and should be repeated.
c. findings suggest infection or inflammation in the throat or neck area.
d. recording of the information is complete because it includes temperature and tenderness.

27. The nurse recognises that an assessment finding of the head and neck that does not need referral is:
a. head lag before 6 months of age.
b. hyperextension of the head with pain on flexion.
c. palpable thyroid gland including isthmus and lobes.
d. closure of the anterior fontanel at the age of 9 months.

28. Normal findings on examination of the pupils may be recorded as PERRLA, which means: _____
_____

29. Which of the following assessments is an expected finding in the child's eye examination?
a. Opaque red reflex of the eye
b. Ophthalmoscopic examination reflecting veins that are darker in colour and about one-fourth larger in size than the arteries
c. Strabismus in the 12-month-old infant
d. shining a light into the eyes and observing the child does not follow the light to midline.

30. When palpating the abdomen of a 7-year-old who is complaining of pain, what is the most appropriate nursing action?
a. Palpate the painful area first.
b. Palpate the painful area last.
c. Palpate for rebound tenderness.
d. Use percussion instead of palpation.

31. On auscultation of 8-year-old Tammie's lung fields, the nurse hears inspiratory sounds that are described as crackles. These sounds reflect which of the following:
a. a lung tumour.
b. passage of air through moisture or fluid.
c. a narrowed passageway.
d. reduced lung volumes.

32. Closure of the pulmonic and aortic valves:
a. S_1.
b. S_2.
c. S_3.
d. S_4.

33. In performing an examination for scoliosis, the nurse understands that which of the following is an incorrect method?
a. The child should be examined in only in their undergarments.
b. The child should stand erect with the nurse observing from behind.
c. The child should squat down with hands extended forward so that the nurse can observe for asymmetry of the shoulder blades.
d. The child should bend forward so that the back is parallel to the floor and the nurse can observe from behind.

34. The most important procedure for examining the heart includes:
a. inspection.
b. palpation.
c. auscultation.
d. percussion.

35. Which of the following organs is located in the lower right quadrant of the abdomen?
a. Bladder
b. Liver
c. Stomach
d. Appendix

III. THINKING CRITICALLY

1. Describe the differences between the ear canal of an infant and the ear canal of a school-age child.

2. Compare and contrast the differences in skin colour changes between light-skinned and dark-skinned individuals when cyanosis, pallor, erythema and petechiae occur.

Chapter **33** **Pediatric Health Assessment**

34 Pain Assessment and Management

I. LEARNING KEY TERMS

MATCHING: Match each term with its corresponding definition or description.

1. _____ Constellation of behaviours that may be present in response to pain.

2. _____ Collection of strategies that include distraction, relaxation, and guided imagery that may help decrease pain perception.

3. _____ Strategy to assist an infant return to calm state after a painful procedure which includes holding the infant's extremities flexed and contained close to the trunk.

4. _____ Eutectic mixture of local anesthetics.

5. _____ Pain not relieved with the usual scheduled dose of pain medication.

6. _____ A multidimensional pain instrument to assess patient and parental perceptions of the pain experience in a manner appropriate for the cognitive-developmental level of children and adolescents.

7. _____ A multidimensional pain instrument for children and adolescents that is used to assess three dimensions of pain: location, intensity, and quality.

8. _____ Uses descriptors along a 10cm line anchored by numbers or word descriptors ranging from 'no pain' to 'worst pain'.

9. _____ A pain assessment tool that uses six cartoon faces ranging from a smiling face to a tearful face that to help a child describe their pain.

10. _____ Measures pain by quantifying behaviours in five categories: facial expression (F), leg movement (L), activity (A), cry (C), and consolability (C); commonly used in children ages 2 months to 7 years.

11. _____ A Likert-style pain scale for children 8 years and older that uses numbers 0 to 10 to denote intensity of pain.

12. _____ Pain that persists or recurs for more than 3 months beyond the expected period of healing.

13. _____ Drugs which may be used alone or with opioids for pain management and to reduce opioid side effects.

a. Facilitated tucking

b. Coanalgesic drugs or adjunct analgesics

c. Distress behaviours

d. Chronic pain (persistent pain)

e. Nonpharmacologic techniques

f. Paediatric Pain Questionnaire (PPQ)

g. Wong-Baker Faces Pain Rating Scale

h. Adolescent Paediatric Pain Tool (APPT)

i. Visual Analog Scale (VAS)

j. FLACC Postoperative Pain Tool

k. Numeric Rating Scale (NRS)

l. EMLA

m. Breakthrough pain

II. REVIEWING KEY CONCEPTS

1. Pain management:
   a. requires a multidisciplinary approach.
   b. requires ongoing pain assessment following pain treatments and procedures.
   c. requires consideration for acute and chronic (persistent) pain experiences.
   d. all of the above.

2. When using patient-controlled analgesia (PCA) with children, the:
   a. drug of choice is meperidine.
   b. drug can be administered through the IM route.
   c. the nurse or parent can never use the PCA device for the child.
   d. drug of choice is morphine.

3. The anaesthetic cream EMLA is applied:
   a. eliminates or reduces pain from most procedures involving skin puncture.
   b. as preoperative oral sedation.
   c. for chronic cancer pain.
   d. postoperatively.

4. For postoperative or cancer pain control, analgesics should be administered:
   a. as needed.
   b. around the clock.
   c. before the pain escalates.
   d. after the pain peaks.

5. The most common side effect from opioid therapy is:
   a. respiratory depression.
   b. pruritus.
   c. nausea and vomiting.
   d. constipation.

6. T F Children can usually achieve comfort with a combination of opioids and adjuvant analgesics during end of life care.

7. T F Evidence supports medical cannabinoids for children and adolescents in the management of chemotherapy-induced nausea and vomiting.

8. T F Children cannot tell you where they hurt.

9. T F A 3-year-old child can use a pain scale.

10. T F Children metabolise medications slower than adults and require lower doses of opioids to achieve the same analgesic effect.

11. T F Parents may require reassurance that the advancing disease may lead to death and not medications required to treat the pain associated with the disease.

12. T F Infants do not feel pain.

13. T F Surgery and traumatic injuries generate a catabolic state and lead to increased demands on the cardiorespiratory systems.

14. Epidural analgesia:
    a. cannot be used in postoperative pain management
    b. results from the medication's effect on opiate receptors in the dorsal horn of the spinal cord instead of the brain.
    c. frequently contributes to respiratory depression
    d. delivers opioid medications only as a patient-controlled strategy

15. T F Oral mucositis is associated with different forms of cancer therapies and is difficult to relieve.

16. Most children _____ years and older are able to use the 0 to 10 numeric rating scale because of its easy use.

17. Mothers, _____ are important sources of information to aid in understanding and identifying pain behaviours.

18. The Noncommunicating Children's Pain Checklist is a pain measurement tool designed for caregivers to assess pain in non-verbal children or children with

    _____.

19. NSAIDs are suitable to manage mild to moderate pain, _____ are needed to treat moderate to severe pain.

20. List the five classifications of complementary and alternative medicine (CAM) therapies and give an example of each.

III. THINKING CRITICALLY

1. Recurrent headaches in children are caused by several factors. Outline three common factors children may experience and describe two behavioural approaches to headache management.

2. Describe 'first pass effect' and the role the intra-nasal medication route may contribute in delivering care in the emergency department.

35 Promoting Optimum Health During Childhood

I. LEARNING KEY TERMS

MATCHING: Match each term with its corresponding definition.

1. _____ An inflammatory and degenerative condition involving the gums and tissues supporting the teeth.

2. _____ Soft bacterial deposits that adhere to the teeth and cause dental decay and periodontal disease.

3. _____ The destruction of teeth resulting from the process of bathing the teeth in a cariogenic environment for a prolonged period; most often affects the maxillary incisor and the molars.

4. _____ The manifestation of decreased nutritional needs along with a decreased appetite, usually seen around 18 months of age.

5. _____ Exarticulation; "knocked out."

6. _____ The most desirable complete diet for the infant during the first 6 months.

7. _____ Partial arousal from a deep, nondreaming sleep.

8. _____ Scary dreams that are followed by full waking.

9. _____ Condition said to exist when a child's BMI is equal to or greater than the 95th percentile.

10. _____ Vaccination; responsible for the decline of infectious diseases over the past 60 years.

11. _____ Infectious disease that has declined greatly since the advent of immunizations and the use of antibiotics and antitoxins.

12. _____ Occur between early manifestations of a disease and its overt clinical syndrome.

13. _____ Serious form of physical abuse caused by violent shaking of infants and young children.

14. _____ The infliction of harm on a child caused by a parent or other person who fabricates or induces illness in the child.

15. _____ The use, persuasion, or coercion of any child to engage in sexually explicit conduct.

16. _____ Failure to meet the child's need for affection, attention, and emotional nurturance.

17. _____ Deliberate infliction of bodily injury on a child, usually by the child's caregiver.

a. Prodromal period

b. Immunisation

c. Communicable disease

d. Early childhood caries

e. Plaque

f. Obesity

g. Avulsed tooth

h. Weaning

i. Lactovegetarians

j. Physiological anorexia

k. Unintentional injuries

l. Human milk

m. Sleep terrors

n. Malocclusion

o. Health promotion

p. Nightmares

q. Munchausen syndrome by proxy

r. Sexual abuse

s. Periodontal disease

t. Physical abuse

u. Emotional neglect

v. Abusive head trauma

18. _____ The complete cessation of breast or bottle feeding or refer to the process of introducing complementary foods while a child continues to breast-feed.

19. _____ The process of enabling people to increase control over, and to improve, their health.

20. _____ Diet that excludes meat and eggs but includes milk

21. _____ When teeth of the upper and lower dental arches do not approximate in the proper relationships

22. _____ The leading cause of death among children aged 1 to 14.

II. REVIEWING KEY CONCEPTS

1. Which of the following statements is *true* in regard to nutritional changes from the infant to the toddler years?
   a. Protein and energy requirements remain high to meet demands for muscle growth.
   b. The needs for minerals such as iron and calcium are easy to meet.
   c. Toddlers enjoy being fed by an adult caretaker.
   d. Toddlers like to experience new tastes and foods.

2. Which of the following methods is most effective for plaque removal?
   a. Brushing and flossing
   b. Annual fluoride treatments
   c. Allowing the child to brush his or her own teeth
   d. Using a large stiff toothbrush

3. Physiological anorexia in toddlers is characterised by:
   a. strong taste preferences.
   b. extreme changes in appetite from day to day.
   c. heightened awareness of social aspects of meals.
   d. weight loss and thinner appearance.

4. Which of the following statements about injuries in childhood is false?
   a. The majority of injury-related deaths are preventable.
   b. The use of car restraints, bicycle helmets, and smoke detectors have significantly decreased fatalities for children.
   c. During infancy, more boys die from aspiration or suffocation than do girls
   d. Children ages 3 to 6 years old are at greatest risk of bicycling fatalities.

5. A nurse should withhold a vaccine if the child:
   a. has a common cold.
   b. is currently taking antibiotics.
   c. has a severe febrile illness.
   d. was born prematurely.

6. Honey should be avoided in infants younger than 12 months of age because of its association with the occurrence of:
   a. SIDS.
   b. Food allergy.
   c. Infant botulism.
   d. Pertussis.

7. Healthy ways of serving food to toddlers include:
   a. Requiring the child to sit at a table for meals.
   b. Permitting nutritious grazing between meals.
   c. Discouraging between-meal snacking.
   d. Providing rewards for foods consumed.

8. A mother of a 4-month-old tells the clinic nurse that her infant son sleeps approximately 20 hours per day, combining naps and nighttime sleep. The nurse recognises that this pattern of sleep in infancy is:
   a. a normal sleep pattern for this age.
   b. an abnormal sleep pattern for this age.

9. Which of the following is the current recommendation regarding car seat safety?
   a. All infants and toddlers should be rear facing until they weigh a minimum of 10 kg and are able to walk on their own.
   b. All infants and toddlers should be rear facing until they reach the age of 2 years or height recommended by the car seat manufacturer.
   c. All infants and toddlers who have outgrown their car seats may be switched to a booster seat in the back seat of the car.
   d. Manual shoulder belts are appropriate to use for toddlers.

10. The parents should consider moving the toddler from the crib to a bed after the toddler:
    a. reaches the age of 2 years.
    b. will stay in bed all night.
    c. reaches a height of 90 cm.
    d. is able to sleep through the night.

11. Which of the following nutritional requirements remains relatively high during the toddler years?
    a. Calories
    b. Minerals
    c. Proteins
    d. Fluids

12. Which of the following are recommended dietary guidelines for adolescents?
    a. Reduction of saturated fat and avoidance of trans-fat.
    b. Increase in daily dietary fibre.
    c. Inclusion of essential minerals such as zinc, calcium, and iron during periods of rapid growth.
    d. All of the above are correct.

13. When educating the preschool child about injury prevention, the parents should:
    a. set a good example.
    b. help children establish safety habits.
    c. be aware that pedestrian/motor vehicle injuries increase in this age group.
    d. do all of the above.

14. Studies indicate that toddlers up to 24 months of age are safer riding in _____ in the _____ position.

15. Give an example of an item that could cause aspiration, burns, or suffocation for each of the following categories of items hazardous to the toddler.
    a. Foods
    b. Play objects
    c. Common household objects
    d. Electrical items

16. T F Sleep terrors can be described as a partial arousal from a very deep nondreaming sleep.

17. T F Television viewing before bedtime may cause bedtime resistance.

18. T F Preschoolers can independently brush and floss their teeth.

19. T F Preschoolers are more prone to falls than toddlers.

20. T F Children can be offered low fat milk after that age of 12 months

21. T F 2-year old children should be offered 250 mL of milk with each meal.

MATCHING: Match each term with its corresponding definition or description.

22. _____ This vaccine is administered in early fall and is repeated yearly for ongoing protection; may be given to infants as young as 6 months.

23. _____ Vaccine protects against a number of serious infections caused by *Haemophilus influenzae* type b, especially bacterial meningitis, epiglottitis, bacterial pneumonia, septic arthritis, and sepsis.

24. _____ Vaccine protects against Streptococcal pneumococci, which are responsible for a number of bacterial infections in children under 2 years; these include generalised infections such as septicemia and meningitis or localised infections such as otitis media, sinusitis, and pneumonia.

25. _____ This vaccine is administered at 2, 4, and 6 months to protect from pertussis, diphtheria, and tetanus.

26. _____ Vaccine is administered to protect against severe diarrhoea in infants and young children.

27. _____ Vaccine given to protect against muscle paralysis.

a. Inactivated poliovirus vaccine (IPV)

b. Hib

c. Prevnar

d. DTaP

e. Influenza vaccine

f. Rotavirus vaccine

III. THINKING CRITICALLY

1. Develop a teaching plan for parents of a 4-year old who is a picky eater.

2. List two dietary supplements that should be given in infancy and briefly explain the rationale for administration of each in this age group.

3. Develop a strategy in providing care for parents who are hesitant to have vaccines administered to their child.

4. Parents ask a nurse whether to use fluoride with their 3-year-old child. What teaching would be provided? What further information is required?

5. Develop a teaching plan for parents of an infant regarding the use of a car seat across the child's life span.

36 The Infant and Family

I. LEARNING KEY TERMS

MATCHING: Match each term with its corresponding definition or description.

1. _____ Between ages 4 and 8 months, the infant progresses through the first stage of separation-individuation and begins to have some awareness of self and mother as separate beings.

2. _____ Orderly sequence of acquisition of skills from head to toe.

3. _____ The unexpected and abrupt death of an infant under 1 year of age that remains unexplained after a complete postmortem examination, including an investigation of the death scene and a review of the case history.

4. _____ A sign of inadequate growth resulting from inability to obtain or use calories required for growth.

5. _____ A major accomplishment of cognitive development that develops at approximately 9 to 10 months of age; the realisation that objects continue to exist after they leave one's visual field.

6. _____ Significant amounts are received that provide immunity for approximately 3 months after birth.

7. _____ Fusion of two ocular images that begins to develop at 6 weeks and should be well established by age 4 months.

8. _____ Paroxysmal abdominal pain manifested by a duration of more than 3 hours more than 3 days per week and for more than 3 weeks in a healthy infant.

9. _____ Begins to develop by age 7 to 9 months but may not be fully mature until 2 or 3 years of age, thus increasing the infant's and younger toddler's risk of falling.

10. _____ An acquired condition that occurs as a result of cranial moulding during infancy; incidence has increased dramatically since implementation of the Back to Sleep campaign.

11. _____ Not an instinctual ability but a learned acquired process.

a. Binocularity

b. Object permanence

c. Positional plagiocephaly

d. Parenting

e. Maternal immunoglobulin G (IgG)

f. Stereopsis (depth perception)

g. Failure to thrive

h. Separation anxiety

i. Colic

j. Sudden infant death syndrome (SIDS)

k. Cephalocaudal

II. REVIEWING KEY CONCEPTS

1. An infant is brought to the clinic for their 1-year well-child visit. The infant weighed 3.4 kg. at birth. Based on normal growth and development what would an appropriate weight be at this visit?
   a. 5.7 kg
   b. k6.6 kg.
   c. 10.1 kg
   d. 10.7 kg

2. The age at which most infants can roll from back to abdomen is:
   a. 3 months.
   b. 6 months.
   c. 9 months.
   d. 12 months.

3. The child's anterior fontanel usually closes by:
   a. 3 to 6 months.
   b. 7 to 9 months.
   c. 12 to 18 months.
   d. 24 months.

4. Which of the following characteristics of vision begins to develop by 6 weeks of age and should be well established by age 4 months?
   a. Corneal reflex
   b. Stereopsis
   c. Binocularity
   d. Strabismus

5. Which of the following assessment findings would be considered most abnormal?
   a. The infant who displays head lag at 3 months of age
   b. The infant who displays head lag at 6 months of age
   c. The infant who begins to roll from front to back at 4 months
   d. The infant who begins to roll from front to back at 6 months

6. At what age would the fine pincer grasp typically be seen in an infant following normal growth and development patterns?
   a. 2 months
   b. 4 months
   c. 6 months
   d. 10 months

7. Reactive attachment disorder stems from:
   a. crying and vocalising to the mother.
   b. clinging to the mother.
   c. crying when the mother leaves the room.
   d. maladaptive or absent attachment.

8. If a parent is concerned about the fact that their 14-month-old infant is not walking, the nurse would particularly want to evaluate whether the infant:
   a. pulls up to the furniture.
   b. uses a pincer grasp.
   c. transfers objects.
   d. has developed object permanence.

9. Colic is said to be more common in the infant who:
   a. is between 3 and 6 months of age.
   b. has a difficult temperament.
   c. has other congenital abnormalities.
   d. has signs of failure to thrive.

10. T F Maternal smoking during and after pregnancy has been implicated as a contributor to SIDS.

11. T F Parents should be advised to position an infant on their abdomen to prevent SIDS.

12. T F Failure to thrive (growth failure) occurs almost exclusively in developing countries where food shortage and poverty are prevalent.

13. T F Placing a healthy term infant who spits up part of their feedings on their side to sleep will reduce the risk for aspiration and further complications.

III. THINKING CRITICALLY

1. Describe the fine motor and gross motor, language, and social developmental milestones to assess in a 7-month-old infant who is coming to the well-child clinic.

2. A nurse is providing education to new parents regarding the prevention of SIDS.

   a) List five risk factors the nurse will teach the parents.

   b) List three topics the nurse will teach to protect against SIDS.

c) The family members state they feel comfortable with this information and will ensure their baby is always on their back to prevent SIDS. What further teaching is required related to this statement?

3. Parents of a 6-month old infant come to the well-baby clinic and state their parents tell them they are spoiling their infant by going to the child whenever it cries and picking the baby up. What teaching can a nurse provide to the parents?

37 The Toddler and Family

I. LEARNING KEY TERMS

MATCHING: Match each term with its corresponding description.

1. _____ The need to maintain sameness and reliability.

2. _____ One of the major tasks of toddlerhood.

3. _____ Imitating household activities

4. _____ The developmental stage in which the toddler relinquishes dependence on others.

5. _____ A necessary assertion of self-control in the toddler.

6. _____ Characterised by the child playing alongside, but not with, other children.

7. _____ The retreat from one's present pattern of functioning to past levels of behaviour.

8. _____ Achievements that mark the child's expressions of their individual characteristics in the environment

a. Autonomy

b. Negativism

c. Ritualism

d. Domestic mimicry

e. Toilet independence

f. Individuation

g. Regression

h. Parallel play

II. REVIEWING KEY CONCEPTS

1. Regression in toddlers occurs when there is:
   a. stress.
   b. a threat to their autonomy.
   c. a need to revert to dependency.
   d. a, b, and c.

2. The nurse is conducting an assessment of fine motor development in a 3-year-old. Which of the following is the expected drawing skill for this age?
   a. Holds the writing instrument with his or her fist
   b. Can draw a complete stick figure
   c. Can copy a triangle
   d. Can copy a circle

3. The usual number of words acquired by the age of 2 years is about:
   a. 50.
   b. 100.
   c. 300.
   d. 500.

4. Which of the following types of play increases in frequency as the child moves through the toddler period?
   a. Parallel play
   b. Imitative play
   c. Tactile play
   d. Solitary play

5. Which of the following statements is *false* in regard to toilet independence?
   a. Bowel training is usually accomplished after bladder training.
   b. Nighttime bladder training is usually accomplished after bowel training.
   c. The toddler who is impatient with soiled diapers is demonstrating readiness for toilet learning.
   d. Fewer wet diapers signal that the toddler is physically ready for toilet learning.

6. Which of the following strategies is appropriate for parents to use to prepare a toddler for the birth of a sibling?
   a. Explain the upcoming birth as early in the pregnancy as possible.
   b. Move the toddler to their own new room.
   c. Provide a doll for the toddler to imitate parenting.
   d. Tell the toddler that a new playmate will come home soon.

7. The best approach for extinguishing a toddler's attention-seeking behaviour of a temper tantrum with head banging is to:
   a. ignore the behaviour.
   b. provide time-out.
   c. offer a toy to calm the child.
   d. protect the child from injury.

8. Which of the following statements about stress in toddlers is *true*?
   a. Toddlers are rarely exposed to stress or the results of stress.
   b. Any stress is destructive because toddlers have a limited ability to cope.
   c. Most children are exposed to a stress-free environment.
   d. Small amounts of stress help toddlers develop effective coping skills.

III. THINKING CRITICALLY

1. Describe four areas that the nurse should assess to obtain the information necessary to give adequate anticipatory guidance to the parents of a 14-month-old toddler.

2. A nurse is assessing the development of a 2-year old.

   a) Describe three gross motor developmental milestones that a 2-year-old toddler should have accomplished.

   b) Describe three fine motor developmental milestones that a 2-year-old toddler should have accomplished.

   c) Describe three language developmental milestones that a 2-year-old toddler should have accomplished.

3. Describe how negativism contributes to the toddler's acquisition of a sense of autonomy.

4. The parents of an 18-month old asks a nurse how they will know when their child is ready to learn to use the potty. What should the nurse teach the parents?

38 The Preschooler and Family

I. LEARNING KEY TERMS

MATCHING: Match each term with its corresponding definition or description.

1. _____ Imitating the behaviour of significant others.

2. _____ An invented companion that serves many purposes in the preschooler's development.

3. _____ Group activities that have no rigid organisation or rules; typical of the preschool period.

4. _____ A feeling of accomplishment in one's activities; a psychosocial developmental task of the preschool period.

5. _____ Preschool-aged children have difficulty understanding the concept of tomorrow, yesterday, or next week.

6. _____ A type of speech pattern that occurs normally in children during the preschool period, when children are using their rapidly growing vocabulary faster than they can produce the words.

7. _____ Ascribing lifelike qualities to inanimate objects.

8. _____ The superego; development in this area is a major task for the preschooler.

9. _____ The result of a preschooler's transductive reasoning; the belief that thoughts are all powerful.

10. _____ Behaviour that attempts to hurt a person or destroys property; differs from anger.

11. _____ Articulation problems that occur when children are pressured to produce sounds ahead of their developmental level.

a. Sense of initiative

b. Conscience

c. Concept of time

d. Dyslalia

e. Magical thinking

f. Animism

g. Associative play

h. Modelling

i. Imaginary playmates

j. Aggression

k. Stuttering (stammering)

II. REVIEWING KEY CONCEPTS

1. The approximate age range for the preschool period is

   from age _____ years to _____ years.

2. The average annual weight gain during the preschool

   years is _____ kg.

3. Which of the following statements about the average preschooler's physical proportions is *true*?
   a. Preschoolers have a squat and potbellied frame.
   b. Preschoolers have a slender but sturdy frame.
   c. The muscle and bones of the preschooler have reached full maturity.
   d. Sexual characteristics can be differentiated in the preschooler.

4. During the preschool years, anticipatory guidance shifts to a focus on:
   a. protection rather than education.
   b. education and correcting dysfluency in speech patterns.
   c. education with an emphasis on reasoning.
   d. protection and safeguarding the immediate environment.

5. The moral and spiritual development of the preschooler is characterised by:
   a. concern for why something is wrong.
   b. actions that are directed toward satisfying the needs of others.
   c. thoughts of loyalty and gratitude.
   d. a very concrete sense of justice.

6. According to Erikson, the preschooler's primary psychosocial task of this period is acquiring a sense of:
   a. trust.
   b. autonomy.
   c. initiative.
   d. belonging.

7. T F Preschoolers have a concrete concept of a God or other diety with physical characteristics, often similar to an imaginary friend.

8. Which of the following gross motor skills would NOT be expected for a 4-year-old child?
   a. Ride a tricycle
   b. Hop on one foot
   c. Jump rope
   d. Throw a ball reliably

9. The nurse is conducting an assessment of fine motor development in a 3-year-old. Which of the following is the expected drawing skill for this age?
   a. Holds the writing instrument with his or her fist
   b. Can draw a complete stick figure
   c. Can copy a diamond
   d. Can copy a circle

III. THINKING CRITICALLY

1. Use the following scenario to respond to questions a through d.

Imagine that you are a nurse on the staff of a paediatric group practice. A mother comes in to discuss her son, who is 37 months old. He will attend the preschool programme at a local school this year. He has attended a home day care programme since he was a baby, while his mother worked in her own interior decorating business.

An older woman runs the day care that the child has attended until now. The woman and her helper both treat the 12 children in the programme as if they were family. The programme is very structured regarding schedule and routines.

The child's mother tells you that she is looking forward to Jacob's new environment. His teacher is very creative and approaches the classroom from the perspective of the child's development. There will be a lot of choices for activities during the day.

a. Based on the information, analyse the data presented in relation to the child's needs and the concerns for a smooth transition.

b. Develop an expected outcome that is reasonable to establish for this mother and her child.

c. Describe interventions and strategies that are appropriate for you to suggest to this mother and her child.

d. Explain to the mother the characteristics that indicate the child is ready for preschool.

2. The parent of a 4-year old asks a nurse about their child watching television. They are concerned they child is watching too much TV. Develop teaching topics for this parent.

39 The School-Age Child and Family

I. LEARNING KEY TERMS

MATCHING: Match each term with its corresponding definition.

1. _____ One of the most important socialising agents in the school-age years.

2. _____ Any recurring activity that intends to cause harm, distress, or control toward another in which there is a perceived imbalance of power between the aggressor (s) and the victim.

3. _____ The child's ability to relate a series of events to mental representations that can be expressed both verbally and symbolically.

4. _____ An awareness of oneself regarding personal attributes and the idea of self in relation to others

5. _____ Elementary school children who are left to care for themselves before or after school without supervision of an adult.

6. _____ Involuntary urination.

7. _____ Absence of one X chromosome.

8. _____ Presence of one or more additional X chromosome.

a. Enuresis

b. Self-concept

c. Turner syndrome

d. Latchkey children

e. Peer group

f. Bullying

g. Concrete operations

h. Klinefelter syndrome

II. REVIEWING KEY CONCEPTS

1. The middle childhood is also referred to as "school age" or the "school years." What ages does this period represent?
   a. 5 to 12 years
   b. 4 to 14 years
   c. 5 to 11 years
   d. 6 to 13 years

2. T F The heart is smaller in relation to the rest of the body during the middle years.

3. T F During the middle years, the immune system develops little immunity to pathogenic microorganisms.

4. T F Middle childhood is the period of development where children develop skills needed to become useful, contributing members of their social communities.

5. T F Physical maturity correlates well with emotional and social maturity during the middle years.

6. Generally, the earliest age at which puberty begins is

   age _____ for girls and age _____ for boys, but

   it can be normal for either sex after the age of _____ years.

7. T F In the middle school years, children want to spend more time in the company of peers, and they often prefer peer group activities to family activities.

8. Middle childhood is the time when children:
   I. learn the value of doing things with others.
   II. learn the benefits derived from division of labour in accomplishing goals.
   III. achieve a sense of industry and accomplishment.
   IV. expand interests and engage in tasks that can be carried to completion.
      a. I, II, III, and IV
      b. I, III, and IV
      c. I and IV
      d. II and III

9. A 6-year-old boy is starting in a new neighbourhood school. On the first day of school he says he has a headache and tearfully tells his mother he does not want to go. His mother takes him to school, and the nurse is consulted. The nurse recognises that this is a slow-to-warm-up child and suggests which of the following?
   a. Put him in the classroom with the other children and leave him alone.
   b. Insist that he join and lead the class song.
   c. Include him in activities without assigning him tasks until he willingly participates in activities.
   d. Send him home with his mother because he has a headache.

10. During the school-age years, children learn valuable lessons from peers. How is this accomplished?
   a. The child learns to appreciate the varied points of view that are within the peer group.
   b. The child becomes sensitive to the social norms and pressures of the group.
   c. The child's interactions among peers lead to the formation of intimate friendships between same-sex peers.
   d. All of the above are correct.

11. Children's self-concepts are composed of:
   a. their own critical self-assessment.
   b. their idea of self in relation to others.
   c. their body image awareness.
   d. all of the above.

12. Which of the following factors influences the amount and manner of discipline and limit setting imposed on school-age children:
   a. psychosocial maturity of the parent.
   b. parents child rearing experiences
   c. response of the child to rewards and punishments.
   d. a, b, c

13. To assist school-age children in coping with stress in their lives, the nurse should:
   I. be able to recognise signs that indicate the child is undergoing stress.

II. teach the child how to recognise signs of stress in her or himself.
III. help the child plan a means for dealing with any stress through problem solving.
IV. reassure the child that the stress is only temporary.
   a. I, II, III, and IV
   b. I, II, and III
   c. I, II, and IV
   d. I and III

14. T F Previously well-behaved children may engage in lying, stealing, and cheating during the school-age years.

15. Bullying which uses force and most often used by boys is referred to as _____ _____ and bullying using methods such as gossip, rumors, and exclusion and used mainly by girls is referred to as _____ _____.

III. THINKING CRITICALLY

1. Use the following scenario to respond to questions a to d below.

A 9-year-old boy is brought to the clinic by his mother for a physical examination. His mother is concerned, because the child wants to join the school soccer team this year. On physical examination, the nurse discovers that since last year there has been an increase of 5 cm in height and a 4.5 kg weight gain. Health history is unchanged from the previous year. The young boy tells the nurse that he rides his bike more now than last year because he has a new best friend to go riding with.

a. Describe the areas of assessment that the nurse should expand upon.

b. Describe an appropriate response to the mother's concern about her son playing soccer.

c. Describe an educational session that would most benefit this child and his mother.

d. Describe how the mother of this 9-year-old boy can foster his development.

2. A 7-year-old boy and his parent attend the clinic for a wellness check. The parent tells the nurse the child wets his bed at least 3 times per week. The parent states that they have tried yelling and pleading with the child and they do not know what else to do.

a. What further assessments should be done?

b. What would you teach the parent about their response to the bedwetting?

c. Develop a plan with the child and the parent related to the enuresis.

40 The Adolescent and Family

I. LEARNING KEY TERMS

MATCHING: Match each term with its corresponding definition.

1. _____ The masculinising hormones; secreted in small and gradually increasing amounts up to about 7 or 9 years of age, then followed by a rapid increase in both sexes, the level of androgens in males increasing over that in females with the onset of testicular function.

2. _____ Development of sexual identity in adolescents

3. _____ The hormone that increases with the onset of testicular function.

4. _____ Pattern of sexual arousal or romantic attraction toward persons of the same sex, opposite sex or both sexes.

5. _____ Single greatest cause of death in the adolescent age group, claiming more lives than all other causes combined.

6. _____ The initial appearance of menstruation; occurs about 2 years after the appearance of the first pubescent changes.

7. _____ The feminising hormone; found in low quantities during childhood; increasing in quantity in early puberty.

8. _____ Temporary breast enlargement and tenderness; common during midpuberty in boys.

9. _____ Are strongly influenced by interpersonal relationships with peers as well as adults in their environment.

10. _____ A period of transition between childhood and adulthood—a time of rapid physical, cognitive, social, and emotional maturation.

11. _____ The first period of puberty; occurs about 2 years immediately before puberty, when the child is developing preliminary physical changes that herald sexual maturity.

12. _____ The maturational, hormonal, and growth process that occurs when the reproductive organs begin to function and the secondary sex characteristics develop.

a. Puberty

b. Prepubescence

c. Adolescence

d. Oestrogen

e. Androgens

f. Testosterone

g. Menarche

h. Gynecomastia

i. Peer group

j. Sexual orientation

k. Identity formation

l. Injuries

II. Reviewing Key Concepts

1. The normal age range for menarche is usually _____

   to _____ years, with the average age being _____

   years, _____ months.

2. Which of the following secretes sex hormones?
   a. Ovaries
   b. Testes
   c. Adrenals
   d. a, b, c

3. The adolescent growth spurt is characterised as beginning:
   a. sooner in boys.
   b. between the ages of 9.5 and 14.5 years in boys.
   c. sooner in girls.
   d. between the ages of 10.5 and 16 years in girls.

4. Girls may be considered to have _____ _____ if

   breast development has not occurred by age _____.

197

5. The first pubescent change in boys is:
   a. appearance of pubic hair.
   b. testicular enlargement with thinning, reddening, and increased looseness of the scrotum.
   c. penile enlargement.
   d. temporary breast enlargement and tenderness.

6. Which one of the following statements about pattern of growth during adolescence is *true*?
   a. Knowing the correct sequence of the growth pattern is useful only when assessing abnormal growth patterns versus normal growth patterns.
   b. Boys start an increase of muscle mass during early puberty that lasts throughout adolescence.
   c. Boys usually begin puberty and reach maturity about 2 years earlier than girls.
   d. Girls and boys have an increase in linear growth that begins for both during mid-puberty.

7. On the average, girls gain _____ to _____ cm in height and _____ to _____ kg during adolescence, whereas boys gain _____ to _____ cm and _____ to _____ kg.

8. Which of the following best describes the formal operational thinking that occurs between the ages of 11 and 14 years?
   a. Thought process includes thinking in concrete terms.
   b. Thought process includes information obtained from the environment and peers.
   c. Thought process includes thinking in abstract terms, possibilities, and hypotheses.
   d. All of the above.

9. T F There is evidence that greater levels of religiosity and spirituality in adolescence are associated with fewer high risk behaviours and more health-promoting behaviours.

10. According to Erikson, adolescence is described as:
    a. the period of formation of a sense of identity.
    b. the period where adolescents see themselves as distinct individuals
    c. the period adolescents may experience times of confusion, depression, and discouragement as they develop their personal identity.
    d. a, b, c

11. The formation of sex-role identity during adolescence usually involves which of the following?
    a. Shift from relationships with same-sex peers to intimate relationships with members of the opposite sex during middle adolescence
    b. Usually involves forming close friendships with same-sex peers.
    c. Developing emotional and social identities separate from those of families
    d. All of the above

12. Advances in cognitive development bring which of the following changes for adolescents?
    a. Their beliefs become more concrete and less rooted in general ideological principles.
    b. They show an increasing emotional understanding and acceptance of parents' beliefs as their own.
    c. They develop a personal value system distinct from that of significant adults in their lives.
    d. They encounter few new situations or opportunities for decisions because of their past experiences.

13. Compared with school-age children, adolescent peer groups are:
    a. more likely to include peers of the opposite sex.
    b. less autonomous.
    c. less likely to influence members' socialisation roles.
    d. more likely to require parental supervision.

14. Of the following male reproductive problems, the one most likely to be identified in an adolescent male is:
    a. hypospadias.
    b. cryptorchidism.
    c. testicular tumour.
    d. urethritis.

15. T F Growth in height in girls typically ceases 2 to 2.5 years after menarche begins and around ages 18 to 20 for boys.

III. THINKING CRITICALLY

1. Explain the principles of physical growth that are important for adolescent girls to understand if they are concerned about their weight.

2. Explain how a peer group contributes to the development of a sense of identity in the adolescent and why peer groups are an important influence during the adolescent years.

3. Describe three guiding principles to offer to parents of adolescents to help them better communicate with their adolescent child.

4. Explain how an adolescent can benefit from participating in sports.

5. A nurse is asked to do a presentation to a high school class on the risks of body art and tanning. What content would be included?

6. A 15-year old male patient comes to the clinic asking questions about testicular cancer. What should the nurse teach the teen?

199

41 Caring for the Child With a Chronic Illness and at the End of Life

I. LEARNING KEY TERMS

MATCHING: Match each term with its corresponding description.

1. _____ A concept that reflects the efforts of family members to create a normal family life, the perceived consequences and meanings attributed to the efforts.

2. _____ Actions carried out by a person other than the patient to end the life of the patient suffering from a terminal condition.

3. _____ Coping mechanisms that result in movement away from adjustment; maladaptation to the crisis.

4. _____ A multidisciplinary approach to the care of children living with or dying from chronic, complex or life-limiting conditions with a primary focus on symptom relief, supportive care, and quality of life.

5. _____ Provision of palliative care in an alternative, homelike setting.

6. _____ Coping mechanisms that result in movement toward adjustment and resolution of the crisis.

7. _____ Feelings of sorrow and loss that recur in waves over time.

8. _____ An emotional response that may occur when death is the expected or possible outcome of a disorder.

9. _____ A process of recognizing, promoting, and enhancing competence for families and/or children living with complex medical needs.

10. _____ Behaviours aimed at reducing the tension caused by a crisis.

11. _____ A defence mechanism that enables the prevention of disintegration and is a normal response to grieving for any type of loss.

a. Coping mechanisms

b. Normalisation

c. Approach behaviours

d. Chronic sorrow

e. Avoidance behaviours

f. Anticipatory grief

g. Palliative care

h. Euthanasia

i. Hospice care

j. Denial

k. Empowerment

II. REVIEWING KEY CONCEPTS

1. Which of the following can be used to assist families in coping with stress and periodic crises they may be experiencing due to their child's chronic condition, disability, or end-of-life care decisions?
   a. Providing anticipatory guidance
   b. Working collaboratively with families in developing problem-solving strategies
   c. Providing emotional support
   d. All of the above

2. A goal that is considered appropriate for family-centred care is for the nurse to:
   a. Form partnerships with family.
   b. Engage in active listening.
   c. Accept differences.
   d. Respect the family as the constant in the child's life.
   e. All of the above.

200

3. Identify one strategy a nurse can use to help break patterns of unrewarding or unproductive interaction in parents of a child with special needs.

4. Describe the adaptive tasks of parents who have a child with a chronic condition.

5. The sibling of a child with a chronic disabling condition may experience:
   a. responsibility for caregiving of the sibling with a chronic condition.
   b. differential treatment by parents.
   c. limitations in family resources.
   d. all of the above.

6. When the parents of a child with special needs experience chronic sorrow, the process:
   a. of grief is pronounced and self-limiting.
   b. involves social reintegration after grieving.
   c. is characterised by realistic expectations.
   d. may include new caregiving demands.

7. List three common phases of families' adaptation and emotional responses to a chronic illness or disability or complex condition.

8. When the parent of a child who is dying tells the nurse the child is in pain even when the child appears comfortable, the nurse should be sure that:
   a. as needed (prn) pain control measures are instituted.
   b. pain control is administered on a regular schedule.
   c. parents understand that dying is a physical process and that physical symptoms do not always reflect pain.
   d. parents understand that the child is probably in less pain than he or she appears to be.

9. Pain control is often a concern of dying children and their parents. Which of the following strategies should the nurse use to help them deal with this fear?
   a. Assure the parents that the pain will be relieved.
   b. Use heavy sedation to help the child cope with this phase.
   c. Adopt a medication schedule that will prevent the pain from escalating.
   d. Give pain medications intravenously only when the child is near death.

10. List at least five physical signs of approaching death.

11. When death is the expected outcome of a disorder, the child and family members may experience anticipatory grief which can include:
    a. depression.
    b. denial
    c. psychologic or physical symptoms
    d. all of the above.

12. Complicated grief reactions include symptoms of:
    a. denial.
    b. anger.
    c. pangs of severe emotion.
    d. depression.

13. Which of the following symptoms is considered normal acute grief behaviour?
    a. Feeling the need to have friends and relatives around
    b. Feeling an emotional closeness to friends and relatives
    c. Hearing the dead person's voice
    d. a, b, and c

14. To ensure families receive support and guidance after their child's death, the minimum standard includes:
    a. A list of grief support groups for siblings
    b. An online survey to complete a needs assessment
    c. Meeting with the family at the time of death
    d. A follow-up telephone call or meeting

1. Outline one key principle associated with the following themes in the care of children with special needs:

   Developmental focus

   Family-centred care

   Shared Decision Making

   Normalisation

2. Describe the phenomenon of becoming the 'perfect child' after the death of a sibling.

3. Outline strategies nurses can employ to maintain effective functioning in the clinical setting.

42 Impact of Intellectual Disability or Sensory Impairment on the Child and Family

I. LEARNING KEY TERMS

MATCHING: Match each term with its corresponding description.

1. _____ Also known as nearsightedness, able to see objects at close range but not at a distance.

2. _____ Refers to a person whose hearing disability precludes successful processing of linguistic information through audition, with or without a hearing aid.

3. _____ Encompasses both partial sight and legal blindness.

4. _____ Refers to a person who, with the use of a hearing aid, has residual hearing sufficient to enable successful processing of linguistic information through audition.

5. _____ A disability that may range in severity from slight to profound hearing loss

6. _____ Inability to express ideas in any form, either written or verbally.

7. _____ Most common genetic cause of intellectual disability and autism spectrum disorders; caused by an abnormal gene on the lower end of the long arm of the X chromosome.

8. _____ The inability to interpret sound correctly.

9. _____ Systematic programme of therapy, exercises, and activities intended to address developmental delays and subsequently assist children in achieving optimal cognitive development.

10. _____ Difficulty in processing details or discrimination among sounds.

11. _____ Special decoding device in which the transmission of the audio portion of a television programme is translated into subtitles that appear on the screen.

12. _____ Important in prenatal care, may help decrease occurrence of neural tube defects.

13. _____ A unit of sound intensity measured at various frequencies; used to express the degree of hearing impairment.

14. _____ Most common chromosomal abnormality of a generalised syndrome.

15. _____ Equipment used to help people who are hearing impaired to communicate with each other over the telephone.

16. _____ Most common eye infection.

17. _____ The measurement of an individual's hearing impairment by means of an audiometer.

a. Intellectual disability

b. Autism spectrum disorders

c. Conjunctivitis

d. Down syndrome

e. Folic acid supplements

f. Early intervention programmes

g. Fragile X

h. Hearing impairment

i. Severe to profound hearing loss

j. Slight to moderate hearing loss

k. Aphasia

l. Agnosia

m. Dysacusis

n. Decibel

o. Hearing threshold level

p. American Sign Language (ASL)/ British Sign Language (BSL)

q. Amblyopia

r. Teletypewriters/telecommunications devices for the deaf (TDD)

s. Closed captioning

t. Visual impairment

u. Myopia

v. Hyperopia

w. Astigmatism

x. Strabismus

18. _____ Complex neurodevelopmental disorders of unknown aetiology with impairments in social communication, unusual sensory sensitivities or interests, and repetitive or restricted patterns of behaviour.

19. _____ A visual-gestural language using hand signals that roughly correspond to specific words and concepts in the English language.

20. _____ Also known as farsightedness; ability to see objects at a distance

21. _____ A general term for any type of mental difficulty or deficiency; term is used in place of cognitive impairment.

22. _____ Known as "lazy eye," reduced visual acuity in one eye.

23. _____ "Squint" or cross-eye; malalignment of eyes.

24. _____ Unequal curvatures in refractive apparatus.

II. REVIEWING KEY CONCEPTS

1. Acquiring social skills for the cognitively impaired child includes:
   a. Teaching socially acceptable sexual behaviour.
   b. Exposing the child to strangers to practise manners.
   c. Responding to and greeting others.
   d. a, b, and c.

2. Define task analysis and describe its use when teaching a cognitively impaired child.

3. Trisomy 21 is also known as:
   a. Jacob syndrome.
   b. Turner syndrome.
   c. Down syndrome.
   d. Klinefelter syndrome.

4. Which of the following could be early signs suggestive of intellectual disability?
   a. Gross motor delay
   b. speech development delay
   c. Behaviour difficulties
   d. a, b, and c

5. Parents of a child with fragile X syndrome should optimally receive _____ _____.

6. Conductive hearing defects respond to:
   a. antibiotic therapy for acute otitis media.
   b. tympanostomy tubes for chonic otitis media.
   c. hearing aid if conductive loss is permanent.
   d. all of the above.

7. While screening an infant for suspected hearing impairment, the nurse should be alert for:
   a. absent cry.
   b. consistent lack of the startle reflex to a loud sound.
   c. a louder than usual cry.
   d. absence of babble or voice inflections by age 4 months.

8. In the assessment of a child to identify whether a hearing impairment has developed, the nurse would look for:
   a. monotone speech.
   b. consistent lack of the startle reflex.
   c. a high level of social activity.
   d. attentiveness, especially when someone is talking.

9. Which of the following strategies could facilitate lipreading for a child who is hearing impaired?
   a. Touching the child lightly to signal presence of a speaker
   b. Face directly or move to a 45-degree angle
   c. Using facial expressions to assist in conveying messages
   d. a, b, and c

10. If a child has a penetrating injury to the eye, the parent should:
    a. apply an eye patch.
    b. attempt to remove the object.
    c. irrigate the eye.
    d. take the child to the emergency department.

11. Clinical manifestations of autism spectrum disorders (ASD) include:
    a. social interaction deficits
    b. communication deficits
    c. behaviour deficits
    d. a, b, and c.

204

12. List at least eight of the strategies that the nurse can use during hospitalisation with a child who has lost his or her sight.

13. Which of the following statements is correct about eye care and sports?
    a. Glasses may interfere with the child's ability in sports.
    b. Eye protection gear should be worn for golfing.
    c. Corrective lenses provide less visual acuity than glasses for sports.
    d. Corrective lenses improve visual acuity so children are able to compete more effectively in sports.

14. T F The most common cause of impaired hearing loss is acute otitis media.

III. THINKING CRITICALLY

1. Outline three recommendations a nurse can suggest to help parents prepare the school setting to support the social integration of their hearing impaired child.

2. List three strategies nurses can implement to support a child with autism spectrum disorder who requires hospitalisation.

3. List three aspects of discharge teaching that families need when their child has undergone enucleation because of retinoblastoma.

43 Family-Centred Care of the Child During Illness and Hospitalization

I. LEARNING KEY TERMS

MATCHING: Match each term with its corresponding description.

1. _____ An effective, nondirective modality for helping children deal with their concerns and fears; often helpful to the nurse in gaining insights into children's needs and feelings.

2. _____ Provides an expressive outlet for creative ideas and interests; An effective tool for managing a child's stress.

3. _____ A psychologic technique reserved for use by trained and qualified therapists as an interpretive method with emotionally disturbed children.

4. _____ The major stress from middle infancy throughout the preschool years, especially for children ages 6 to 30 months, also called anaclitic depression.

5. _____ One of the most traumatic hospital experiences for the child and parents.

6. _____ Health care providers with extensive knowledge of child growth and development and of the special psychosocial needs of hospitalised children.

a. Separation anxiety

b. Play

c. Emergency admission

d. Child life specialists

e. Play therapy

f. Therapeutic play

II. REVIEWING KEY CONCEPTS

1. Major stressors of hospitalisation in children include:
   a. loss of control.
   b. separation.
   c. fear of bodily injury.
   d. pain.
   e. all of the above.

MATCHING: Match each phase of separation anxiety with the behaviours that are typical of that phase.

2. _____ Inactive; withdraws from others; uninterested in environment, play, or food.

3. _____ Becomes more interested in surroundings and plays with others; resulting from resignation to the situation.

4. _____ Cries and screams; refuse attention of anyone else; inconsolable.

a. Protest

b. Despair

c. Detachment

5. T F Preschoolers may demonstrate separation anxiety by refusing to eat, experiencing difficulty in sleeping, crying quietly for their parents, continually asking when the parents will visit, or withdrawing from others.

6. T F Parents of a hospitalised child may experience a sense of helplessness, question the skill level of the staff yet seek reassurance from caregivers.

7. What age group is more likely to experience increased stress to hospitalisation and loss of peer group contact?
   a. Preschooler
   b. Middle school-age child
   c. Adolescent
   d. Early school-age child

8. Which of the following risk factors make a child more vulnerable to the stressors of hospitalisation?
   a. Male gender
   b. Strong support network
   c. Female gender
   d. Passive temperament

9. Describe at least three posthospital stay behaviours commonly observed in young children.

10. Siblings who visit their brother or sister in the hospital have an increased tendency to exhibit which of the following behaviours?
    a. Resentment
    b. Anger
    c. Guilt
    d. Acceptance
    e. a, b, and c

11. To help the parents deal with the issues related to separation while their child is hospitalised, the nurse should suggest that parents:
    a. quietly leave while the child is distracted or asleep.
    b. make the surroundings familiar with the child's toys from home.
    c. encourage infrequent parental visits to help decrease the child's frequency of disappointment.
    d. visit over one extended time if rooming-in is impossible.

12. One technique used during hospitalisation that can minimise the disruption in the routine of the school-age child who is not critically ill is:
    a. stop school activities.
    b. wear hospital scrubs.
    c. encourage self-care.
    d. watch television.

13. Preparing children for intrusive procedures usually increases their:
    a. ability to cooperate.
    b. fear.
    c. stress.
    d. misconceptions.

14. Whenever performing a painful procedure on a child, the nurse should attempt to:
    a. perform the procedure in the playroom.
    b. perform the procedure in the child's hospital room.
    c. perform the procedure as quickly as possible.
    d. request the parents leave during the procedure.

15. Which of the following reactions to surgery is most typical of an adolescent's reaction to fear of bodily injury?
    a. Concern about the pain
    b. Concern about the procedure itself
    c. Concern about the scar
    d. Understanding explanations literally

16. Identify three factors that affect parents' reactions to their child's illness.

17. Describe techniques for modifying procedural techniques for children in each age group which may assist in minimising fear of bodily injury.

III. THINKING CRITICALLY

1. Six-year old Abhijeet experienced several injuries from a motor vehicle collision that required admission to CCU. After 3 weeks in CCU, Abhijeet is ready for transfer to the Orthopaedics unit. Discuss the strategies that a critical care nurse can implement to help families transition from the ICU setting to a regular unit setting.

2. Three-year old Siobhan required day surgery to repair an inguinal hernia. Outline aspects of discharge teaching the nurse will provide for the family when Siobhan goes home.

44 Pediatric Variations of Nursing Interventions

I. LEARNING KEY TERMS

MATCHING: Match each term with its corresponding description.

1. _____ Provides for total nutritional needs when feeding by way of the gastrointestinal tract is impossible, inadequate, or hazardous.

2. _____ A noninvasive method of providing continual monitoring of partial pressure of oxygen in arterial blood that uses an electrode that is attached to the skin.

3. _____ Precautions designed for the care of all patients to reduce the risk of transmission of microorganisms from both recognised and unrecognised sources of infection.

4. _____ Designed to reduce the risk of transmission of droplets suspended in the air for long periods of time.

5. _____ Designed to reduce the risk of transmission of infectious agents generated from the source person primarily during coughing, sneezing, or talking and during the performance of certain procedures such as suctioning and bronchoscopy.

6. _____ No longer dependent on parents or legal guardians.

7. _____ A continuous, noninvasive method of determining oxygen saturation; used to guide oxygen therapy.

8. _____ Designed to reduce the risk of transmission by direct or indirect contact through patients known or suspected to be colonised with microorganisms.

9. _____ A noninvasive measurement of exhaled carbon dioxide.

10. _____ An alternative device to keeping an intravenous line intact when extended venous access is required for intermittent use.

11. _____ Refers to the legal requirement of ensuring the patient and their legal surrogate receive appropriate and sufficient information regarding treatment plans, have decision-making capacity and make decisions voluntarily.

12. _____ Different types of catheters inserted into and positioned within a vein in the body; may include tunnelled or non-tunnelled catheters.

a. Informed consent

b. Emancipated minor

c. Routine Precautions

d. Airborne precautions

e. Droplet precautions

f. Contact precautions

g. Intermittent infusion device

h. Central venous access device

i. End-tidal carbon dioxide monitoring

j. Pulse oximetry

k. Transcutaneous oxygen monitoring

l. Total parenteral nutrition

II. REVIEWING KEY CONCEPTS

1. Which of the following routes is the preferred method of medication administration in children?
   a. Intravenous
   b. Intramuscular
   c. Oral
   d. Otic

2. The nurse is preparing to administer an oral medication to a young child. The nurse's best approach to involve the child's cooperation is reflected in which statement?
   a. "Do you want to take this medicine now? It tastes yummy."
   b. "It's time for your pain medicine. Would you like water or juice to drink with it?"
   c. "Here's your medicine. Do you want me to give it to you or would you rather your mother give it?"
   d. "Here is your pain medicine. Please take it or you will have lots of pain."

3. If a child needs support during an invasive procedure, what should the nurse do?
   a. Inform the parents about how the child did after the procedure.
   b. Ask the parents to stay in the room, where they can have eye contact with the child.
   c. Determine parent and child's preference related to parental presence during procedure.
   d. Encourage the parents to stay close by to console the child immediately following the procedure.

4. List at least five strategies the nurse can use to support the child during and after a procedure.

5. Describe at least one play activity for each of the following procedures.
   a. Ambulation
   b. Range of motion
   c. Injections
   d. Deep breathing
   e. Extending the environment
   f. Soaks
   g. Fluid intake

6. T F When administering eye drops and eye ointment, the eye drops should be administered first, followed by the eye ointment 3 minutes later.

7. T F When administering a medication via the rectum, if the suppository must be halved it should be cut lengthwise and inserted with the apex first.

8. T F The angle for injection for a subcutaneous medication is typically 90 degrees.

9. Which of the following examples of provides optimal documentation of a child's food intake?
   a. Child ate about a cup of cereal with ½ cup of milk.
   b. Child ate an adequate breakfast.
   c. Child ate 80% of the breakfast served.
   d. Parent states that child ate an adequate breakfast.

10. The best positioning technique for a lumbar puncture in a child is a:
    a. side-lying position with neck flexion.
    b. sitting position.
    c. side-lying position with modified neck extension.
    d. side-lying position, head flexed with knees to chest.

11. The most frequently used site for bone marrow aspiration in children is the:
    a. femur.
    b. sternum.
    c. tibia.
    d. iliac crest.

12. To avoid the complication of necrotizing osteochondritis when performing infant heel puncture, the puncture should be:
    a. no deeper than 4 mm and on the inner aspect of the heel.
    b. no deeper than 2 mm and on the outer aspect of the heel.
    c. no deeper than 2 mm and on the inner aspect of the heel.
    d. no deeper than 4 mm and on the outer aspect of the heel.

13. To obtain a sputum specimen for RSV in an infant, the nurse would optimally:
    a. have the infant cough.
    b. obtain mucus from the throat.
    c. insert a suction catheter into the back of the throat.
    d. instil 1–3 ml of sterile normal saline into a nostril

14. Of the following choices for measuring 5 ml of medication at home, the best device for the nurse to instruct the parent to use at home is the:
    a. household soup spoon.
    b. household measuring spoon.
    c. hospital's USP standard dropper.
    d. calibrated hollow-handled medicine spoon.

15. All of the following techniques for medication administration to an infant are acceptable except:
    a. adding the medication to the infant's bottle of formula.
    b. allowing the infant to sit in the parent's lap during administration.
    c. allowing the infant to suck the medication from an empty nipple.
    d. inserting the needleless syringe into the side of the mouth while the infant nurses.

16. T F The needle length needed for intramuscular injections will vary depending on the amount of subcutaneous fat a child has. The needle length must be long enough to penetrate the subcutaneous fat and deposit the medication into the body of the muscle.

17. The preferred site for intramuscular injection in an infant is the:
    a. deltoid muscle.
    b. dorsolateral.
    c. vastus lateralis.
    d. ventrolateral.

18. Total parenteral nutrition (TPN) is infused through a central venous access device because:
    a. other medications need to be infused with the TPN.
    b. several attempts to administer it peripherally have probably occurred.
    c. there is less risk of infection.
    d. the concentration of glucose in the solution is irritating to the smaller veins.

19. To instil eye drops in an infant whose eyelids are clenched shut, the nurse should:
    a. apply finger pressure to the lacrimal punctum.
    b. place the drops in the nasal corner where the lids meet and wait until the infant opens the lid.
    c. administer the eye drops before nap time.
    d. do all of the above.

20. During intermittent or continuous enteral feedings, the nurse could:
    a. push the formula gradually through the feeding tube.
    b. use a parenteral burette to calibrate the feeding times.
    c. give the infant a pacifier for non-nutritive sucking.
    d. hang the feeding container from an IV pole.

21. A 3-year-old with cystic fibrosis has a gastrostomy feeding device to supplement nutritional intake. The parent notes moist and beefy red tissue around the insertion site but there is no evidence of foul odour, bleeding, or formula leakage. The nurse reassures the parent this finding is consistent with:
    a. a skin infection.
    b. normal granulation tissue.
    c. a reason to change the device.
    d. a reason to discontinue using this device.

22. One of the major advantages of the recently developed skin-level feeding devices is that the button device:
    a. does not clog as easily as other devices.
    b. eliminates the need for frequent burping.
    c. is less expensive than the traditional devices.
    d. allows the child more mobility.

23. A 7-year-old child is being prepared for bowel surgery. The best agent for bowel cleansing in this child is:
    a. a paediatric Fleet enema.
    b. a commercially prepared hypertonic enema solution.
    c. an oral or nasogastric tube administration of polyethylene glycol–electrolyte solution.
    d. plain water enemas.

24. In order to protect the pouch and stoma site, a young child with an ostomy may need to:
    a. wear a loose-fitting one-piece outfit.
    b. begin toilet training at a later than usual age.
    c. limit activity to avoid skin damage.
    d. use elbow restraints at all times.

25. In an infant with an unpouched colostomy, optimal skin care around the stoma would include:
    a. a barrier substance such as zinc oxide.
    b. a larger diaper than the one usually worn.
    c. stoma powder mixed with skin barrier substance.
    d. a, b, and c.

III. THINKING CRITICALLY

1. Discuss the purpose, rationale, and requirements for the use of physical, chemical, and environmental restraints in children.

2. Discuss the current evidence as well as best practise for verifying NG tube placement in a young (18-month-old) paediatric patient.

3. Carson, a 10 year old patient, recently required bowel surgery and was admitted to ICU after a complex operation, requiring mechanical ventilation. The nurse notes a sudden change in Carson's vital signs including pulse oximetry and end-tidal carbon dioxide monitoring. Outline the details of the DOPE pneumonic the nurse and health care team will employ.

45 Respiratory Conditions

I. LEARNING KEY TERMS

MATCHING: Match each term with its corresponding description.

1. _____ A measurement of the maximum flow of air that can be forcefully exhaled in 1 second.

2. _____ Provide an objective method of evaluating the presence and degree of lung disease, as well as the response to therapy.

3. _____ Cessation of breathing for more than 20 seconds or for a shorter period of time when associated with cyanosis, pallor or bradycardia; may be central, obstructive or mixed in nature.

4. _____ A medical emergency that can result in respiratory failure and death if untreated.

5. _____ Involves stimulating the production of sweat with a special device (stimulation with 3-mA electric current), collecting the sweat on filter paper, and measuring the sweat electrolytes; used in the diagnosis of cystic fibrosis.

6. _____ Inability of the respiratory system to maintain adequate oxygenation of the blood, with or without carbon dioxide retention.

7. _____ A serious obstructive inflammatory process supraglottic.

8. _____ In general, applies to two conditions: increased work of breathing with near normal gas exchange function or the inability to maintain normal blood gas tensions that develops from carbon dioxide retention with subsequent hypoxemia and acidosis.

9. _____ Broad term referring to a group of acute and infectious processes that are characterised by a bark-like or brassy cough; may be associated with hoarseness, inspiratory stridor and varying degrees of respiratory distress.

10. _____ The earliest manifestation of cystic fibrosis where the small intestine is blocked with thick, puttylike, tenacious, mucilaginous meconium in the newborn.

11. _____ The child insists on sitting upright and leaning forward with the chin thrust out, mouth open, and tongue protruding to facilitate breathing.

12. _____ occur when the immune system becomes sensitive and reacts to elements in the environment e.g. house dust mites, tobacco smoke, mold, or pets.

13. _____ An infection of the mucosa of the upper trachea with features of both croup and epiglottitis; may cause serious airway obstruction.

a. Bacterial tracheitis

b. Croup

c. Tripod position

d. Acute epiglottitis

e. Status asthmaticus

f. Pulmonary function tests (PFTs)

g. Peak expiratory flow rate (PEFR)

h. Allergen

i. Meconium ileus

j. Respiratory insufficiency

k. Respiratory failure

l. Pertussis

m. Sweat chloride test

n. Direct observation therapy (DOT)

o. Airway clearance therapies

p. Apnea

213

14. _____ Essential part of CF management and includes several modalities that require individualization to determine optimal impact of the patient.

15. _____ Health care worker or delegate is present when medications are administered to the patient.

16. _____ Highly contagious acute respiratory tract infection; symptoms may last for 6 to 10 weeks or longer.

II. REVIEWING KEY CONCEPTS

1. Most respiratory infections in children are caused by:
   a. pneumococci.
   b. viruses.
   c. streptococci.
   d. *Haemophilus influenzae*.

2. The most likely reason that the respiratory infection rate increases drastically in the age range from 3 to 6 months is that the:
   a. infant's exposure to pathogens is greatly increased during this time.
   b. viral agents that are mild in older children are extremely severe in infants.
   c. maternal antibodies have decreased and the infant's own antibody production is immature.
   d. diameter of the airways is smaller in the infant than in the older child.

3. Children exposed to passive (secondhand) or environmental tobacco smoke have:
   a. an increased number of respiratory illnesses.
   b. increased respiratory symptoms.
   c. reduced performance on PFTs.
   d. all of the above.

4. Which of the following is the best choice for the child with acute respiratory infections?
   a. IV fluid restriction
   b. Maintenance of patient comfort
   c. Insist that the child play quietly in bed.
   d. Use of hot steam vapouriser

5. The best means for prevention of the spread of nasopharyngitis is:
   a. prompt immunization.
   b. frequent hand washing and avoiding touching one's eyes andnose.
   c. mist vaporization.
   d. to ensure adequate fluid intake.

6. Group A β-hemolytic streptococcal (GABHS) infection is usually a:
   a. serious infection of the upper airway.
   b. common cause of pharyngitis in children over the age of 15 years.

c. brief illness that places the child at risk for serious sequelae, including rheumatic fever.
d. disease of the heart, lungs, joints, and central nervous system.

7. In the postoperative period following a tonsillectomy, the child should be:
   a. placed in the Trendelenburg position.
   b. encouraged to cough and deep breathe.
   c. suctioned vigorously to clear the airway.
   d. placed on abdomen or side to facilitate drainage of secretions.

8. The best pain medication administration regimen for a child in the initial postoperative period following a tonsillectomy is:
   a. at regular intervals.
   b. as needed.

9. Of the foods listed, the most appropriate selection to offer first to an alert child who is in the postoperative period following a tonsillectomy is:
   a. strawberry ice cream.
   b. red cherry-flavored gelatin.
   c. an apple-flavored ice pop.
   d. cold diluted orange juice.

10. Which of the following signs is an early indication of haemorrhage in a child who has had a tonsillectomy?
    a. continuous swallowing
    b. decreasing blood pressure
    c. restlessness
    d. a, b, and c

11. During influenza epidemics, it is generally believed the age group that provides a major source of transmission is the:
    a. infant.
    b. school-age child.
    c. adolescent.
    d. preschool-age child.

12. Which of the following is not a typical clinical manifestation of the influenza virus?
    a. Nausea and vomiting
    b. Fever and chills
    c. dry throat and nasal mucosa
    d. Photophobia and myalgia

13. The diagnosis of acute otitis media is made if:
    a. the tympanic membrane reveals a purulent discoloured effusion.
    b. a bulging or full, opacified tympanic membrane.
    c. acute onset of ear pain.
    d. all of the above.

14. Risk factors for otitis media include:
    a. a higher prevalence in the summer months.
    b. preschool age girls.
    c. exposure to passive cigarette smoking.
    d. none of the above.

15. The nurse should prepare for an impending emergency situation to care for the child with suspected:
    a. spasmodic croup.
    b. laryngotracheobronchitis.
    c. acute spasmodic laryngitis.
    d. acute supraglottitis.

16. The nurse should suspect epiglottitis if the child has:
    a. cough, sore throat, and agitation.
    b. cough, drooling, and retractions.
    c. absence of cough in the presence of fever, drooling of saliva and painful swallowing.
    d. absence of cough, hoarseness, and retractions.

17. In the child who is suspected of having epiglottitis, the nurse should:
    a. have intubation equipment available.
    b. visually inspect the child's oropharynx with a tongue blade.
    c. obtain a throat culture.
    d. prepare to immunise the child for *Haemophilus influenzae.*

18. Since the advent of immunisation for *Haemophilus influenzae*, there has been a decrease in the incidence of:
    a. laryngotracheobronchitis.
    b. epiglottitis.
    c. influenza (seasonal).
    d. croup.

19. The nurse may anticipate intubation as the care management for the young child diagnosed with:
    a. acute spasmodic laryngitis.
    b. bacterial trachealis.
    c. acute laryngotracheobronchitis.
    d. acute laryngitis.

20. Respiratory syncytial virus (RSV) is:
    a. an uncommon virus that causes severe bronchiolitis.
    b. an uncommon virus that usually does not require hospitalisation.
    c. a common virus that usually occurs primarily in winter and early spring.
    d. a common virus that usually does not require hospitalisation.

21. The use of palivizumab is given in high-risk populations because:
    a. it helps prevent RSV
    b. it is an antiviral agent
    c. it helps treat patients at low risk for mortality
    d. it can be used for any infant

22. Nursing care management of the 6-month-old infant with RSV bronchiolitis might include:
    a. maintain adequate oxygenation as measured by pulse oximetry.
    b. periodic superficial suctioning if abundant nasal secretions present.
    c. small, frequent feeds to maintain hydration.
    d. a, b, and c.

23. General signs of bacterial pneumonia include:
    a. gradual onset
    b. clear breath sounds and foul-smelling sputum.
    c. fever and rapid, shallow respirations.
    d. accompanied with diarrhea.

24. Which of the following is the most common bacterial pathogen responsible for community-acquired pneumonia in newborns to age 4 years?
    a. *Haemophilus pneumoniae*
    b. *Mycoplasma pneumoniae*
    c. *Staphylococcus aureus pneumoniae*
    d. *Streptococcus pneumoniae*

25. The best test to screen for tuberculosis infection is the:
    a. chest radiograph.
    b. tuberculin skin test (TST).
    c. sputum culture.
    d. DNA blood test.

26. The child who has active tuberculosis infection is treated with:
    a. isoniazid.
    b. rifampin.
    c. pyrazinamide.
    d. ethambutol
    e. a combination of the above drugs.

27. Severity of a foreign body aspiration is determined by:
    a. location of the object in the airway.
    b. the type of object aspirated.
    c. the extent of obstruction.
    d. a, b, and c.

28. The term *latent tuberculosis infection* (LTBI) is used to indicate infection in a person with:
    a. positive TST.
    b. absence of physical findings of disease.
    c. a normal chest radiograph.
    d. a, b, and c.

29. The nurse examines a 6-year-old child with asthma and notes there are intercostal and substernal retractions. Breath sounds reveal a loud pan-expiratory and inspiratory wheeze and oxygen saturations remain at 90% in room air. His peak flow versus personal best is 80%. Based on these findings, the nurse suspects that there is:
   a. moderate asthma.
   b. severe asthma.
   c. mild asthma.
   d. impending respiratory failure.

30. Which of the following principles should be a part of the home self-management programme for a child with asthma?
   a. Individuals must learn not to abuse their medications so that they will not become addicted.
   b. It is easy to treat an asthmatic episode as long as the child knows the symptoms.
   c. Although quite uncommon, asthma is very treatable.
   d. Children with asthma are usually able to participate in the same activities as nonasthmatic children.

31. The principal treatment for the pancreatic insufficiency which occurs in cystic fibrosis is the administration of:
   a. enemas.
   b. corticosteroids.
   c. antibiotics.
   d. enzymes.

32. Which of the following strategies would be used cautiously as an acute management strategy for cystic fibrosis?
   a. Forced expiration
   b. Aerobic exercise
   c. Supplemental oxygen
   d. Percussion and postural drainage

33. Dietary supplements are given in cystic fibrosis in the form of:
   a. multivitamins.
   b. water-miscible form of vitamins.
   c. pancreatic enzymes.
   d. a, b, and c.

34. List the four cardinal signs of impending respiratory failure.

35. Which of the following represent the early subtle signs of hypoxia?
   a. Peripheral cyanosis
   b. Central cyanosis
   c. Hypotension
   d. Change in level of consciousness

MATCHING: Match each drug used for paediatric emergency care with its appropriate use during resuscitation.

36. _____ β-adrenergic agonist used as an inhaled bronchodilator for acute exacerbations of bronchospasm.

37. _____ Intravenous antibiotic of choice in otitis media when causative organism is a highly resistant pneumococcus.

38. _____ A long-acting β2-agonist (bronchodilator) that is used twice a day (no more frequently than every 12 hours) for long-term prevention of asthma symptoms.

39. _____ A potent intravenous muscle relaxant that acts to decrease inflammation and improves pulmonary function and peak flow rate among paediatric patients with severe asthma.

40. _____ First-line drug for pulmonary tuberculosis infection.

41. _____ anti-inflammatory agent used as a key management strategy for treatment of asthma.

42. _____ Leukotriene modifier that blocks inflammatory and bronchospasm effects of asthma; long term oral agent.

43. _____ Anticholinergic that acts as a bronchodilator to relieve acute asthma symptoms; does not elicit CNS effects.

a. Inhaled corticosteroid

b. Ceftriaxone

c. Magnesium sulphate

d. Singulair

e. Salmeterol

f. Amoxicillin

g. Dornase alpha (Pulmozyme)

h. Albuterol

i. Ipratropium

j. Omalizumab (Xolair)

k. Hypertonic saline

l. Isoniazid

44. _____ When nebulised it has been shown to be effective in improving airway hydration and increasing mucous clearance in patients with CF.

45. _____ A monoclonal antibody that blocks the binding of IgE to mast cells; inhibits the inflammation that is associated with asthma and it is used in patients with moderate to persistent asthma who have confirmed perennial aeroallergen sensitivity.

46. _____ Nebulised agent that acts to decrease the viscosity of mucus to improve airway clearance for management of cystic fibrosis.

47. _____ First-line choice oral antibiotic for the treatment of acute otitis media.

III. THINKING CRITICALLY

1. Describe the parameters that the nurse should assess to recognise status asthmaticus.

2. Explain the rationale for each of the following clinical manifestations of cystic fibrosis.

   a. Pulmonary

   b. Restricted growth and development

   c. Future reproduction potential

3. Describe the instructions the nurse should give to a mother of a child with tuberculosis infection about returning to school.

46 Gastrointestinal Conditions

I. LEARNING KEY TERMS

MATCHING: Match each term with its corresponding description.

1. _____ Inflammation of the blind sac at the end of the caecum, the most common cause of abdominal surgery in childhood.

2. _____ A protrusion of a portion of an organ or organs through an abnormal opening.

3. _____ Characterised by extremely long intervals between defecation.

4. _____ Alteration in the frequency, consistency, or ease of passing stool.

5. _____ Absence of ganglion cells in the affected intestine resulting in mechanical obstruction from inadequate motility.

6. _____ Transfer of gastric contents into the oesophagus occurring throughout the day most frequently after meals and at night.

7. _____ Complications arising from transfer of gastric contents into the oesophagus (e.g., failure to thrive, respiratory problems, dysphagia).

8. _____ Trace elements with a daily requirement of less than 100 mg; exact role in nutrition unclear.

9. _____ Constipation with faecal soiling.

10. _____ Chronic inflammatory process involving any part of the GI tract from the mouth to the anus, most often affecting the terminal ileum.

11. _____ Essential nutrients with daily requirements greater than 100 mg (e.g., calcium, phosphorus, magnesium, sodium, potassium, chloride, and sulfur).

12. _____ Inflammation of the colon and rectum with distal colon and rectum most severely affected.

a. Macrominerals

b. Microminerals

c. Gastroesophageal reflux

d. Hernia

e. Appendicitis

f. Ulcerative colitis

g. Crohn disease

h. Gastroesophageal reflux disease

i. Hirschsprung disease

j. Constipation

k. Obstipation

l. Encopresis

II. REVIEWING KEY CONCEPTS

1. Malnutrition may occur when:
   a. gastroenteritis is a major factor in general daily life.
   b. diversity of food consumed is unlimited.
   c. neighbourhoods have access to affordable food.
   d. the diet consists mainly of starch grains.

2. Kwashiorkor occurs when:
   a. the food supply is inadequate.
   b. the food supply is adequate for fat requirements.
   c. food preparation occurs in unsanitary conditions.
   d. the diet consists mainly of starch grains with subsequent high-quality protein deficiency.

3. Marasmus occurs when:
   a. the child develops generalised edema.
   b. fat metabolism is grossly impaired.
   c. the adults eat first, leaving insufficient food for children.
   d. the diet consists mainly of starch grains with subsequent high-quality protein deficiency.

4. Which of the following diagnostic strategies is considered the most definitive for identifying a cow's milk allergy?
   a. Stool analysis for blood
   b. Serum IgE levels
   c. milk elimination from diet with subsequent resolution of symptoms followed by challenge testing
   d. Skin prick or scratch testing

5. A child with extreme sensitivity related to food allergies:
   a. stay home from school.
   b. rarely 'outgrow' their food allergy.
   c. should carry injectable epinephrine.
   d. typically present with hives and flushing.

6. Treatment of diagnosed cow's milk allergy in infants ideally involves changing the formula to:
   a. soy-based formula.
   b. goat's milk.
   c. casein hydrolysate milk formula.
   d. whole milk.

7. Infants are at high risk for fluid and electrolyte imbalance. Which of the following factors contributes to this vulnerability?
   a. Decreased body surface area
   b. Lower metabolic rate
   c. Mature kidney function including stable glomerular filtration rate
   d. Increased body fluid contained in extracellular fluid volume

8. _____ dehydration occurs when electrolyte and water deficits are present in approximately balanced proportion.

9. _____ dehydration occurs when the electrolyte deficit exceeds the water deficit. There is a greater loss of extracellular fluid, and plasma sodium concentration is usually _____ than 130 mmol/L.

10. _____ dehydration results from water loss in excess of electrolyte loss. This is often caused by a larger _____ of water and/or a larger _____ of electrolytes. Plasma sodium concentration is _____ than 150 mmol/L.

11. Which of the following choices most accurately describes dehydration or fluid loss in infants and young children?
    a. As a percentage of body weight lost
    b. In millilitres per kilogramme of body weight
    c. By the amount of oedema present
    d. By the degree of skin elasticity

12. List eight assessment findings that may be used to determine dehydration in a child.

13. A priority goal in the management of acute diarrhoea is:
    a. determining the cause of the diarrhoea.
    b. preventing the spread of the infection.
    c. rehydration of the child.
    d. managing the fever associated with the diarrhea.

14. To confirm the diagnosis of Hirschsprung disease, the nurse prepares the child for:
    a. endoscopy.
    b. sonogram.
    c. rectal biopsy.
    d. oesophagostomy.

15. The nurse would expect to see which of the following clinical manifestations in the child diagnosed with Hirschsprung disease?
    a. History of bloody diarrhea, fever, and vomiting
    b. Irritability, severe abdominal cramps, and faecal soiling
    c. Increased serum lipids and positive stool for O&P (ova and parasites)
    d. Constipation (failure to pass meconium as newborn), abdominal distention, may appear quite unwell if presenting in infancy.

16. The parents of a 2-month-old with gastroesophageal reflux are counselled by the nurse to include which of the following in the infant's care?
    a. Spread out the feeding intervals to reduce the total number of feedings.
    b. After feeding and burping, position the infant prone when awake and observed, or carry in an upright position
    c. After feeding and burping, position the infant on the back with the head turned to the side.
    d. Increase feeding volume right before bedtime.

17. Which of the following would alert the nurse to possible peritonitis in a child suspected of having appendicitis?
    a. Colicky abdominal pain with guarding of the abdomen
    b. Periumbilical pain that progresses to the lower right quadrant of the abdomen with an elevated WBC
    c. Low-grade fever with the child having difficulty walking and assuming a side-lying position with the knees flexed toward the chest
    d. Fever, progressive abdominal distention, tachycardia and sudden relief from acute abdominal pain

18. The most common clinical manifestations expected with Meckel diverticulum include:
    a. fever, vomiting, and constipation.
    b. weight loss, hypotension, and obstruction.
    c. painless rectal bleeding, abdominal pain, or signs of intestinal obstruction.
    d. abdominal pain, bloody diarrhea, and foul-smelling stool.

219

19. A common occurrence of Crohn disease is:
   a. growth delay.
   b. chronic constipation.
   c. obstruction.
   d. burning epigastric pain.

20. Which clinical manifestation would be the most suggestive of acute appendicitis?
   a. Abdominal pain relieved by eating
   b. Red, currant jelly–like stools
   c. Ribbon like, foul-smelling stools
   d. Abdominal pain most intense at McBurney point

21. The single most effective strategy to prevent the spread of viral hepatitis is _____.

22. _____ is the most important cause of serious gastroenteritis among children and a significant health care-associated pathogen; most severe in children 3 to 24 months of age.

MATCHING: Match each viral hepatitis type with its corresponding description.

23. _____ Particularly prevalent in developing countries with poor living conditions, inadequate sanitation, crowding, and poor personal hygiene practices; spread associated with improper food handling.

24. _____ Transmission usually through exchange of blood or body fluids; universal vaccination recommended for all children.

25. _____ Endemic in Asia, South America, the Middle East and Western and Northern Africa; does not cause chronic liver disease.

26. _____ Rare in North America; requires the helper function Hepatitis B.

27. _____ Transmitted from mother to child, blood or blood product transfusion, organ/tissue transplant or sharing of used needles; may become a chronic condition.

a. Hepatitis A
b. Hepatitis B
c. Hepatitis C
d. Hepatitis D
e. Hepatitis E

28. The definition of *biliary atresia* is:
   a. persistent jaundice with elevated direct bilirubin levels.
   b. progressive inflammatory process causing bile duct fibrosis and obstruction.
   c. absence of bile pigment.
   d. hepatomegaly and palpable liver.

29. The most common early symptom of biliary atresia is:
   a. projectile vomiting.
   b. bloody stools.
   c. alcoholic stools.
   d. jaundice.

30. _____ is often a significant problem in children with biliary atresia that is addressed by drug therapy or comfort measures such as baths in colloidal oatmeal compounds.

31. To assess for the presence of a cleft palate, the nurse should:
   a. assess the infant's ability to swallow.
   b. assess the colour of the infant's oral mucosa.
   c. palpate the hard palate with a gloved finger.
   d. flick the infant's foot and make it cry.

32. One of the major problems for infants born with cleft lip and palate is related to:
   a. rejection by the mother.
   b. feeding problems despite normal swallowing.
   c. apnea and bradycardia.
   d. aspiration pneumonia.

33. Postoperative care for the infant with a cleft lip and palate repair would *not* include the strategy of:
   a. applying bilateral elbow immobilizers.
   b. application of petroleum jelly to surgical site.
   c. placing child in the upright infant seat position.
   d. vigorously suctioning the infant's mouth for secretions.

34. Feeding the infant with surgical repair of either a cleft lip or palate postoperatively includes:
   I. Adequate pain analgesia
   II. use of an upright position or infant seat
   III. cleft palate repair feedings include the use of spoons.
   IV. feeding is resumed when tolerated, using a blenderized or soft diet
   a. I and II
   b. I, II, III, and IV
   c. I and III
   d. I, II and IV

35. A segment of the bowel invaginates into a more distal segment of the bowel, pulling the mesentery with it is called:
    a. intussusception.
    b. pyloric stenosis.
    c. tracheoesophageal fistula.
    d. Hirschsprung disease.

36. A 5-month-old infant suspected of having intussusception would most likely have what clinical manifestations?
    a. Crying, vomiting, and currant jelly–appearing stools
    b. Fever, diarrhea, vomiting, and decreased WBC
    c. Weight gain, constipation, and refusal to eat
    d. Abdominal distention, periodic pain, and hypotension

37. A 5-month-old infant's intussusception is treated with conservative treatment with radiology imaging guidance. The nurse should expect care after the reduction to include:
    a. administration of antibiotics.
    b. enema administration to remove remaining stool.
    c. close observation of stool patterns and passage of any contrast material.
    d. blood pressure every 4 hours.

38. The nurse observes frothy saliva in the mouth and nose of the neonate who is a few hours old. When fed, the infant swallows normally, but suddenly the fluid returns through the nose and mouth of the infant. The nurse suspects:
    a. esophageal atresia.
    b. pyloric stenosis.
    c. anorectal malformation.
    d. biliary atresia.

39. A 1-month-old infant is brought to the clinic by his mother. The nurse suspects pyloric stenosis because the mother gives a history of:
    a. diarrhea.
    b. projectile nonbilious vomiting.
    c. fever.
    d. abdominal distention.

40. The preoperative nursing plan for an infant with pyloric obstruction should include:
    a. restoration of hydration and electrolyte balance by intravenous fluids.
    b. nasogastric (NG) tube placement to decompress the stomach.
    c. parental support and reassurance.
    d. a, b, and c.

41. The assessment finding that is most likely to indicate an anorectal malformation is:
    a. abdominal distention and vomiting.
    b. a normal-appearing perineum.
    c. passage of meconium stool after 24 hours.
    d. failure to pass meconium through the anal opening.

42. The most important therapeutic management for the child with celiac disease is:
    a. eliminating corn, rice, and millet from the diet.
    b. adding iron, folic acid, and fat-soluble vitamins to the diet.
    c. eliminating wheat, rye, and barley from the diet.
    d. educating the child's parents about the short-term effects of the disease and the necessity of reading all food labels for content until the disease is in remission.

43. The prognosis for children with short bowel syndrome has improved as a result of:
    a. dietary supplemental vitamin B12 additions.
    b. improvement in surgical procedures.
    c. improved home care availability to reduces episodes of sepsis.
    d. advances in parenteral nutrition and understanding the importance of enteral feeding.

44. A common long-term complication after surgical repair of esophageal atresia is:
    a. pneumonia.
    b. feeding difficulties.
    c. pneumothorax.
    d. short bowel syndrome.

45. Describe the 3 phases of parenteral rehydration therapy for the child diagnosed with moderate dehydration.

III. THINKING CRITICALLY

1. Baby Rory was born at 36 weeks in good condition, birthweight 3.2 kg. On day of life 3, Rory developed bilious emesis with abdominal distension and blood was noted in the stool. As Rory's nurse you understand the importance of communicating Rory's change in condition immediately. An upper GI study was completed and a malrotation was evident. Explain why malrotation is a serious obstruction and requires urgent attention.

2. Differentiate between ulcerative colitis and Crohn disease in relation to pathology, rectal bleeding, diarrhoea, pain, anorexia, weight loss, and growth restriction.

47 Cardiovascular Conditions

I. LEARNING KEY TERMS

MATCHING: Match each term with its corresponding description.

1. _____ Abnormally fast heart rate.

2. _____ The consistent elevation of blood pressure beyond values considered to be the upper limits of normal.

3. _____ Abnormally slow heart rate.

4. _____ Refers to abnormalities of the myocardium in which the cardiac muscles' ability to contract is impaired; relatively rare in children.

5. _____ Refers to excessive cholesterol in the blood; believed to play an important role in atherosclerosis development.

6. _____ A general term for excessive lipids (fat) and fatlike substances; believed to play an important role in atherosclerosis development.

7. _____ Strategies to terminate supraventricular tachycardia (SVT); may include applying ice to the face, massaging one carotid artery, or having the child exhale against a closed glottis.

8. _____ A thickening and flattening of the tips of the fingers and toes; thought to be a result of chronic tissue hypoxemia and polycythemia.

9. _____ Cardiovascular efficiency diminished; microcirculatory perfusion marginal despite compensatory adjustments; outcomes include tissue hypoxia, metabolic acidosis, and impairment of organ systems function.

10. _____ Procedure in which a radiopaque catheter is inserted through a peripheral blood vessel into the heart; contrast material injected; films taken of the dilution and circulation of the contrast material; used for diagnosis, treatment of valves/vessels, and electrophysiology studies.

11. _____ Slower than normal heart rate.

12. _____ Condition in which damage to vital organs that death occurs even if therapeutic intervention stabilises cardiovascular measurements.

13. _____ The inability of the heart to pump an adequate amount of blood to the systemic circulation to meet the metabolic demands of the body; often secondary to increases in blood volume and pressure within heart from cardiac anomalies; may also result from impaired ventricular contractility.

14. _____ Faster than normal heart rate.

15. _____ An increased number of red blood cells.

16. _____ Includes primarily anatomic abnormalities present at birth that result in abnormal cardiac function, the consequences of which are hypoxemia and heart failure.

a. Congenital heart disease
b. Acquired cardiac disorders
c. Tachycardia
d. Bradycardia
e. Cardiac catheterisation
f. Heart failure
g. Hypoxemia
h. Hypoxia
i. Cyanosis
j. Polycythemia
k. Clubbing
l. Hyperlipidemia
m. Hypercholesterolemia
n. Bradydysrhythmias
o. Tachydysrhythmias
p. Cardiomyopathy
q. Vagal manoeuvres
r. Systemic hypertension
s. Compensated shock
t. Decompensated shock
u. Irreversible shock

17. _____ Refers to an arterial oxygen tension (or pressure) that is less than normal and can be identified by a decreased arterial saturation or a decreased PaO_2.

18. _____ Vital organ function is maintained by intrinsic compensatory mechanism; blood flow is usually normal or increased, but generally uneven or maldistributed in the microcirculation.

19. _____ Disease processes or abnormalities that occur after birth and can be seen in the normal heart or in the presence of congenital heart defects resulting from factors such as infection, autoimmune responses, environmental factors, and familial tendencies.

20. _____ A reduction in tissue oxygenation that results from low oxygen saturation and PaO_2 and results in impaired cellular processes.

21. _____ A blue discolouration in the mucous membranes, skin, and nail beds of the child with reduced oxygen saturation; results from the presence of deoxygenated haemoglobin (haemoglobin not bound to oxygen); determined subjectively.

II. REVIEWING KEY CONCEPTS

1. During foetal life, oxygenated blood travels from the right atrium into the left atrium through a structure known as the:
   a. truncus arteriosus.
   b. foramen ovale.
   c. sinus venosus.
   d. ductus venosus.

2. In foetal circulation only a small amount of blood flows through the nonfunctioning:
   a. pulmonary circulation.
   b. ductus arteriosus.
   c. hepatic circulation.
   d. ductus venosus.

3. When an abnormal connection exists between the heart chambers (e.g., a septal defect), blood will flow from an area of higher pressure (left side) to one of lower pressure (right side). This is called a:
   a. left-to-right shunt.
   b. right-to-left shunt.

4. When preparing a child for cardiac catheterisation the nurse should:
   a. ask about allergies.
   b. assess and mark distal pulses.
   c. review current status for signs and symptoms of infection.
   d. provide information about the procedure to the child and parents.
   e. a, b, c, and d.

5. Coarctation of the aorta should be suspected when the:
   a. blood pressure is higher in the arms than in the legs.
   b. blood pressure in the right arm is different from the blood pressure in the left arm.
   c. apical pulse is greater than the radial pulse.
   d. point of maximum impulse is shifted to the right.

6. The test in which a transducer is placed in the oesophagus behind the heart to obtain images of posterior heart structures or used in patients with poor images from chest approach is the:
   a. electrocardiogram (EKG)
   b. echocardiogram (Echo)
   c. transesophageal echocardiogram (TEE)
   d. two-dimensional echocardiogram.(2-D Echo)

7. Priority nursing responsibilities after cardiac catheterisation in children includes:
   I. monitoring IV fluid intake and subsequently oral fluid intake.
   II. checking pulses below the site of catheterization.
   III. Assessing the temperature and colour of the affected extremity.
   IV. checking vital signs including blood pressure every 15 minutes.
   V. monitoring blood glucose levels in infants.
   VI. checking the dressing for bleeding.
   a. I, II, III, IV
   b. I, II, III, IV, and V
   c. I, II, III, IV, V, and VI
   d. II, III, IV, V, and VI

8. List possible complications following a cardiac catheterisation in an infant or young child.

9. If bleeding occurs at the insertion site after a cardiac catheterisation, the nurse should apply:
   a. warmth to the unaffected extremity.
   b. pressure below the insertion site.
   c. warmth to the affected extremity.
   d. pressure above the insertion site.

10. Signs and symptoms of supraventricular tachycardia (SVT) in an infant or young child may include:
    a. pallor.
    b. irritability.
    c. poor feeding.
    d. a, b, and c

11. A 4-year-old would be diagnosed as hypertensive with a systolic or diastolic blood pressure that:
    a. falls above the 99th percentile one time.
    b. consistently falls at or over the 95th percentile plus 5 mm Hg.
    c. falls between the 95th and 99th percentiles one time.
    d. falls below the 99th percentile one time.

12. The nurse is teaching a mother how to administer digoxin (Lanoxin) at home to her 3-year-old child. The nurse tells the mother that as a general rule, digoxin should not be administered to the younger child whose pulse is:
    a. 125.
    b. 115.
    c. 105.
    d. 85.

13. The nurse is assessing a 6-month-old with heart failure. Which of the following is a clinical manifestation of systemic congestion which can occur with HF?
    a. Tachypnea
    b. Bradycardia
    c. Peripheral oedema
    d. Intercostal retractions

14. The two main angiotensin-converting enzyme (ACE) inhibitors most commonly used for children with congestive heart failure are:
    a. digoxin and captopril.
    b. enalapril and captopril.
    c. enalapril and furosemide.
    d. spironolactone and captopril.

15. The electrolyte most commonly depleted with diuretic therapy is:
    a. sodium.
    b. chloride.
    c. potassium.
    d. magnesium.

16. The nutritional needs of the infant with heart failure are usually:
    a. the same as an adult's.
    b. less than a healthy infant's.
    c. the same as a healthy infant's.
    d. greater than a healthy infant's.

17. The calories are usually modified for an infant with heart failure by:
    a. feeding every 2 hours.
    b. increasing the volume of each feeding.
    c. increasing the caloric density of the formula.
    d. increasing the feeding duration to 1 hour.

18. Which of the following clinical manifestations is a sign of chronic hypoxemia in a child?
    a. Fatigue with feeding
    b. Tachypnea
    c. Clubbing
    d. a, b, and c

19. Prostaglandin is administered to the newborn with a congenital heart defect to:
    a. keep the ductus arteriosus open.
    b. close the ductus arteriosus.
    c. keep the foramen ovale open.
    d. close the foramen ovale.

20. Dehydration must be prevented in children who are hypoxemic because dehydration places the child at risk for:
    a. infection.
    b. cerebral vascular accident.
    c. fever.
    d. air embolism.

MATCHING

Match each specific disorder with its corresponding type of defect. (Defects may be used more than once.)

21. _____ Patent ductus arteriosus

22. _____ Coarctation of the aorta

23. _____ Ventricular septal defect

24. _____ Subvalvular aortic stenosis

25. _____ Hypoplastic left heart syndrome

26. _____ Atrioventricular canal defect

27. _____ Pulmonic stenosis

28. _____ Tetralogy of Fallot

29. _____ Aortic stenosis

30. _____ Tricuspid atresia

31. _____ Valvular aortic stenosis

32. _____ Truncus arteriosus

33. _____ Atrial septal defect

34. _____ Transposition of the great vessels

a. Defects with decreased pulmonary blood flow

b. Mixed defects

c. Defects with increased pulmonary blood flow

d. Obstructive defects

35. Which of the following sets of assessment findings are the most frequent clinical manifestations of an atrial septal defect in an infant or child?
   a. Decreased cardiac output and low blood pressure
   b. Heart failure and a murmur
   c. Increased blood pressure and pulse
   d. Dyspnea and bradycardia

36. Parents of the infant with a congenital heart defect should know the signs of heart failure, which may include:
   a. poor feeding.
   b. sudden weight gain.
   c. increased efforts to breathe.
   d. a, b, and c.

37. Tetralogy of Fallot consists of these defects:
   I. VSD
   II. ASD
   III. right ventricular hypertrophy
   IV. pulmonic stenosis
   V. overriding aorta
   VI. patent ductus arteriosus
      a. II, III, IV, and VI
      b. I, III, IV, and V
      c. II, IV, V, and VI

38. Because an incision is made through muscle, most children consider the most painful part of cardiac surgery to be the:
   a. thoracotomy incision site.
   b. graft site on the leg.
   c. sternotomy incision site.
   d. intravenous insertion sites.

39. An infant who weighs 7 kg has just returned to the intensive care unit following cardiac surgery. The chest tube has drained 40 mL in the past hour. In this situation, what is the first action for the nurse to take?
   a. Notify the surgeon immediately.
   b. Identify any other signs of haemorrhage.
   c. Suction the patient.
   d. Identify any other signs of renal failure.

40. Following cardiac surgery, fluid *intake* calculations for a child would include:
   a. intravenous fluids.
   b. arterial and CVP line flushes.
   c. fluid used to dilute medications.
   d. a, b, and c.

41. Following cardiac surgery, in addition to hourly recordings of urine, fluid *output* calculations in a child should include:
    a. nasogastric secretions.
    b. blood drawn for analysis.
    c. chest tube drainage.
    d. a, b, and c.

42. One of the most important factors in preventing infective endocarditis is:
    a. administration of prophylactic antibiotic therapy before procedures known to increase the risk of entry of organisms.
    b. surgical repair of the defect.
    c. administration of prostaglandin to maintain patent ductus arteriosus.
    d. administration of antibiotics after dental work to high-risk patients.

43. The most reliable test to provide evidence of recent streptococcal infection in children suspected of having acute rheumatic fever is the:
    a. throat culture.
    b. mantoux test.
    c. liver enzymes test.
    d. antistreptolysin O test.

44. The peak age for the incidence of Kawasaki disease is in the:
    a. infant age group.
    b. toddler age group.
    c. school-age group.
    d. adolescent age group.

45. Discharge teaching for a child with Kawasaki disease who received IVIG should include:
    a. temperature should be taken daily for the first 1-2 weeks; occurrence of fever should be communicated to the primary health care provider.
    b. arthritis, especially in the weight-bearing joints, although temporary, may persist for several weeks.
    c. defer any live vaccines such as measles, mumps, and rubella (MMR) vaccine for 11 months.
    d. all of the above.

46. Elevated cholesterol:
    a. can predict the long-term risk of heart disease for the individual.
    b. can predict the risk of hypertension in adulthood.
    c. plays an important role in causing atherosclerosis.
    d. plays an important role in causing congestive heart failure.

III. THINKING CRITICALLY

1. List risk factors associated with an increased incidence of congenital heart disease.

2. Describe how to prepare families when their child requires surgery to correct a congenital heart defect.

48 Hematological and Immunological Conditions

I. LEARNING KEY TERMS

MATCHING: Match each term with its corresponding definition or description.

1. _____ Nosebleed.

2. _____ The peripheral blood smear demonstrates the triad of profound anaemia, thrombocytopenia, and leukopenia.

3. _____ The process that stops bleeding when a blood system vessel is injured.

4. _____ Bleeding into a joint space; most frequent type of internal bleeding.

5. _____ A condition in which the number of red blood cells or haemoglobin concentration is reduced below normal; oxygen-carrying capacity of the blood is diminished; less oxygen is available to the tissues.

6. _____ Bleeding and clotting that occurs simultaneously; characterised by fibrin deposition in the microvasculature, consumption of coagulation factors and endogenous production of thrombin and plasmin

7. _____ Malignant diseases of the bone marrow and lymphatic system. An unrestricted proliferation of immature white blood cells in the blood-forming tissues of the body.

8. _____ A chemical agent which may cause severe cellular damage to tissues if even minute amounts of the drug infiltrate surrounding tissue; sclerosing agent

9. _____ Malignancy primarily involving the lymph nodes and usually metastasizes to non-nodal or extra lymphatic sites e.g. spleen, lungs, liver.

10. _____ A procedure used to establish healthy haemopoiesis with viable blood stem cells in both malignant and nonmalignant disease.

11. _____ A heterogeneous cancer commonly staged by the St. Jude Staging system; relapse after 2 years is rare

12. _____ Removal of blood from an individual, separation of the blood into its components and reinfusing the remainder of the blood into the individual.

13. _____ Hereditary haemoglobinopathy that partly or completely replaces HgbA with HgbS

14. _____ A retrovirus transmitted by lymphocytes and monocytes and found in all bodily fluids causing immunosuppression.

15. _____ Diagnostic test for detecting homozygous and heterozygous forms of sickle cell anaemia that separates various Haemoglobin by high voltage

a. Non-Hodgkin Lymphoma

b. Sickle cell anaemia

c. Pancytopenia

d. Disseminated intravascular coagulation

e. Haemoglobin electrophoresis

f. Hemarthrosis

g. Human Immunodeficiency Virus

h. Vesicant

i. Hodgkin Disease

j. Hematopoietic Stem Cell Transplantation

k. Hemostasis

l. Apheresis

m. Anaemia

n. Leukaemia

o. Epistaxis

II. REVIEWING KEY CONCEPTS

1. A common term used in describing an abnormal CBC is shift to the left, which refers to the:
   a. presence of immature neutrophils in the peripheral blood.
   b. elevated white blood cell count.
   c. under-function of the bone marrow
   d. increased risk of bleeding during sepsis.

2. Poverty, food insecurity, diminishing access to iron-rich foods, increasing access to low-iron "convenience foods" and other factors contribute to the development of_____ _____ anaemia in childhood.

3. At birth the healthy full-term newborn has maternal stores of iron sufficient to last:
   a. the first 6 months.
   b. 2 to 3 months.
   c. 8 months.
   d. less than 1 month.

4. List three essential guidelines for the effective administration of oral iron supplements to small children.

5. A 5-year-old with sickle cell anaemia is admitted because of diminished RBC production triggered by a viral infection. The episode is characterised by ischemia and pain of the distal extremities. The crisis the child is most likely to be experiencing is:
   a. vasoocclusive crisis.
   b. splenic sequestration crisis.
   c. aplastic crisis.
   d. hyperhemolytic crisis.

6. Therapeutic management of sickle cell crisis generally includes:
   a. long-term oxygen use to enable the oxygen to reach the sickled RBCs.
   b. an increase in activity to promote circulation in the affected area.
   c. a diet high in iron to decrease anaemia.
   d. oral or intravenous hydration.

7. In controlling severe pain related to vasoocclusive sickle cell crisis, the plan of care will most likely include:
   a. administration of long-term oxygen.
   b. application of cold compresses to the area.
   c. appliscation of warm compresses to the area.
   d. intravenous or oral opioids.

8. Treatment for the child with aplastic anaemia will most likely include:
   a. administration of testosterone.
   b. administration of iron-chelating agents.
   c. irradiation.
   d. bone marrow transplant.

9. Primary prophylaxis in haemophilia patients involves the infusion of factor VIII:
   a. at the emergency department when joint damage occurs.
   b. regularly, before the onset of joint or muscle damage.
   c. whenever bleeding into a joint occurs.
   d. when bleeding begins to impair joint function.

10. Carson, previously diagnosed with haemophilia A, is being admitted with hemarthrosis. The nurse knows that which of the following would most likely be included in the plan of care?
    I. Ice packs to the affected area
    II. Affected joint is elevated and immobilised
    III. Teaching Carson to self-administer antihaemophilic factor
    IV. Administration of aspirin or aspirin-containing compounds
    V. Administration of factor replacement therapy
    VI. Active range-of-motion exercises after the acute episode
      a. I, III, and VI
      b. II, III, IV, and VI
      c. I, IV, and V,
      d. I, II, V, and VI

11. An acquired hemorrhagic disorder characterised by thrombocytopenia, absence/minimal bleeding and normal bone marrow with normal or increased number of immature platelets and eosinophils is

_____ _____.

12. T   F   Thalassemia is an inherited blood disorder characterised by deficiencies in the rate of production of specific globin chains in Hgb.

13. Transfusions are the foundation of medical management in children with thalassemia with the goal of maintaining the Hgb level above _____ g/L.

14. In children and adolescents, HIV is most likely to be transmitted:
    a. mother-to-child.
    b. risky sexual behaviours
    c. to adolescents engaged in IV drug use.
    d. via all of the above.

15. Immunisation against common childhood illnesses is recommended for children exposed to and infected with HIV, but the nurse recognises that children with HIV who are receiving intravenous gamma-globulin (IVGG) prophylaxis may not respond to the:
    a. varicella vaccine.
    b. poliovirus vaccine.
    c. measles-mumps-rubella vaccine.
    d. pneumococcal vaccine.

16. _____ _____ _____ is the most common opportunistic infection of children infected with HIV; it occurs most frequently between 3 and 6 months of age.

17. Which of the following is not a clinical manifestation of HIV in children?
    a. Oral candidiasis
    b. Chronic diarrhoea
    c. Failure to thrive
    d. Frequent URIs

18. Diagnosis of severe combined immunodeficiency disease (SCID) is primarily based on:
    a. failure to thrive.
    b. delayed development.
    c. feeding problems.
    d. recurrent, severe infections from early infancy.

19. In Wiskott-Aldrich syndrome, the most notable effect of the disease at birth is:
    a. bloody diarrhoea.
    b. infection.
    c. eczema.
    d. malignancy.

20. T F Prophylaxis treatment for *Pneumocystis* pneumonia is provided with administration of trimethoprim-sulfamethoxazole during the first year of life for children infected with HIV.

21. The administration of _____ may be used to reduce the incidence of infection secondary to neutropenia.

22. Children with ITP and a platelet count _____ should avoid activities that may cause injury or bleeding such as riding a bike, skateboarding, or playing at the playground.

23. What treatment strategy has been found to be beneficial in decreasing the nausea and vomiting associated with chemotherapy and radiotherapy for children?

24. Identify interventions for mouth care in infants and toddlers who may have developed mucosal ulcers as a side effect of chemotherapy.

25. T F Viscous lidocaine is an acceptable medication to use in decreasing the pain from mucosal ulcers in young children.

26. Identify three strategies to possibly decrease the side effect of haemorrhagic cystitis.

27. A 4-year-old girl is receiving steroids as part of her treatment plan. Which of the following would be important to educate the family regarding steroid administration?
    a. The child may experience mood changes.
    b. The child may experience physical changes such as a rounded face.
    c. The child may experience an increase in appetite.
    d. All of the above may occur.

28. T F An immunosuppressed child should receive all immunizations as scheduled, including live, attenuated vaccines to ensure they are protected from childhood diseases.

29. List the three main consequences of the bone marrow dysfunction seen in leukemia.

30. T F Leukemic cells invading the periosteum can lead to severe pain and possible fractures in the child.

31. Which of the following is the gold standard test for a definitive diagnosis in children with leukemia?
    a. MRI
    b. CT scan
    c. Peripheral blood smear
    d. Bone marrow aspiration

32. Children diagnosed with leukaemia are at risk for invasion of the _____ and therefore receive _____.

33. Hodgkin disease is characterised by which of the following clinical manifestations?
    a. Painless enlargement of lymph nodes
    b. Firm, nontender irregular mass in the thoracic cavity
    c. Painless swelling in the abdomen
    d. A whitish glow in the pupil

III. THINKING CRITICALLY

1. Outline pain management strategies for acute vaso-occlusive pain management for children with sickle cell anaemia.

2. Identify proactive strategies families with a child diagnosed with haemophilia can use to prevent serious bleeding episodes.

3. Seth was diagnosed with Acute Lymphoid Leukaemia (ALL) 8 months ago and requires occasional blood transfusions as part of the established treatment plan. As the nurse caring for plan, please outline the core nursing responsibilities associated with administering blood transfusions.

4. Annalise was born with Severe Combined Immunodeficiency Disease (SCID) and the family has learned that a bone marrow transplant is recommended. Family members are seeking confirmation of their understanding about how bone marrow transplants work. As their nurse, what general principles related to Hematopoietic Stem Cell Transplantation would you reinforce?

231

49 Genitourinary Conditions

I. LEARNING KEY TERMS

MATCHING: Match each term with its corresponding description.

1. _____ Procedure of separating colloids and crystalline substances whereby blood filtrate is circulated by hydrostatic pressure exerted across a semipermeable membrane with simultaneous infusion of a replacement solution.

2. _____ Presence of bacteria in the urine.

3. _____ Fluid accumulation in the abdominal cavity.

4. _____ Fluid accumulation in the interstitial spaces and body cavities.

5. _____ Meatal opening located on dorsal surface of penis.

6. _____ A reduction in the serum albumin level.

7. _____ Inflammation of the bladder.

8. _____ Procedure in which colloids and crystalline substances are separated by using the abdominal cavity as a semipermeable membrane through which water and solute of small molecular size move by osmosis and diffusion based on concentrations on either side of the membrane.

9. _____ One of the most frequent causes of acute renal failure; clinical features include acquired haemolytic anaemia, thrombocytopenia, renal injury, and CNS symptoms.

10. _____ Inflammation of the urethra.

11. _____ Procedure in which colloids and crystalline substance are separated by circulating the blood outside the body through artificial membranes, which permits a similar passage of water and solutes.

12. _____ Opening of urethral meatus below the glans penis or anywhere along the ventral surface of penis.

13. _____ Inflammation of the upper urinary tract and kidneys.

14. _____ The most immediate threat to the life of a child with acute kidney injury; excess potassium in the blood; treated with an ion-exchange resin such as Kayexalate and dialysis.

15. _____ A condition in which there is an abnormal retrograde flow of urine from the bladder, through the ureters to the kidneys.

16. _____ Febrile urinary tract infection coexisting with systemic signs of bacterial illness; blood culture reveals presence of urinary pathogen.

a. Bacteriuria

b. Cystitis

c. Urethritis

d. Pyelonephritis

e. Urosepsis

f. Hypospadias

g. Vesicoureteral reflux

h. Hypoalbuminemia

i. Oedema

j. Ascites

k. Hemolytic uremic syndrome

l. Epispadias

m. Hyperkalemia

n. Haemodialysis

o. Peritoneal dialysis

p. Hemofiltration

II. REVIEWING KEY CONCEPTS

1. Which of the following are measures of UTI prevention?
   a. Good perineal hygiene
   b. Avoiding constipation
   c. Emptying bladder frequently and completely
   d. a, b, and c

2. _____ male infants have been reported to have a higher incidence of urinary tract infection in their first several months of their life than other males or females.

3. Clinical manifestations of urinary tract infection in the first month of life include all but which of the following?
   a. Fever
   b. Poor feeding
   c. vomiting
   d. Anaemia

4. For the child with nephrotic syndrome, one aim of the therapy is to reduce:
   a. excretion of urinary protein.
   b. excretion of fluids.
   c. serum albumin levels.
   d. urinary output.

5. Acute glomerulonephritis may be suspected when the child presents with the clinical manifestations of:
   a. normal blood pressure, generalised oedema, and oliguria.
   b. oedema, hematuria, and oliguria.
   c. fatigue, elevated serum lipid levels, and elevated serum protein levels.
   d. temperature elevation, circulatory congestion, and normal creatinine serum levels.

6. The nurse caring for the child with acute glomerulonephritis would expect to:
   a. enforce complete bed rest.
   b. regular monitoring of vital signs.
   c. perform peritoneal dialysis.
   d. ensure a diet low in protein.

7. The nurse caring for a child with minimal-change nephrotic syndrome can expect to administer a _____ as the first-line drug therapy.

8. Clinical manifestations of nephrotic syndrome include:
   a. hyperlipidemia, hypoalbuminemia, oedema, and proteinuria.
   b. hematuria, hypertension, periorbital oedema, and flank pain.
   c. oliguria, hypocholesterolemia, and hyperalbuminemia.
   d. hematuria, generalised oedema, hypertension, and proteinuria.

9. When teaching the family of a child with nephrotic syndrome about prednisone therapy, the nurse includes the information that:
   a. corticosteroid therapy begins after BUN and serum creatinine elevation.
   b. prednisone is administered orally in a dosage of 4 mg/kg of body weight.
   c. steroid therapy will occur over several months and restarted if a relapse occurs.
   d. the drug is discontinued as soon as the urine is free from protein.

10. Renal injury, acquired hemolytic anaemia, central nervous system symptoms, and thrombocytopenia are characteristic clinical manifestations of the disorder known as:
    a. minimal-change nephrotic syndrome.
    b. Wilms tumor.
    c. hemolytic-uremic syndrome.
    d. vesicoureteral reflux.

11. The most frequent cause of transient renal failure in infants and children is:
    a. nephrotoxic agents.
    b. obstructive uropathy.
    c. severe dehydration.
    d. burn shock.

12. The primary manifestation of acute kidney injury is:
    a. oedema.
    b. oligoanuria.
    c. metabolic acidosis.
    d. weight gain and proteinuria.

13. The most immediate threat to the life of the child with acute kidney injury is:
    a. hyperkalemia.
    b. anaemia.
    c. hypertensive crisis.
    d. cardiac failure from hypovolemia.

14. The drug therapy used for the removal of elevated serum potassium is:
    a. furosemide.
    b. vasopressin.
    c. ion exchange resin.
    d. calcium gluconate.

15. In general, during the oliguric phase of acute renal failure, which electrolytes are withheld?
    a. Sodium
    b. Potassium
    c. Chloride
    d. a and b only
    e. a, b, and c

233

16. Which of the following manifestations would not be an expected finding in the child with acute renal failure?
    a. Anaemia
    b. Hypertension
    c. Hypernatremia
    d. Cardiac failure with pulmonary oedema

17. Which of the following features contribute to urinary tract infections:
    a. acidic urine pH
    b. decreased fluid intake
    c. frequent emptying of the bladder
    d. dietary intake of cranberry juice

18. Which of the following is included in dietary regulation of the child with chronic kidney disease?
    a. Restricting protein intake below the recommended daily allowance
    b. Dietary protein intake is limited only to the reference daily intake (Recommended Dietary Allowance [RDA]) for the child's age.
    c. Restricting potassium when creatinine clearance falls below 50 mL/min
    d. Giving vitamin A, E, and K supplements

19. Methods of dialysis for management of renal failure are _____,

    _____, and

    _____.

20. _____ is the preferred method of dialysis for children with life-threatening hyperkalemia that needs to be rapidly corrected.

21. _____ dialysis is usually recommended for small children.

22. A child, age 12, had a renal transplant 5 months ago. He now presents to the outpatient clinic with fever, tenderness over the graft area, decreased urinary output, and a slightly elevated blood pressure. The nurse's priority at this time is to:
    a. Recognise that the child is probably undergoing acute rejection and to notify the health care provider immediately.
    b. Recognise that this is an episode of increased inflammation within the donor kidney because the child has probably been noncompliant with his immunosuppressant drugs.
    c. Obtain urine for culture and sensitivity and a blood count to quickly identify the child's infection before alerting the health care provider.
    d. Recognise that the child is in chronic rejection and that no present therapy can halt the progressive process.

III. THINKING CRITICALLY

1. Describe the nursing interventions to provide proper nutrition for the child who has minimal-change nephrotic syndrome.

2. The parents of 2 month old baby Kia have been told that Kia has vesicoureteral reflux (VUR). As their nurse, explain what routine aspects of daily life are necessary to preserving the health of Kia's kidneys.

3. Dimitri, a 6 month old infant, has had an orchiopexy procedure to reposition his undescended testicle. As his nurse, outline essential postoperative care instructions that Dimitri's care-providers require.

234

Chapter **49** Genitourinary Conditions

Copyright © 2022, Elsevier Inc. All rights reserved.

50 Neurological Conditions

I. LEARNING KEY TERMS

MATCHING: Match each term with its corresponding definition or description.

1. _____ A severe reduction in LOC; arouses with very strong stimulus but is close to a comatose state.

2. _____ Rigid flexion with the arms held tightly to the body; flexed elbows, wrists, and fingers; plantar flexed feet; legs extended and internally rotated; and possibly the presence of fine tremors or intense stiffness

3. _____ Caused by excessive and disorderly neuronal discharges in the brain; most frequently observed neurologic disorder in children; clinical manifestations determined by the site of origin and may include unconsciousness or altered consciousness, involuntary movements, and changes in perception, behaviours, sensations, and posture.

4. _____ A sign of dysfunction at the level of the midbrain or lesions to the brainstem. It is characterised by rigid extension and pronation of the arms and legs, flexed wrists and fingers, a clenched jaw, an extended neck, and possibly an arched back.

5. _____ The most common head injury in which there is a transient disturbance of brain function often traumatically induced that involves a complex pathophysiologic process.

6. _____ Determined by observations of the child's responses to the environment; the earliest indicator of improvement or deterioration in neurologic status.

7. _____ Limited spontaneous movement, sluggish speech, drowsy, falling asleep quickly.

8. _____ An imbalance in the production and absorption of the cerebral spinal fluid in the ventricular system.

9. _____ No motor or verbal response or extension posturing to painful stimuli.

10. _____ An individual who is awake, alert, and oriented to time, place, and person; demonstrating behaviour appropriate for age.

11. _____ Altered state of consciousness that reflects depressed cerebral function; the inability to respond to sensory stimuli and to have subjective experiences.

12. _____ Causes an acute inflammation of the meninges and CSF.

13. _____ A high-fat, low-carbohydrate, and adequate protein diet that has been shown to be an efficacious and tolerable treatment for medically refractory seizures.

a. Full consciousness

b. Bacterial meningitis

c. Unconsciousness

d. Coma

e. Level of consciousness

f. Decorticate posturing/Flexion posturing

g. Decerebrate posturing/Extension posturing

h. Ketogenic diet

i. Lethargy

j. Obtunded

k. Seizure

l. Hydrocephalus

m. Concussion

II. REVIEWING KEY CONCEPTS

1. The most common solid tumour in children and the second most common childhood cancer is:
   a. Wilms tumour.
   b. brain tumour.
   c. osteosarcoma.
   d. Ewing sarcoma.

2. The sign which can be used to indicate increased intracranial pressure in the infant but not in the older child is:
   a. projectile vomiting.
   b. headache.
   c. bulging fontanel.
   d. pulsating fontanel.

3. The earliest indicator of improvement or deterioration in neurologic status is:
   a. motor activity.
   b. level of consciousness.
   c. reflexes.
   d. vital signs.

4. Which of the following would be most important when caring for a child during a seizure:
   a. intervene to halt the seizure.
   b. restrain the child.
   c. protect the child from injury.
   d. place a solid object between the teeth.

5. Which of the following nursing observations would usually indicate pain in a comatose child?
   a. Increased flaccidity
   b. Increased oxygen saturation
   c. Decreased blood pressure
   d. Increased agitation

6. The activity that has been shown to increase intracranial pressure is:
   a. using earplugs to eliminate noise.
   b. gentle range-of-motion exercises.
   c. suctioning.
   d. osmotherapy and sedation.

7. The most important nursing observation following head trauma is assessment of the child's:
   a. head for bruises or lacerations.
   b. level of consciousness.
   c. neurologic signs.
   d. vital signs.

8. Epidural haemorrhage is less common in children under 2 years of age than in adults because:
   a. the middle meningeal artery is embedded in the bone surface of the skull until approximately 2 years of age.
   b. fractures are less likely to lacerate the middle meningeal artery in children less than 2 years of age.

   c. separation of the dura from bleeding is more likely to occur in children than in adults.
   d. there is an increased tendency for the skull to fracture in children less than 2 years of age.

9. The outcome of craniocerebral trauma:
   a. depends on the extent of the injury and the complications
   b. has a prognosis more favourable for children than for adults
   c. shows more than 90% of children with concussions or simple linear fractures recover without symptoms after the initial period
   d. a, b, and c

10. The epidemiology of bacterial meningitis has changed in recent years because of the:
    a. diphtheria, pertussis, and tetanus vaccine.
    b. rubella vaccine.
    c. *Haemophilus influenzae* type B and pneumococcal conjugate vaccines.
    d. hepatitis B vaccine.

11. The most common mode of transmission for bacterial meningitis is:
    a. vascular dissemination of an infection elsewhere.
    b. direct implantation from an invasive procedure.
    c. direct extension from an infection in the mastoid sinuses.
    d. direct extension from an infection in the nasal sinuses.

12. _____ _____ occurs in epidemic form and is the only type readily transmitted by droplet infection from nasopharyngeal secretions; it occurs predominantly in school-age children and adolescents.

13. Secondary outcomes from bacterial meningitis are most likely to occur in the:
    a. school-aged child.
    b. infant under 6 months of age.
    c. infant over 6 months of age.
    d. child with *H. influenzae* meningitis.

14. Which of the following types of meningitis is self-limiting and least serious?
    a. meningococcal meningitis
    b. tuberculous meningitis
    c. *H. influenzae* meningitis
    d. nonbacterial (aseptic) meningitis

15. The type of seizure, also known as a petit mal seizure, that occurs more often in children between the ages of 4 and 12 years is the:
    a. generalised absence seizure.
    b. absence seizure.
    c. atonic seizure.
    d. jackknife seizure.

16. The risk factors associated with recurrence of seizures include:
    a. older age at onset.
    b. numerous seizures before control is achieved.
    c. presence of a neurological dysfunction.
    d. a, b, and c.

17. Fosphenytoin may be given IV to treat childhood seizures instead of phenytoin because the former drug:
    a. is compatible with glucose and saline solutions.
    b. has fewer complications.
    c. may be given IM.
    d. may be administered at a faster rate.
    e. may involve all of the above.

18. Risk factors for febrile seizures include:
    a. family history of febrile seizures.
    b. viral infections.
    c. family history of epilepsy.
    d. a and b.
    e. a, b, and c.

19. When a child has a febrile seizure, it is important for the parents to know that the child will:
    a. not likely develop epilepsy.
    b. most likely develop epilepsy.
    c. most likely develop neurologic damage.
    d. usually need tepid sponge baths to control fever.

20. A 6-year-old child is seen in the urgent care unit for a history of seizures at home. They begin to have seizures in the urgent care unit that last more than 5 minutes. IV access has not been successful. The nurse caring for this child is knowledgeable that which medications may be given to stop the child's seizures?
    a. IM phenytoin
    b. Rectal diazepam
    c. Buccal midazolam
    d. a and c
    e. b and c

21. Clinical manifestations of hydrocephalus in children outside of the infancy phase include:
    a. headache.
    b. irritability.
    c. lethargy.
    d. vomiting.
    e. a, b, and d.
    f. a, b, c, and d.

22. A 12-month-old infant with a history of hydrocephalus and ventriculoperitoneal shunt (VP) placement is brought to the ED by a family member who states that the baby refuses to eat, is afebrile but extremely fussy, and does not engage in playful activity. The diagnostic evaluation for this child will most likely include:
    a. urinary catheterisation.
    b. upper GI series.
    c. skull radiographs.
    d. head CT or brain MRI.

III. THINKING CRITICALLY

1. Describe the parameters to assess and the interventions to maintain a stable intracranial pressure in an 8-year-old child who has been unconscious for 3 days.

2. Describe the assessment data that would be most helpful to obtain from the family of a 4-year-old child who is admitted for possible seizure disorder.

3. Describe indications for inserting an intracranial pressure (ICP) monitor in a child with a head injury.

51 Endocrine Conditions

I. LEARNING KEY TERMS

MATCHING: Match each term with its corresponding definition or description.

1. _____ Protruding eyeballs; occurs in hyperthyroidism.

2. _____ Ketone bodies in the urine.

3. _____ Excessive thirst.

4. _____ Elevation of the blood glucose; usually caused by illness, growth, or emotional upset.

5. _____ Occurs when serum glucose level exceeds the renal threshold (10mmol/L) and glucose "spills" into the urine.

6. _____ low blood glucose; caused by an imbalance of food intake, insulin and activity.

7. _____ The condition produced by the presence of ketone bodies in the blood; strong acids lower serum pH.

8. _____ Excessive urination.

9. _____ Hyperventilation that is characteristic of metabolic acidosis; occurs as a result of the respiratory system attempting to eliminate excess carbon dioxide by increased depth and rate of respirations.

10. _____ Carpal spasm elicited by pressure applied to nerves of the upper arm.

11. _____ Early maturation and development of the gonads with secretion of sex hormones, development of secondary sex characteristics, and sometimes production of mature sperm and ova.

12. _____ Carpopedal spasm, muscle twitching, cramps, seizures, and sometimes stridor; indicative of disorders of parathyroid function.

13. _____ Caused by excess growth hormone occurring after epiphyseal closure; characterised by facial features such as overgrowth of the head, lips, nose, tongue, jaw, and paranasal and mastoid sinuses.

14. _____ Facial muscle spasm elicited by tapping the facial nerve in the region of the parotid gland.

a. Acromegaly

b. Central precocious puberty

c. Polyuria

d. Polydipsia

e. Exophthalmos

f. Chvostek sign

g. Trousseau sign

h. Tetany

i. Glycosuria

j. Ketonuria

k. Ketoacidosis

l. Kussmaul respirations

m. Hypoglycaemia

n. Hyperglycemia

II. REVIEWING KEY CONCEPTS

1. In a child with hypopituitarism, the hormone abnormalities may lead to:
   a. diarrhoea.
   b. stunted somatic growth.
   c. early establishment of sexual maturation.
   d. weight gain out of keeping with dietary intake and activity level.

2. The best time to administer a growth hormone replacement injection is:
   a. midmorning.
   b. at the afternoon nap.
   c. at bedtime.
   d. before breakfast.

3. _____ _____ delay refers to individuals (usually boys) with delayed linear growth, generally beginning as a toddler, and skeletal and sexual maturation that is behind that of age-mates.

4. Explain the difference between acromegaly and pituitary hyperfunction that would not be considered acromegaly.

5. Recent data suggest that precocious puberty evaluation for a pathologic cause should be performed for

   White females younger than _____ years of age or

   for Black girls younger than _____ years of age; manifestations of sexual development before the age of

   _____ years in boys would suggest precocious puberty.

6. Parents of the child with precocious puberty need to know that:
   a. dress and activities should be aligned with the child's sexual development.
   b. heterosexual interest will usually be advanced.
   c. the child's mental age is congruent with the chronologic age.
   d. overt manifestations of affection represent sexual advances.

7. The most common cause of thyroid disease in children and adolescents is:
   a. Hashimoto disease (lymphocytic thyroiditis).
   b. Graves disease.
   c. goiter.
   d. thyrotoxicosis.

8. A common cause of secondary hyperparathyroidism is:
   a. maternal hyperparathyroidism.
   b. chronic renal disease.
   c. adenoma.
   d. renal rickets.

9. Pheochromocytoma is a tumour characterised by:
   a. secretion of insulin.
   b. secretion of catecholamines
   c. adrenal crisis.
   d. myxedema.

10. The parents of a child who has Addison disease should be instructed to:
    a. use extra hydrocortisone cautiously in times of crises.
    b. discontinue the child's cortisone if side effects develop.
    c. decrease the cortisone dose during times of stress.
    d. report signs of acute adrenal insufficiency to the primary practitioner.

11. Which of the following tests, which yields immediate results, is particularly useful in diagnosing congenital adrenal hyperplasia?
    a. Chromosome typing
    b. Pelvic ultrasound
    c. Pelvic X-ray
    d. Testosterone level

12. Definitive treatment for pheochromocytoma consists of:
    a. Surgical removal of the thyroid.
    b. Administration of potassium.
    c. Surgical removal of the tumor.
    d. Administration of beta blockers.

13. The primary pathologic defect in children with type 1 DM is:
    a. insulin resistance in which the body fails to use insulin properly.
    b. destruction of pancreatic βcells resulting in absolute insulin deficiency.

14. The pathologic defect in type 1 DM is the basis for

    the lifelong need for _____ administration.

15. What are characteristics often seen in type 1 DM:
    a. abrupt onset
    b. child is often underweight
    c. low to no serum insulin levels
    d. a, b, and c.

16. Glycated haemoglobin (A_1C) is an acceptable method to:
    a. diagnose diabetes mellitus.
    b. assess the control of diabetes.
    c. assess oxygen saturation of the haemoglobin.
    d. determine blood glucose levels most accurately.

17. The most common acute complication of diabetes that a young child may encounter is:
    a. retinopathy.
    b. ketoacidosis.
    c. hypoglycaemia.
    d. hyperosmolar nonketotic coma.

18. Exercise for the child with diabetes mellitus:
    a. is restricted to noncontact sports.
    b. may require a decreased intake of carbohydrate.
    c. may necessitate an increased insulin dose.
    d. may require the provision of extra snacks.

19. List the three cardinal signs/clinical symptoms of type 1 DM.

20. Conventional management of type 1 DM has consisted of a twice-daily insulin regimen of a combination of _____ and _____ insulin drawn up into the same syringe and injected _____ and before _____.

21. The nurse is teaching 15-year-old Mario about the management of type 1 DM. The management of type 1 DM for the prevention of complications is based on:
      I. a daily insulin regimen.
     II. a periodic insulin regimen.
    III. blood glucose self-monitoring.
     IV. a regular exercise regimen.
      V. a balanced diet.
     VI. limited physical exercise.
        a. I, III, and IV
        b. II, IV, and V
        c. I, III, IV, and V

22. Problems of adjustment to diabetes are most likely to occur when it is diagnosed in:
    a. infancy.
    b. adolescence.
    c. the toddler years.
    d. the school-age years.

III. THINKING CRITICALLY

1. Describe the clinical manifestations usually seen in a child with hypopituitarism.

2. Describe the following as they relate to a child with diabetes insipidus (DI):

    a. clinical manifestations of DI.

    b. therapeutic management.

3. Identify the symptoms of hypoglycaemia in a child with type 1 DM.

4. Describe the interventions to treat hypoglycaemia in the child with type 1 DM.

52 Integumentary Conditions

I. LEARNING KEY TERMS

1. _____ Layer of skin consisting of connective tissue comprised of collagen and elastic fibres, blood and lymph vessels, nerves, hair follicles, and sweat glands.

2. _____ Glands that produce sebum for skin lubrication and minimise fluid loss.

3. _____ Itching sensation which varies in intensity.

4. _____ excessive sensitivity.

5. _____ Layer of skin tissue containing melanocytes that pigments the skin, and blood vessels that tint the skin pink.

6. _____ diminished sensation.

7. _____ abnormal sensation, such as burning or prickling.

8. _____ absence of sensation.

9. _____ Localised red or purple discolourations caused by extravasation of blood into dermis and subcutaneous tissues.

10. _____ pinpoint, tiny, and sharp circumscribed spots in the superficial layers of the epidermis.

11. _____ inflammatory reaction of the skin to natural or synthetic chemical substances that cause a hypersensitivity response or irritation.

12. _____ An abscess on the inner or outer part of the eyelid caused by a bacterial infection.

13. _____ Insect that leads to a localised red, itchy, flat or raised lesions that often occur linear in a group of three.

14. _____ caused by prolonged and repetitive contact with an irritant, most commonly urine or feces.

15. _____ Caused by testosterone which stimulates the sebaceous glands to enlarge and increase in number or produce oil and plug the pores.

16. _____ Tissue damage caused when excessive heat loss to local tissues leads to ice crystal formation in tissues; affected area appears white or blanched and is without sensation

17. _____ A reddened area caused by increased amounts of oxygenated blood in the dermal vasculature

18. _____ Type of pruritic eczema associated with a hereditary tendency; dermatological manifestations appear subsequent to scratching from the intense pruritus

19. _____ Infestation of the scalp caused by a parasite; itching is typically the only symptom

20. _____ Redness and swelling of the skin when exposed to cold temperatures and moisture; usually occurs on the hands

a. Pruritus

b. hyperesthesia

c. paresthesia

d. anaesthesia

e. Dermis

f. Sebaceous glands

g. hypoesthesia

h. ecchymoses

i. contact dermatitis

j. Epidermis

k. Sty

l. Pediculosis capitis

m. Cimicidae (Bed bug)

n. Atopic dermatitis

o. Petechiae

p. Acne

q. Chilblain

r. Erythema

s. Diaper dermatitis

t. Frostbite

II. REVIEWING KEY CONCEPTS

1. A type of pruritic fungal infection is localised to the medial proximal aspect of the thigh and crural fold, and may involve the scrotum in males:
   a. Tinea capitis
   b. Tinea corporis
   c. Tinea cruris
   d. Tinea pedis

2. Baby Levi, a preterm infant born with jejunal atresia, underwent bowel surgery two days ago and has a new onset of elevated temperature. The nurse observes Levi's peri-incisional skin to be intensely red, oedematous and is firm on palpation. These symptoms are consistent with a new onset of:
   a. Staphylococcal scalded skin syndrome
   b. Cellulitis
   c. Candidiasis
   d. None of the above

3. Healing wounds and incisions may cause significant pruritus. As part of discharge teaching, the nurse can suggest which of the following to protect the wound and relieve the itch sensation:
   a. Cool compresses
   b. Bathing the wound with baking soda preparations
   c. Ensure the child's fingernails are kept trimmed and clean
   d. All of the above

4. The primary function of human skin is:
   a. To protect against the external environment
   b. To reduce sensory input to the cerebral cortex
   c. To promote water loss and regulate fluid balance in the intravascular compartment
   d. None of the above

5. Scar tissue may form:
   a. When the epidermal layer of skin is injured
   b. When a bandage is not provided to protect an abrasion
   c. When tissue comprised of muscle and nerve cells is injured
   d. When significant bleeding occurs at the time of tissue injury

6. Treatment for Tinea corporis, also known as ringworm, may include
   a. Oral griseofulvin
   b. Oral antiviral agent
   c. Topical antibiotic
   d. Corticosteroids

7. A child who is taking an extended treatment course of oral Griseofulvin for their skin disorder requires
   a. A low-fat diet
   b. Monitoring for leucopenia
   c. Monitoring of cardiac function
   d. Monitoring for excessive weight gain

8. A child who has become sensitised to hymenopteran (bees, wasps) bites may experience:
   a. Skin pallor
   b. Hypertension
   c. Laryngeal oedema
   d. Euphoria

9. To minimise flare-ups or treat exacerbations the family of a child with atopic dermatitis can:
   a. Encourage bubble baths to promote hydration of dry skin
   b. Avoid swimming in pools
   c. Bathe in tepid water followed with a colloid-based emollient
   d. None of the above

10. T F Topical immunomodulators, nonsteroidal treatment for actopic dermatitis, accelerate the cells of the immune system in the skin.

11. T F Seborrhoeic dermatitis may occur on eyelids, nasolabial folds and the inguinal region.

12. T F Acne can create feelings of depression and self-harm.

13. T F Adolescents using Tretinoin for acne management are encouraged to avoid the sun and use sunscreen daily to reduce the possible occurrence of severe sunburn.

14. T F Young women using oral contraceptive pills may experience exacerbations of their mild acne.

15. T F The severity of a burn injury is assessed on the basis of the percentage of total body surface area burned and the amount of pain experienced by the child.

III. THINKING CRITICALLY

1. Three-year-old Sheeba, who attends daycare regularly, has a red, irregularly demarcated macular rash with ruptured vesicles and has been diagnosed with the bacterial skin infection, Impetigo. As the clinic nurse, please outline core principles recommended for Sheeba's family to reduce the spread of the infection.

2. Wilson has experienced a generalised upper body skin rash from a bed bug infestation that developed in the family home. Along with providing specific treatment interventions for Wilson's rash, please outline suggestions for Wilson's family regarding how to eliminate Cimicidae from their home.

53 Musculoskeletal or Articular Conditions

I. LEARNING KEY TERMS

MATCHING: Match each term with its corresponding definition or description.

1. _____ Produced by compression of porous bone; appears as a raised or bulging projection at the fracture site; occurs in the most porous portion of the bone; more common in young children.

2. _____ Occurs when the bone is bent but not broken; a child's flexible bone can be bent 45 degrees or more before breaking.

3. _____ Occurs when a bone is angulated beyond the limits of bending, one side bending and the other side breaking.

4. _____ applied directly to skeletal structure by a pin, wire or tongs inserted into or through the diameter of the bone distal to the fracture.

5. _____ Fractures in which small fragments of bone break off from the fractured shaft and lie in the surrounding tissue.

6. _____ A fracture in which bone fragments cause damage to other organs or tissues such as the lung or bladder.

7. _____ Fracture that divides the bone fragments.

8. _____ Applied directly to skin surface and indirectly to skeletal structures.

9. _____ Fracture with an open wound through which the bone is protruding or has protruded.

10. _____ Applied to the body part by the hands placed distal to the fracture site.

11. _____ To reduce or realign a fracture site by attaching weight to the distal bone fragment.

12. _____ Black and blue discoloration; the escape of blood into the tissues.

13. _____ A fracture that does not produce a break in the skin.

a. Ecchymosis

b. Simple or closed fracture

c. Compound or open fracture

d. Complicated fracture

e. Comminuted fracture

f. Plastic deformation

g. Buckle or torus fracture

h. Greenstick fracture

i. Complete fracture

j. Traction

k. Manual traction

l. Skin traction

m. Skeletal traction

II. REVIEWING KEY CONCEPTS

1. An appropriate nursing intervention for the care of a child with an extremity in a new hip spica plaster cast is:
   a. keeping the cast covered with a sheet.
   b. using the fingertips when handling the cast to prevent pressure areas.
   c. using heated fans or dryers to circulate air and speed the cast-drying process.
   d. turning the child at least every 2 hours to minimise prolonged pressure.

2. Bone healing is characteristically more rapid in children because:
   a. children have less constant muscle contraction associated with the fracture.
   b. children's fractures are less severe than adults.
   c. children have an active growth plate that helps speed repair with deformity less likely to occur.
   d. children have thickened periosteum and more generous blood supply.

3. When caring for a 7-year-old child after application of skeletal traction, the nurse should *not*:
   a. gently massage over pressure areas to stimulate circulation.
   b. release the traction when repositioning the child in bed.
   c. inspect pin sites for bleeding or infection.
   d. assess for alterations in neurovascular status.

MATCHING: Match each type of traction with its corresponding description.

4. _____ A type of running traction in which the pull is only in one direction; skin traction is applied to the legs, which are flexed at a 90-degree angle at the hips. The child's trunk (with the buttocks raised slightly off the bed) provides counter traction.

5. _____ Uses a system of wires, rings, and telescoping rods that permits limb lengthening to occur.

6. _____ Complication of cervical traction.

7. _____ Uses skin traction on the lower leg and a padded sling under the knee.

8. _____ A type of skin traction with the leg in an extended position; used primarily for short-term immobilization.

9. _____ Skeletal traction in which the lower leg is supported by a boot cast or a calf sling and a pin or wire is placed in the distal fragment of the femur; used for unstable fracture

10. _____ Used with or without skin or skeletal traction; suspends the leg in a flexed position to relax the hip and hamstring muscles.

11. _____ Consists of a steel halo attached to the head by four screws inserted into the outer skull; several rigid bars connect the halo to a vest that is worn around the chest, thus providing greater mobility of the rest of the body while avoiding cervical spinal motion altogether.

12. _____ The process of separating opposing bone to encourage regeneration of new bone in the created space to correct leg discrepancies.

a. Cranial nerve deficits

b. Buck extension

c. Russell traction

d. 90-degree–90-degree traction

e. Balance suspension traction

f. Halo vest or brace

g. Distraction

h. Bryant traction

i. Ilizarov external fixator (IEF)

13. To prevent infection, skeletal pin site cleaning requires diligence and may occur:
   a. when scabs have fallen off.
   b. only when skeletal traction is released.
   c. with an antiseptic cleaner or normal saline.
   d. with soap and water.

14. An appropriate intervention for a child with phantom limb pain is to:
   a. reassure the child the sensation will go away about 1 month after amputation.
   b. recommend a psychiatric consult with a paediatric specialist.
   c. acknowledge the child's feelings and allow open expression.
   d. encourage the child to ignore the feelings.

15. Stress fractures occur as a result of repeated _____

   _____ and are seen most often in _____

   such as _____, _____ and _____.

16. Developmental dysplasia of the hip may occur:
   a. in utero.
   b. in infancy.
   c. in childhood.
   d. in all of the above.

17. What is the most common management device used for the newborn with hip dysplasia?
   a. Hip spica cast
   b. Pavlik harness
   c. Buck extension traction
   d. Denise-Brown splint

18. Clubfoot may occur as an isolated deformity or in association with other disorders or syndromes such as:
   a. chromosomal abnormalities
   b. arthrogryposis.
   c. spina bifida
   d. a, b. and c.

19. The priority in teaching parents about a 1-week-old infant being treated for clubfoot is:
    a. compliance with regular cast changes.
    b. care of the Pavlik harness.
    c. traction care.
    d. passive range of motion.

20. A 7-year-old child is diagnosed with Legg-Calvé-Perthes disease. The manifestation that would *not* be consistent with this diagnosis is:
    a. intermittent appearance of a limp on the affected side.
    b. hip soreness, ache, or stiffness that can be constant or intermittent.
    c. pain and limp most evident on arising and at the end of a long day of activities.
    d. specific history of injury to the area.

21. The cause of slipped capital femoral epiphysis is multifactorial and includes:
    I. obesity.
    II. pubertal hormone changes.
    III. physeal architecture and orientation.
    IV. overuse injury.
        a. I, II, and IV
        b. I, II, and III

22. Slipped capital femoral epiphysis is suspected when an adolescent or preadolescent:
    a. begins to limp and complains of pain in the hip continuously or intermittently.
    b. has pain without restriction of abduction and internal rotation.
    c. complains of referred pain in the groin.
    d. a and c.

23. An accentuation of the cervical or lumbar curvature beyond physiologic limits is termed _____.
    An abnormally increased convex angulation in the curvature of the thoracic spine is termed _____.

24. Diagnostic evaluation is important for early recognition of scoliosis. The correct procedure for the health clinic nurse conducting this examination would be to view the child:
    a. standing and walking fully clothed to look for uneven hanging of clothing.
    b. from the front to evaluate bone maturity.
    c. from the left and right side while the child is completely undressed.
    d. from behind while the child is bending forward and is wearing only underpants.

25. Nursing implementation directed toward nonsurgical management in an adolescent with scoliosis primarily includes:
    a. promoting self-esteem and positive body image.
    b. promoting immobilisation of the legs.
    c. promoting adequate nutrition.
    d. preventing infection.

26. Postoperative priorities of nursing care for the adolescent who has undergone spinal arthrodesis with instrumentation include:
    I. evaluation of incision site.
    II. monitoring vital signs.
    III. assessment of neurologic function.
    IV. monitoring urine output.
    V. observation for features of acute bowel obstruction.
    VI. pain management.
    VII. traction care.
        a. I, II, III, IV, and VII
        b. I, II, III, IV, V, and VI

27. A hospitalised adolescent with scoliosis is 4 days postop and is being prepared for ambulation; when she is helped to a sitting position she suddenly turns pale and complains of shortness of breath and chest pain. The nurse recognises the symptoms and *immediately*:
    a. calls out for rapid medical assistance.
    b. reapplies the pulse oximeter probe to ensure accurate measurement.
    c. takes a peripheral blood pressure.
    d. allows the patient to rest before ambulating.

28. The nurse recognises the adolescent's condition in the previous question as a probable:
    a. orthostatic hypotension.
    b. pulmonary embolism.
    c. fluid volume deficit.
    d. tension pneumothorax.

29. A 3-year-old with suspected acute osteomyelitis in the lower leg is likely to exhibit a recent onset of:
    a. a history of pain in the affected limb
    b. a warm, erythematous affected limb
    c. decreased range of motion in the affected limb
    d. all of the above.

30. The nurse can anticipate that the plan of care for the child during the acute phase of osteomyelitis includes:
    I. encouragement of adequate nutritional intake.
    II. attention to comfortable positioning with affected limb supported.

III. isolation of the child.
IV. administration of intravenous antibiotics.
V. weight-bearing exercises for the affected area.
VI. pain management.
   a. I, II, IV, and VI
   b. II, III, IV, and VI
   c. III and IV

31. Nursing considerations for the patient diagnosed with osteogenesis imperfecta include:
   a. preventing fractures by careful handling.
   b. encouraging the parents to seek genetic counseling.
   c. providing guidelines to the parents to promote optimum development.
   d. a, b, and c.

32. The goal that is most appropriate for the child with juvenile arthritis is for the child to be able to exhibit signs of:
   a. adequate joint function.
   b. improved skin integrity.
   c. weight loss and improved nutritional status.
   d. adequate respiratory function.

33. To promote adequate joint function in the child with juvenile arthritis, the nurse can encourage parents to:
   a. incorporate therapeutic exercises in play activities.
   b. provide heat to affected joints by use of tub baths.
   c. provide written information for all treatments ordered.
   d. explore and develop activities in which the child can succeed.

34. The nurse formulating the plan of care for a 16-year-old who has undergone a limb salvage procedure for osteosarcoma anticipates that:
   a. pain management will be a priority in the patient's care.
   b. stump care will be required.
   c. counselling on coping and psychological adjustment.
   d. a and c.
   e. a and b.

III. THINKING CRITICALLY

1. Outline the instructions parents should receive to care for a 2-month-old infant in a Pavlik harness.

2. List the six Ps of ischaemia from a vascular injury that should always be included in an assessment of the injury.

3. Define compartment syndrome and identify the signs and symptoms of this condition.

54 Neuromuscular or Muscular Conditions

I. LEARNING KEY TERMS

MATCHING: Match each term with its corresponding definition or description.

1. _____ Visible defect on the posterior side of the infant with an external saclike protrusion that contains meninges, spinal fluid, and nerves.

2. _____ Movement disorder characterised by wide-based gait, rapid repetitive movements, performed poorly and disintegration of movements of the upper extremities when the child reaches for objects.

3. _____ Visible defect on the posterior side of the infant with an external saclike protrusion that encases meninges and spinal fluid but no neural elements.

4. _____ Combination of spastic cerebral palsy and dyskinetic cerebral palsy.

5. _____ Type of dyskinetic cerebral palsy characterised by abnormal involuntary movement such as slow, wormlike, writhing movements that usually involve the extremities, trunk, neck, facial muscles, and tongue.

6. _____ Characterised by persistent primitive reflexes, positive Babinski reflex, ankle clonus, exaggerated stretch reflexes, eventual development of contractures.

7. _____ Midline defects involving failure of the osseous spine to close.

a. Spastic cerebral palsy

b. Athetoid

c. Ataxic

d. Mixed-type cerebral palsy

e. Spina bifida

f. Meningocele

g. Myelomeningocele

II. REVIEWING KEY CONCEPTS

1. The aetiology of cerebral palsy (CP) is most commonly related to:
   a. decreased gestational age and birthweight.
   b. maternal obesity.
   c. post term birth.
   d. maternal substance abuse.

2. Factors that may contribute to the development of CP beyond the neonatal period include:
   a. bacterial meningitis.
   b. viral encephalitis.
   c. motor vehicle accidents (MVAs).
   d. traumatic brain injury (shaken baby syndrome).
   e. a, b, c, and d.

3. A child is suspected of having CP because he has clinical manifestations of wide-based gait and rapid repetitive movements of the upper extremities when he reaches for an object. Based on this information, the clinical classification of CP for this child is most likely:
   a. dyskinetic (nonspastic).
   b. ataxic (nonspastic).
   c. mixed-type (spastic and dyskinesia).
   d. spastic (pyramidal).

4. Features of CP may include:
   a. early speech development.
   b. eye cataracts that will need surgical correction.
   c. diminished reflexes.
   d. feeding and swallowing difficulties.

5. While performing a physical examination on a 6-month-old infant, the nurse suspects possible CP, because the infant:
   a. is able to hold on to the nurse's hands while being pulled to a sitting position.
   b. has no Moro reflex.
   c. has no tonic neck reflex.
   d. has an obligatory tonic neck reflex.

6. The goal of therapeutic management for the child with CP is:
   a. assisting with motor control of voluntary muscle.
   b. optimising development.
   c. delaying the development of sensory deprivation.
   d. surgical correction of deformities.

7. Which of the following would be appropriate when caring for an infant with a myelomeningocele preoperatively?
   a. Inspection of the sac for leakage along with frequent dressing changes
   b. Placing the infant in prone position
   c. Placing the infant in an isolette or under a radiant warmer
   d. a, b, and c

8. In order to prevent bladder dysfunction in older children with spina bifida, the child and parents are taught:
   a. clean intermittent catheterization.
   b. Foley catheter care.
   c. oral fluid challenge.
   d. bladder irrigations.

9. There is evidence that rates of serious neural tube defects may be decreased with maternal intake of:
   a. ascorbic acid.
   b. folic acid.
   c. muriatic acid.
   d. probiotics.

10. Children with spina bifida are at high risk for the development of _____ _____ and should be screened before any surgical procedure for _____ _____.

11. An infant had surgical correction of myelomeningocele and is 5 days postop. The nurse includes in the discharge plan for the parents to:
   I. monitor the operative site for redness or leaking.
   II. breastfeed or feed the infant a commercial formula as tolerated.
   III. perform passive range of motion when appropriate.
   IV. place the newborn prone or side-lying if permitted by provider
   V. learn clean intermittent catheterization technique if prescribed.
   a. I, II, III, IV
   b. I, II, III, IV, V
   c. II, III, IV, V

12. The condition inherited only as an autosomal recessive trait and characterised by progressive weakness and wasting of skeletal muscles caused by degeneration of anterior horn cells is:
   a. Spinal muscular atrophy (SMA).
   b. Duchenne muscular dystrophy.
   c. Kugelberg-Welander disease.
   d. Guillain-Barré syndrome.

13. A major goal in the nursing care of children with muscular dystrophy includes:
   a. promoting strenuous activity and exercise.
   b. promoting high calorie intake.
   c. promoting and optimising respiratory and cardiovascular health.
   d. preventing cognitive impairment.

14. Because Duchenne muscular dystrophy is inherited as an X-linked recessive trait, it is important for the parents of an affected child to:
   a. seek psychological counseling.
   b. screen all female offspring for the condition.
   c. receive genetic counseling.
   d. undergo voluntary sterilization.

15. A priority nursing consideration for the child in the acute phase of Guillain-Barré syndrome is:
   a. prevention of respiratory-focused complications including aspiration and atelectasis.
   b. prevention of contractures.
   c. prevention of bowel and bladder complications.
   d. prevention of sensory impairment.

III. THINKING CRITICALLY

1. Outline the social factors for which families and children living with Duchenne Muscular Dystrophy may require support and direction.

2. Describe nursing interventions aimed at preventing the complications of Guillain-Barré syndrome.

3. List the primary nursing goals for the initial stabilisation in the acute phase of care for an adolescent who arrives at the hospital with paraplegia caused by a spinal cord injury.

4. Describe the phenomenon of autonomic dysreflexia, the signs and symptoms, and management of the condition in an adolescent with spinal cord injury.

Caring for the Mental, Emotional, and Behavioural Health Needs of Children and Adolescents

I. LEARNING KEY TERMS

MATCHING: Match each term with its corresponding definition.

1. _____ Eating disorder characterised by turning to food to cope, impulsive or acting out behaviours, and awareness that the eating pattern is abnormal.

2. _____ Substance intended to relieve pain and produces a state of euphoria; withdrawal from use may require gradual tapering doses.

3. _____ Condition characterised by difficulty with sustained focus, wandering off task, low frustration tolerance.

4. _____ Group of disorders with common symptoms including expressing worry most days, trouble concentrating, or being unusually irritable or easily upset or having difficulty sleeping.

5. _____ Treatment strategy for depression that is used to change thought patterns.

6. _____ Mental health state manifested in behavioural, emotional, and mental characteristics that may include withdrawal from daily activities, predominantly sad or slower cognitive processing.

7. _____ Eating disorder characterised by restricting food intake, obsessive-compulsive behaviours and strives to maintain rigid control.

8. _____ Deliberate act of self-injury with intent that injury results in death.

9. _____ Substance that does not produce physical dependence; produces vivid hallucinations and euphoria.

10. _____ Term used to describe a characteristic of visual perceptual deficit; letter reversals.

a. Anorexia Nervosa

b. Anxiety

c. Attention-deficit hyperactivity disorder

d. Cognitive behavioural therapy

e. Depression

f. Suicide

g. dyslexia

h. bulimia

i. Opioid

j. Hallucinogens

II. REVIEWING KEY CONCEPTS

1. T F Suicidal ideation is common in youth.

2. T F Empathetic engagement is a type of collaborative relationship when a young person feels noticed, heard and appreciated.

3. T F Children experience a limited range of mental disorders that primarily involve their stage of neurodevelopment.

4. T F Depression in children can be readily identified because it presents as a response to acute events.

5. T F Copycat suicides may be evident through an increase in suicide after the suicide of one youth is publicized.

6. Substance use in youth
   a. Typically begins through experimentation
   b. Is more prevalent in non-Indigenous youth
   c. Occurs most frequently when away from peers to minimise risk of discovery
   d. most commonly occurs through drinking alcoholic beverages

7. Smoking bans in school help to accomplish more than one goal because they:
   a. Deter students from starting to smoke
   b. Provide opportunities to reinforce health consequences from smoking
   c. promote a smoke-free environment
   d. All of the above

8. Because the hazards of smoking are undisputed, the nurse may profile which alternative products as safe options to cigarette smoking to adolescents:
   a. Smokeless tobacco (chewing tobacco)
   b. Cannabis
   c. Electronic cigarettes
   d. none of the above
   e. all of the above

9. While working with a family whose child has been diagnosed with Attention Deficit Hyperactivity Disorder (ADHD), the nurse will help them to understand:
   a. ADHD is a serious, usually irreversible disorder
   b. the child will outgrow their behavioural health needs
   c. a focus on developing the child's strengths helps to build a family's self-esteem
   d. that education professionals are primarily responsible for coordinating the services required

10. The nurse who is providing a school-based health promotion session related to adolescent substance use will note the short-term effects of alcohol are most likely to:
    a. Cause changes in judgement, memory and learning
    b. Produce a state of euphoria
    c. Lead to neglect of self-care needs including dental care, general cleanliness
    d. All of the above

III. THINKING CRITICALLY

1. Outline the 3 major treatment and management goals for youth experiencing an eating disorder. List 3 questions to help facilitate an assessment of eating related behaviours.

2. Describe possible warning signs that may be present in a young person who may consider death by suicide.

Answer Key

CHAPTER 1: CONTEMPORARY PERINATAL AND PEDIATRIC NURSING IN CANADA

I. Learning Key Terms
1. g   2. c   3. h   4. a   5. e
6. f   7. b   8. d
9. Perinatal nursing
10. Public Health Agency of Canada
11. Sustainable Development Goals (SDG's)
12. Integrative healing
13. Telehealth
14. Health literacy
15. Evidence-informed practise
16. Standards of practise

II. Reviewing Key Concepts
1. See Ethical Issues in Maternal Child Nursing section that identifies the impact of technology on aspects of maternal-child nursing care.
2. a, c; Conventional Western modalities are included, patient autonomy and decision making is encouraged, and the whole patient and not just the disease process is the primary consideration.
3. See separate sections within Health Inequalities within Certain Population for each of the identified vulnerable populations listed to formulate your answer.
4. c

III. Thinking Critically
1. See Social Media section; explain how you could use social media to improve health care you provide to child-bearing families. Identify the precautions you would take to ensure privacy and confidentiality.
2. See sections on Indigenous People and Fig. 1-1 for content to answer the question.
3. See Social Determinants of Health section and Box 1-1- section; address solutions to the identified barriers—be creative and innovative.
4. See sections on Homelessness and Trauma and Violence Informed Care as well as Box 1-2 for strategies in providing care.
5. See Health Literacy section; include therapeutic communication techniques, culturally sensitive approaches, and preparation of bilingual written materials in answer.
6. See Adverse Childhood Experiences section for answers to the question. Discuss the significance of long-term effects of ACE's on a child's development.
7. See Lesbian/Gay/Bisexual/Transsexual/Queer/2-Spirited (LGBTQ2) Health section to help formulate your answer.

CHAPTER 2 THE FAMILY AND CULTURE

I. Learning Key Terms
1. b   2. a   3. d   4. c   5. e
6. b   7. d   8. a   9. c
1. Culture
2. Cultural humility
3. Acculturation
4. Ethnocentrism
5. Cultural competence
6. Future oriented
7. Past oriented
8. Present oriented
9. Personal space
10. Family
11. Nuclear
12. Lone parent
13. Blended
14. Same-sex
15. Multigenerational
16. Consanguineous
17. Genogram
18. Ecomap
19. Spirituality
20. Spiritual assessment

II. Reviewing Key Concepts
1. See Cultural Factors Related to Health section for a discussion of communication, personal space, time orientation, and family roles including how the nurse should consider each area when communicating with and caring for patients in a culturally sensitive manner.
2. b; Providing explanations, especially when performing tasks that require close contact, can help to avoid misunderstandings; touching the patient, making eye contact, and taking away the right to make decisions can be interpreted by patients in some cultures as invading their personal space.
3. d; Choices a, b, and c are incorrect interpretations based on the woman's culture and customs.
4. c; The student should be looking at the patient while speaking and asking questions through the interpreter; a normal tone of voice should be used.
5. a,b, d, and e; Set meals without regard to a patient's cultural background is not culturally sensitive.
6. a, b, d; These are all a part of a spiritual assessment.

III. Thinking Critically
1. Use Providing Culturally Competent Nursing Care; and Family Nursing as Relational Inquiry sections to

253

formulate your answer; consider components of communication, personal space, time orientation, and family roles; identify the degree to which each woman/family follows their cultural beliefs and practices; do not stereotype.
2. Use Multiculturalism in Canada section. Consider the cause of racism and cultural oppression
3. See Communication—Use of Interpreters section and Box 2-6 for the content required to answer this question.
4. Refer to Spirituality section.

CHAPTER 3 – COMMUNITY CARE

I. Learning Key Terms
1. b   2. a   3. h   4. d   5. c
6. f   7. g   8. e
1. Agent, host, and environment
2. Primary prevention
3. Secondary prevention; health screening
4. Walking through a community, participant observation, interviews, focus groups, and analysis of existing data
5. Participant observation
6. Population size, age ranges, sex, racial and ethnic distribution, socioeconomic status, educational level, employment, and housing characteristics

II. Reviewing Key Concepts
1. See Home Care in the Community and Nursing Care sections to formulate your answer. Consider changes in length of hospital stays, portability of technology, and the need to reduce health care costs in your answer; describe the need for nurses to broaden their scope of practice.
2. See Community Health Promotion to formulate your answer.
3. See Phone and On-Line Health Support section; include warm lines, advice lines, and telephonic nursing assessment, consultation, and education.
4. d; Although a and b are appropriate, they are not the most important; gloves are not needed unless the possibility of contacting body substances is present.
5. T   6. F   7. F   8. F   9. T

III. Thinking Critically
1. See Assessing the Community and Community Focus Box for the content required to answer each part of this question.
2. See Nursing Care, Home Visiting sections to answer each component of this exercise, including the approach you would take to prepare, your actions during the visit, safety precautions and infection control measures you would follow, how you would end the visit, and the interventions you would follow after the visit, including documentation of assessments, actions, and responses.

3. See Home Care in the Community—Patient Selection and Referral sections for a and b and Nursing Care section for c.

CHAPTER 4 - PERINATAL NURSING IN CANADA

I. Learning Key Terms
1. c   2. e   3. d   4. g   5. f
6. a   7. b

II. Reviewing Key Concepts
1. See Childbirth-Related Mortality Rate section that identifies many physical and psychosocial factors; consider access to care, improved family planning services and reproductive services for adolescents.
2. a, b, d. Inability to pay is not an option in the Canadian health care system.
3. c
4. See Trends in Fertility and Birth Rate section for answer to question. Answer should include anemia and poor weight gain and twice the risk of giving birth to a preterm or low–birth weight baby.
5. d
6. See Perinatal Health Indicators: The Canadian Perinatal Surveillance System section.

III. Thinking Critically
1. See Perinatal Services in Canada as well as Indigenous Women section for information to answer this question. Consider access to care, culturally safe care, role of elders and family, and socioeconomic status.
2. See Homelessness and Pregnancy section for content to answer this question. Discuss the importance of providing trauma-informed care.
3. See Providing Care in a Culturally Safe Manner and Table 4-1. It is important to acknowledge that one must not make assumptions about different cultures and everyone needs a cultural assessment done first. Nurses are also reminded to reflect on the ways in which their own cultural practises may be interpreted by patients and family members. Nurses may not agree with all cultural practises, but it is important to respect the patient's decisions.
4. See Global Health Section; discuss both female genital cutting (FGC) and human trafficking, consider exploring these issues in greater depth, and investigate media reports regarding these issues.
5. See Care Environment and Midwifery section for information to answer this question. Keep in mind that a person's right to choose where to give birth should be respected.

CHAPTER 5 HEALTH PROMOTION

I. Learning Key Terms
1. Cocaine
2. Methadone
3. Methamphetamine

4. Substance use
5. Addiction
6. Kegel exercise
7. Preconception counselling and care
8. Obesity
9. Anorexia nervosa
10. Bulimia nervosa
11. Intimate partner violence (IPV)
12. Increasing tension, battery, calm and remorse, honeymoon
13. Female genital cutting
14. Human trafficking
1. Cognitive learning
2. Affective learning
3. Psychomotor learning
4. One-on-one discussion
5. Role playing
6. Group teaching
7. Demonstration
8. Health literacy

II. Reviewing Key Concepts

1. See Barriers to Receiving Health Care System section for a full description of each category of issues listed.
2. See Intimate Partner Violence section and Box 5-10.
3. See Nutrition section and Box 5-5 to formulate your answer.
4. See separate section for each of the substances listed in Substance Use section.
5. a; All patients should be screened because abuse can happen to any person; abuse often escalates during pregnancy; the most commonly injured sites are head, neck, chest, abdomen, breasts, and upper extremities. If abuse is suspected the nurse needs to assess further to encourage disclosure and then assist the patient to take action and formulate a plan.
6. a, c, and f; Pap tests are recommended every 3 years for women who are 52 year of age; mammograms should be done every 2 to 3 year for women over 50 years of age and bone mineral density beginning at age 65; clinical breast examinations are not recommended for low risk women (see Table 5-3).
7. a; All patients, not just specific groups, should participate in preconception care 1 year before planning to get pregnant.
8. c and e; Smoking is associated with preterm birth, not postterm pregnancies; smoking can reduce the age for menopause.
9. a, b, d, and e; Asking "why" questions revictimises and blames the victim; the nurse should not talk negatively about the abuser nor talk directly to him about suspicions of abuse. See Box 5-10.
10. b, e, and f; IPV can occur in any family; battering frequently begins or escalates during pregnancy; women may stay even if the battering is bad because of fear and financial dependence, and shelters often have long waiting lists.

III. Thinking Critically

1. See specific sections for each factor.
2. See Intimate Partner Violence section including Boxes 5-9 and 5-12, and Fig. 5-3 for content required to answer all parts of the question.
3. See Preconception Counselling and Care section and Box 5-2 and Fig. 5-1; this nurse should:
   • Define preconception counselling and care and what it entails and stress the importance of both partners participating.
   • Identify the impact of a patient's health status and lifestyle habits on the developing foetus during the first trimester.
   • Describe how preconception counselling can help a couple choose the best time to begin a pregnancy.
4. See Stress and Lack of Exercise sections:
   • Assess for symptoms of stress (Box 5-6) and discuss social support and coping skills that are beneficial in managing stress.
   • Aerobic exercise: Discuss weight-bearing versus non–weight-bearing exercises as well as frequency and duration of exercise sessions for maximum benefit.
5. See Wellness Across the Lifespan – Adolescent section to answer this question.
6. See Cigarette Smoking and Stress section and Box 5-3 to address the woman's concern.
7. See Intimate Partner Violence including *Violence During Pregnancy* sections and Boxes 5-9 and 5-19 and Table 5-2 for content to answer all parts of this question.

CHAPTER 6 HEALTH ASSESSMENT

I. Learning Key Terms

1. f   2. c   3. b   4. e   5. d
6. a

II. Reviewing Key Concepts

1. Guidelines for each component of the procedure are outlined in Box 6-4, Procedure: Papanicolaou Test.
2. Breast self-examination (BSE) is not recommended for women aged 40 to 74 years who do not have a high risk of developing breast cancer. Patients do need to know how their breasts feel and look and to watch for changes, but not on a regular schedule. Some patients may still choose to perform BSE and these patients need to be taught the correct method and the instructions.
3. b; Do not ask questions during the examination because it may distract the patient, interfering with relaxation measures she may be using; only offer explanations as needed during the examination.
4. c; Patients should not use vaginal medications or douche for 24 to 48 hours before the test; OCPs can continue; the best time for the test is midcycle.

255

III. Thinking Critically

1. a. See Box 6-3; explain what will occur and each guideline to follow for preparation and why each is important for the accuracy of the test; tell her to avoid douching, vaginal medications, and intercourse for 24 hours before the examination; she should not be menstruating.

   b. See Internal Structures section; vaginal secretions are usually acidic and protect the reproductive tract from infection; a douche may alter this acidity and injure the mucosa, thereby increasing the risk for infection; gentle and regular front-to-back washing with mild soap and water is all that is necessary to be clean.

2. See Box 6-3 Nurse's Role in Assisting With Pelvic Examination and Box 5-4 Papaniculaou Test.

3. a. Health Assessment: History section and Box 6-1 Health History and Review of Systems for a list and description of components.

   b. Use components of health history as a guide; write questions that are open ended, clear, concise, address only one issue, and progress from general to specific.

   c. See History section.

4. See Cultural Considerations and Communication Variations section and Cultural Awareness box: Communication Variations.
   - Approach the woman in a respectful and calm manner.
   - Consider modifications in the examination to maintain her modesty.
   - Incorporate communication variations such as conversational style, pacing, spacing, eye contact, touch, time orientation.
   - Take time to learn about the woman's cultural beliefs and practises regarding well-woman assessment and care.

5. See Women at Risk for Abuse section including Box 6-2 for content required to answer all parts of the question.

6. See Box 6-3, Nurse's Role in Assisting With Pelvic Examination and Box 6-4 Papanicolaou Test for the content required to answer each part of this question.

7. See Transsexuality Section (and Table 5-3) for the content required to answer this question.

CHAPTER 7 REPRODUCTIVE HEALTH

I. Learning Key Terms

1. Mons pubis
2. Labia majora
3. Labia minora
4. Prepuce
5. Frenulum
6. Fourchette
7. Clitoris
8. Vaginal vestibule
9. Urethra
10. Perineum
11. Vagina; rugae, Skene, Bartholin, hymen
12. Fornices
13. Uterus; cul de sac of Douglas
14. Corpus
15. Isthmus
16. Fundus
17. Endometrium
18. Myometrium
19. Cervix
20. Endocervical; internal os, external os
21. Squamocolumnar junction; transformation
22. Uterine (fallopian) tubes
23. Ovaries; ovulation, estrogen, progesterone, androgen
24. Bony pelvis
25. Breasts
26. Tail of Spence
27. Nipple
28. Areola
29. Montgomery glands (tubercles)
30. Menarche
31. Puberty
32. Climacteric
33. Menopause
34. Perimenopause
35. Menstruation; endometrial, hypothalamic-pituitary, ovarian, 28 days, the first day of bleeding, 5 days, 3 to 6 days
36. Endometrial; menstrual, proliferative, secretory, ischaemic
37. Hypothalamic-pituitary
38. Ovarian; follicular (preovulatory), luteal (post-ovulatory)
39. Gonadotropin-releasing hormone (GnRH); follicle-stimulating hormone (FSH), luteinizing hormone (LH)
40. Follicle-stimulating hormone
41. Luteinizing hormone (LH)
42. Estrogen; spinnbarkeit
43. Progesterone; basal body
44. Mittelschmerz
45. Prostaglandins
46. Amenorrhea
47. Hypogonadotropic amenorrhea
48. Female athlete triad
49. Dysmenorrhea
50. Primary dysmenorrhea
51. Secondary dysmenorrhea
52. Premenstrual syndrome (PMS)
53. Premenstrual dysphoric disorder (PMDD)
54. Endometriosis
55. Oligomenorrhea
56. Hypomenorrhea
57. Menorrhagia
58. Metrorrhagia
59. Abnormal uterine bleeding (AUB)
60. Sexually transmitted infections (STIs)
61. Chlamydia
62. Gonorrhoea

256

63. Syphilis; chancre; symmetric maculopapular rash; lymphadenopathy; condylomata lata
64. Pelvic inflammatory disease (PID)
65. Human papillomavirus (HPV)
66. Herpes simplex virus (HSV)
67. Hepatitis A virus (HAV)
68. Hepatitis B virus (HBV)
69. Hepatitis C virus (HCV)
70. Human immunodeficiency virus (HIV); acquired immunodeficiency syndrome (AIDS)
71. Zika virus
72. Bacterial vaginosis
73. Vulvovaginal candidiasis
74. Trichomoniasis

II. Reviewing Key Concepts

1. b   2. d   3. a   4. f   5. e
6. c
7. Box 7-4 cites many common risk behaviours according to sexual, drug use–related, and blood-related risks.
8. See HIV section and Box 7-6 for a description of risky behaviours and clinical manifestations during seroconversion.
9. See Zika Virus section.
10. See Cancer of the Breast section and Box 7-9 for the content required to answer each part of this question.
11. b; The 13-year-old reflects several of the risk factors associated with this menstrual disorder, namely: presently in a growth period, participating in a sport that is stressful, subjectively scored, requires contour revealing clothing, and success is favoured by a prepubertal body shape.
12. c; Choices a, b, and d interfere with prostaglandin synthesis, whereas acetaminophen has no antiprostaglandin properties; prostaglandins are a recognised factor in the aetiology of dysmenorrhea.
13. b; Caffeine should be avoided; other substances listed can be helpful in relieving discomforts of PMS.
14. b, d, e, and f; Exercise increases endorphins, dilates blood vessels, and helps to reduce ischemia; peaches and watermelon have a natural diuretic effect.
15. c, d, and f; Women taking danazol often experience masculinizing changes; amenorrhea is an outcome of taking this medication; ovulation may not be fully suppressed; therefore, birth control is essential because this medication is teratogenic; danazol is taken orally.
16. a; Dysmenorrhea is painful menstruation; dysuria is painful urination; dyspnea is difficulty breathing.
17. a; Because these infections are often asymptomatic, they can go undetected and untreated causing more damage including ascent of the pathogen into the uterus and pelvis, resulting in PID and infertility; many effective treatment measures are available, including for chlamydia.

18. b; Choice a is indicative of candidiasis; choice c is indicative of HSV-2; choice d is indicative of trichomoniasis.
19. b; Flagyl is used to treat bacterial vaginosis and trichomoniasis; ampicillin is effective in the treatment of chlamydia or gonorrhea; acyclovir is used to treat herpes.
20. d; Recurrent infections commonly involve only local symptoms that are less severe; stress reduction, healthy lifestyle practices, and acyclovir can reduce recurrence rate; nonantiviral ointments, especially those containing cortisone, should be avoided—use lidocaine ointment or an antiseptic spray instead.
21. c, e, and f; Breast cancer is more common among White women; the majority of women do not exhibit the identified risk factors; one in eight women could develop breast cancer in her lifetime.
22. a; Pain is a common finding; it usually begins a week before the onset of menses; leakage from nipples is not associated with this disorder; surgery is unlikely and is only attempted in a few selected cases; overall cancer risk is 5%.
23. d; Fibroadenomas are generally small, unilateral, firm, nontender, moveable lumps located in the upper outer quadrant; borders are discrete and well defined; discharge is not associated with this disorder.
24. b, d; Ginger and black haw are helpful for menstrual cramping; black cohosh root is effective for some of the symptoms of PMS. See Table 7-1.

III. Thinking Critically

1. See Hypogonadotropic Amenorrhea section for the content required to answer each part of this question.
2. See Primary Dysmenorrhea section and Table 7-1 and 7-2 for the content required to answer each part of this question.
3. See PMS section for the content required to answer each part of this question; use assessment findings to determine those that would apply to a particular patient including those that are priority; obtain a detailed history and encourage the patient to keep a diary of physical and emotional manifestations (what occurs, when, contributing circumstances) from one cycle to another.
4. See Endometriosis section for the content required to answer each part of this question.
5. See Infections section, Boxes 7-4, 7-5, 7-6, and 7-7 for the content required to answer each part of this question.
6. See Pelvic Inflammatory Disease section; Patient Teaching Prevention of Genital Tract Infections for the content required to answer each part of this question.
7. See Gonorrhoea section, Patient Teaching Box; Prevention of Genital Tract Infections in Women, and Table 7-3 Sexually Transmitted Infections and Drug Therapies for the content required to answer each part of this question.

8. See HPV section and Figure 7.11.
9. See Herpes simplex virus section for content required to answer each part of this question.
10. See HIV section for content required to answer each part of this question; use Sonya's risky behaviours as a basis for discussing prevention measures, including safer sex practices; discuss impact HIV could have on her health.
11. See Fibrocystic Changes section and Table 7-5 for content required to answer each part of this question.

CHAPTER 8 INFERTILITY, CONTRACEPTION, AND ABORTION

I. Learning Key Terms

1. Infertility
2. Fecundity
3. Assisted human reproduction (AHR)
4. In vitro fertilization-embryo transfer (IVF-ET)
5. Intracytoplasmic sperm injection (ICSI)
6. Gamete intrafallopian transfer (GIFT)
7. Zygote intrafallopian transfer (ZIFT)
8. Therapeutic donor insemination (TDI)
9. Gestational carrier (embryo host)
10. Surrogate motherhood
11. Assisted hatching
12. Donor oocyte
13. Donor embryo (embryo adoption)
14. Therapeutic donor insemination
15. Cryopreservation
16. Semen analysis
17. Hysterosalpingogram
18. Urinary or salivary ovulation predictor kit
19. Hysterosalpingo-contrast sonography
20. Contraception
21. Birth control
22. Family planning
23. Contraceptive failure
24. Long-acting reversible contraception (LARC)
25. Coitus interruptus
26. Fertility awareness methods
27. Natural family planning
28. Calendar day method
29. Standard days method
30. Basal body temperature (BBT)
31. Cervical mucus ovulation detection method
32. Spinnbarkeit
33. Symptothermal
34. Two-day method
35. Lactation amenorrhea method (LAM)
36. Spermicide
37. Condom
38. Diaphragm
39. Cervical cap
40. Contraceptive sponge
41. Combined oral contraceptive (COC)
42. Transdermal contraceptive system (patch)
43. Contraceptive vaginal ring
44. Emergency contraception
45. Intrauterine device (IUD)
46. Sterilization; bilateral tubal ligation; vasectomy
47. Induced abortion; elective abortion; therapeutic abortion

II. Reviewing Key Concepts

1. See Cervical Mucus Ovulation-Detection Method section and Guidelines box, Cervical Mucus Characteristics.
   - Alert couple about reestablishment of ovulation after breastfeeding or discontinuing oral contraceptives.
   - Determine whether cycles are ovulatory at any time including menopause, when planning pregnancy, or for timing infertility treatments and diagnostic procedures.
2. a, c, d, and e; Spermicide should be applied to the surface of the diaphragm and the rim; diaphragm should not be removed for at least 6 hours; it should be washed with warm water and mild soap, and then cornstarch should be applied; it should not be used during menstruation to prevent TSS.
3. b; Spinnbarkeit refers to stretchiness of cervical mucus at ovulation to facilitate passage of sperm; there is an LH surge before ovulation; BBT rises in response to increased progesterone after ovulation; cervical mucus becomes thinner and more abundant with ovulation.
4. a; Oral contraception provides no protection from STIs; therefore, a condom and spermicide are still recommended to prevent transmission; choices b, c, and d reflect appropriate actions and recognition of side effects.
5. a; Although choices b, c, and d are all temporary side effects, the most common is the irregular pattern of vaginal bleeding that occurs; women report that this bleeding is also the most distressing side effect.
6. c; The longer a woman uses DMPA, the more significant the loss of bone mineral density; weight gain not loss can occur.
7. a, d, and e; The string should be checked after menses; a missing string or one that becomes longer or shorter should be checked by a health care professional; A copper IUD contains no hormone; NSAIDs are safe to use for discomfort.
8. d; Clomid is taken orally; therefore, there is no need to teach the patient's partner how to give an IM injection; b refers to nafarelin and c is used as part of treatment with menotropins.

III. Thinking Critically

1. See Nursing Care, Assessment, Psychosocial Implications, and Nonmedical treatment sections and Table 8-1 and Box 8-4 for content required to answer each part of this question.
2. See Assisted Human Reproduction section and Box 8-6 for the content required to answer each part of this question; answer should discuss such issues as

258

- Who should pay? Insurance coverage; wealthy versus poor couples
- Children: Who are their biological parents? What is their medical history?
- Ownership of ovum, sperm, embryos
- Attempt to create the "perfect" child

3. See Contraceptive section including Care Management and Box 8-7 for content required to answer each part of this question.
4. See Combined Oral Contraceptives section, Box 8-9, and Table 8-3 for content required to answer each part of this question.
5. See Box 8-10, Signs of Potential Complications: Intrauterine Devices or Intrauterine Systems, which uses the acronym of PAINS to identify signs of problems; be sure to include in your answer:
   - Teach how and when to check string.
   - Stress importance of appropriate genital hygiene and sexual practices.
   - Inform when IUS needs to be replaced.
6. See Sterilisation section for content required to answer each part of this question.
7. See Fertility Awareness Based Methods section and Guideline boxes for content required to answer each part of this question.
8. See Abortion section and Box 8-11 for content required to answer each part of this question.
9. See Medical Abortion section for a description of the medications used.
10. See Emergency Contraception section for content required to answer each part of this question; be sure to include each of the following in your answer:
    - Explore possibility of pregnancy and options related to continuing pregnancy if it occurs.
    - Explore options for emergency contraception to prevent pregnancy: methods available, how each works, timing, side effects, how administered.
    - Emphasise importance of follow-up to check for effectiveness of method used and occurrence of infection.
    - Discuss methods of contraception and infection prevention measures to prevent recurrence of this situation.

CHAPTER 9 GENETICS, CONCEPTION, AND FETAL DEVELOPMENT

I. Learning Key Terms
1. Conception
2. Gametes; sperm, ovum (egg)
3. Gametogenesis; spermatogenesis, oogenesis
4. Fertilization; ampulla (outer third), zona reaction, diploid (46)
5. Zygote; morula, blastocyst, trophoblast
6. Implantation; chorionic villi, decidua, decidua basalis, decidua capsularis
7. Embryo
8. Foetus
9. Amniotic membranes; chorion, amnion

10. Amniotic fluid
11. Umbilical cord; arteries, vein
12. Wharton's jelly
13. Placenta; hormones, oxygen, nutrients, wastes, carbon dioxide
14. Viability
15. Pulmonary surfactants; lecithin-sphingomyelin
16. Ductus arteriosus
17. Ductus venosus
18. Foramen ovale
19. Hematopoiesis; yolk sac
20. Meconium
21. Dizygotic, fraternal
22. Monozygotic, identical

1. j	2. b	3. m	4. h	5. k
6. c	7. l	8. i	9. q	10. a
11. r	12. f	13. o	14. g	15. s
16. d	17. n	18. p	19. t	20. e

1. Genetic testing
2. Direct or molecular testing
3. Linkage analysis
4. Biochemical testing
5. Cytogenetic testing
6. Predictive testing; presymptomatic; predispositional
7. Carrier screening
8. Homologous
9. Homozygous; heterozygous
10. Genotype
11. Phenotype
12. Karyotype
13. Multifactorial
14. Unifactorial
15. Autosomal dominance
16. Autosomal recessive
17. Inborn error of metabolism

II. Reviewing Key Concepts
1. See individual sections for each of these structures in the Embryo and Foetus section.
2. See Primary Germ Layers section of the Embryo and Fetus, and Fig. 9-8*B*, for identification of tissues and organs that develop from the ectoderm, mesoderm, and endoderm.
3. See Fig. 9-3, a risk factors questionnaire: Ask questions that would elicit information regarding health status of family members; abnormal reproductive outcomes; history of maternal disorders, drug exposures, and illnesses; advanced maternal and paternal age; and ethnic origin.
4. See Genetics—Estimation of Risk section.
5. a; Autosomal dominant inheritance is unrelated to exposure to teratogens; each pregnancy has the same potential for expression of the disorder; there is no reduction if one child is already affected; if the gene is inherited, the disorder is always expressed.
6. b; There is a 25% chance females will be carriers; if males inherit the X chromosome with the defective gene, the disorder will be expressed and they can transmit the gene to female offspring; females are

259

affected if they receive the defective gene from both parents.

7. d; Cystic fibrosis, as an inborn error of metabolism, follows an autosomal recessive pattern of inheritance; two defective genes (one from each parent) are required for the disorder to be expressed; she does not have the disorder and the father does not have the defective gene; therefore, none of their children will have the disorder, but there will be a 50% chance they will be carriers of the defective gene.

8. c, e, and f; The sex of a baby is determined at conception; the heart begins to pump blood by the 3rd week, and a beat can be heard with ultrasound by the 8th week of gestation.

III. Thinking Critically

1. a. See Table 9-1 to formulate your answer; use of illustrations and life-size models would facilitate learning.

   b. See Pulmonary Surfactant section; discuss how the respiratory system develops including the critical factor, surfactant production; describe how surfactant helps the newborn breathe.

   c. See Musculoskeletal and Sensory Awareness section; explain that quickening is the woman's perception of foetal movement that occurs at about 16 to 20 weeks of gestation; it will not hurt but can be uncomfortable and interfere with sleep toward the end of pregnancy; Foetus will develop its own sleep-wake cycle.

   d. Discuss sensory capability of the Foetus using Sensory Awareness section; Foetus can hear sounds such as parents' voices, respond to light and touch, and perceive temperature and taste.

   e. See Reproductive System section; discuss function of X and Y chromosomes; sex of her Foetus will become recognisable around the 9th week of gestation.

   f. See Multifetal Pregnancy—Twins section; discuss monozygotic (identical) and dizygotic (fraternal) twinning and how each occurs; emphasise that fraternal twinning tends to occur in some families.

2. See Genetic Counselling, Genetics and Autosomal Abnormalities sections.

   a. Tay-Sachs is an autosomal recessive disorder that follows a unifactorial pattern of inheritance; the husband needs to be tested because he must also be a carrier to produce a child with the disorder; emphasise the nurse's role in terms of emotional support, facilitation of the decision-making process, and interpretation of diagnostic test results and how they can influence future childbearing decisions.

   b. See Estimation of Risk section: There is a 25% chance the child will be unaffected, a 25% chance that the child will express the disorder, and a 50% chance that the child will be a carrier; this pattern is the same for every pregnancy; there is no reduction in risk from one pregnancy to another. See Fig. 9-2.

   c. Discuss the nature of this disorder, extent of risk, and consequences if the child inherits the disorder; options available include amniocentesis, continuing or not continuing the pregnancy if the child is affected, and use of reproductive technology or adoption; be sensitive to cultural and religious beliefs; encourage expression of feelings; refer for further counselling or support groups as appropriate.

CHAPTER 10 ANATOMY AND PHYSIOLOGY OF PREGNANCY

I. Learning Key Terms

1. Gravidity
2. Parity
3. Gravida
4. Nulligravida
5. Nullipara
6. Primigravida
7. Primipara
8. Multigravida
9. Multipara
10. Viability
11. Preterm
12. Full term
13. Post term
14. Human chorionic gonadotropin (hCG)
15. Presumptive changes
16. Probable changes
17. Positive changes
18. Braxton Hicks contractions
19. Uterine souffle
20. Funic souffle
21. Quickening
22. Supine hypotension
23. Polymorphic eruption of pregnancy (PEP)
24. Pica

25. c	26. p	27. k	28. t	29. s
30. u	31. j	32. n	33. v	34. b
35. g	36. a	37. o	38. i	39. q
40. e	41. m	42. w	43. f	44. h
45. d	46. r	47. l	48. x	

II. Reviewing Key Concepts

1. Manjit (G3-T1-P1-A0-L1); Marsha (G4-T2-P0-A1-L2); Alana (G4-T1-P2-A1-L3).

2. See designated sections in General Body Systems section as well as Table 10-3 & Table 10-5.

3. See Pregnancy Tests section and Community Focus Box: Pregnancy Tests.

4. a. See Table 10-4.

   b. See Circulation and Coagulation Times section of Cardiopulmonary System and Table 10-4.

   c. See Acid-Base Balance section and Table 10-4.

   d. See Renal System section.

5. a. See Renal System section; slowed passage of more alkaline urine and dilation of the ureters as a result of progesterone increases the risk for

UTIs; bladder irritability, nocturia, urinary frequency, and urgency (first and third trimesters after lightening).

b. See Gastrointestinal section; constipation and hemorrhoids; effect of increased progesterone, which decreases peristalsis and intestinal displacement by enlarging uterus.

6. a, c, and e; hCG indicates a positive pregnancy test and is a probable sign of pregnancy along with other changes that can be observed by the examiner; breast tenderness and amenorrhea are presumptive signs; foetal heart sounds are a positive sign of pregnancy.

7. d; Gravida (total number of pregnancies including the present one is 5); para (term birth of daughter at 39 weeks = 1; preterm stillbirth at 32 weeks and triplets at 30 weeks = 4; spontaneous abortion at 8 weeks = 1; total number of living children = 4).

8. c; Although little change occurs in respiratory rate, breathing becomes more thoracic in nature with the upward displacement of the diaphragm; pregnant patients normally experience a greater awareness of their breathing and may even state they have symptoms of dyspnea at rest as pregnancy progresses; supine hypotension syndrome with a decrease in systolic pressure as much as 30 mm Hg occurs as a result of vena cava and aorta compression by the uterus when the patient is in a supine position; baseline pulse rate increases by 10 to 15 beats per minute; systolic and diastolic pressure decreases by approximately 5 to 10 mm Hg beginning in the second trimester, returning to first trimester levels in the third trimester.

9. b; Friability refers to cervical fragility resulting in slight bleeding when scraped or touched; Chadwick sign refers to a deep bluish colour of cervix and vagina as a result of increased circulation; Hegar sign refers to softening and compressibility of the lower uterine segment.

10. a, b, and f; Choices c and e are probably signs and choice d is a positive sign, diagnostic of pregnancy.

III. Thinking Critically

1. a. See Cervical Changes section; discuss cervical and vaginal friability and increased vascularity; makes the vagina and cervix softer and more delicate so spotting after intercourse is expected; caution that any bleeding should be reported so it can be evaluated.

b. See Pregnancy Tests section: emphasise the importance of following directions because each brand of test is slightly different; use first-voided morning specimen for the most concentrated urine and notify health care provider regardless of the test result.

c. See Vagina and Vulva and Renal System sections: discuss impact of increased vaginal secretions and impact of stasis of urine that contains nutrients and has a high pH; review prevention measures at this time.

d. See Breasts section; discuss changes in breasts such as enlargement of Montgomery glands and development of lactation structures resulting in larger breasts that are tender during the first trimester; changes in consistency and presence of lumpiness during BSE; changes are bilateral.

e. See Uteroplacental Blood Flow, BP, and Renal System sections; discuss supine hypotensive syndrome and importance of the lateral position when at rest; also emphasise safety when changing position from supine to upright and to do so slowly as pregnancy progresses to reduce effects of orthostatic hypotension and dizziness.

f. See Respiratory System section; discuss impact of estrogen-stimulated increase in upper airway vascularity, which increases edema, congestion, and hyperemia of the tissue making nosebleeds more common.

g. See Renal System section; explain that the swelling of her ankles is a result of the pressure of the enlarging uterus and the dependent position of her legs; elevating her legs and exercising them helps decrease edema; caution her to never take someone else's medications or to self-medicate.

h. See Musculoskeletal section; lordosis occurs as a result of the enlargement of the uterus, which decreases abdominal muscle tone and increases mobility of the pelvic joints, tilting the pelvis forward and resulting in lower back pain, a change in posture, and a shifting forward of the centre of gravity.

i. See Changes in Contractility section; the woman is describing prelabour contractions because they diminish with activity; these contractions facilitate blood flow and promote oxygen delivery to the fetus; compare these contractions with true labour contractions.

2. See Box 10-1 and Blood Pressure section for content required to answer each part of this question.

CHAPTER 11 NURSING CARE OF THE FAMILY DURING PREGNANCY

I. Learning Key Terms

1. Nägele's rule; 3, last menstrual period (LMP), 7.
2. Trimesters
3. Fundal height
4. Developmental tasks; accepting pregnancy, identifying with role of parent, reordering personal relationships, establishing relationship with foetus preparing for childbirth
5. Emotional lability
6. Ambivalence
7. Supine hypotension; vena cava; abdominal aorta
8. Orthostatic (postural) hypotension
9. Couvade syndrome
10. Prescriptions; proscriptions; taboos
11. Doulas
12. Birth plan

II. Reviewing Key Concepts

1. Use Nägele rule: Subtract 3 months and add 7 days and 1 year to the first day of the last menstrual period.
   a. February 12, 2021
   b. October 26, 2021
   c. April 11, 2021
2. See Variations in Prenatal Care sections.
   a. Consider the following factors: beliefs that conflict with typical Western prenatal practices, lack of money and transportation, communication difficulties, concern regarding modesty and gender of health care provider, fear of invasive procedures, view of pregnancy as a healthy state whereas health care providers imply illness, view pregnancy problems as a normal part of pregnancy.
   b. See separate sections for each area.
3. See Initial Visit and Follow-up Visits in the Nursing Care section.
4. a. See Table 11-2 for signs of potential complications, which lists signs according to the first, second, and third trimesters.
   b. • Discuss the signs, possible causes, when and to whom to report.
      • Present the signs verbally and in written form.
      • Provide time to answer questions and discuss concerns; make follow-up phone calls.
      • Gather full information of signs that are reported; use information as a basis for action.
      • Document all assessments, actions, and responses.
5. See Fundal Height section; consider pregnant patient's position, type of measuring tape used, measurement method (Fig. 11-6), and conditions of the examination such as an empty bladder and relaxed or contracted uterus.
6. a. See Posture and Body Mechanics section, Fig. 11-11, and Patient Teaching box Posture and Body Mechanics.
   b. See Patient Teaching box, Safety During Pregnancy, Fig. 8.17, and prevention measures identified in subsections of Education for Self-Management section such as physical activity, rest and relaxation, employment, clothing, and travel.
7. See Preparation for Breastfeeding the Newborn section.
8. See Paternal Adaptation—Accepting the Pregnancy section for a discussion of each phase.
9. a; Use Nägele rule by subtracting 3 months and adding 7 days and 1 year to the first day of the last menstrual period (September 10, 2020).
10. d; Supine hypotension related to compression of aorta and vena cava is being experienced; the first action is to remove the cause of the problem by turning the patient on their side; this should alleviate the symptoms being experienced, including nausea; assessment of vital signs can occur after the patient's position is changed.
11. a and d; Ambivalence is a common response when preparing for a new role and mood swings or emotional lability is commonly related to hormonal changes; a pregnant patient's partner or the father of the baby is usually the greatest source of support; attachment begins with the pregnancy and intensifies during the second trimester.
12. a, e, and f; Intake of at least 2 to 3 litres per day is recommended; they do not have to abstain from intercourse, but should empty their bladder before and after intercourse and drink a large glass of water; cranberry juice may be helpful, but there is conflicting evidence.
13. d; Continuous support is critical and involves praise, encouragement, reassurance, comfort measures, physical contact, and explanations; the doula does not get involved in clinical tasks; the doula is not a substitute for the partner but rather encourages their participation as a partner along with the doula in supporting the labouring patient.
14. a, b, e, and f; The pregnant patient should assume a lateral position and continue to count for one more hour.

III. Thinking Critically

1. See Initial Visit and Follow-up Visits sections, in Nursing Care section.
   a. • Establish therapeutic relationship with the pregnant patient and their family.
      • Plan time for purposeful communication to gather baseline data related to the patient's subjective appraisal of their health status and to gather objective information based on observation of the patient's affect, posture, body language, skin colour, and other physical and emotional signs.
      • Update information and compare to baseline information during follow-up interviews.
   b. Be sure questions reflect principles of effective questioning; consider the need to ask follow-up questions to clarify and gather further information when a problem is identified.
   c. Focus on updating baseline information and asking questions related to anticipated events and changes for the patient's gestational age at the time of the visit.
2. See Variations in Prenatal Care – Adolescents and the Nursing Care Plan for Adolescent Pregnancy; answer should emphasise the following:
   • Establishing a therapeutic, trusting relationship so the woman will feel comfortable continuing with prenatal care
   • Teaching the woman about the importance of prenatal care for her health and that of her baby
   • Involving her boyfriend in the care process so he will encourage her participation in prenatal care
   • Following guidelines for health history interview, physical examination, and laboratory testing; ensure privacy and comfort during the examination

and teach her about how her body is changing and will continue to change with pregnancy
- Evaluating the couple's reaction (e.g., same or different) to pregnancy and the need for community agency support

3. a. Reliability depends on the accuracy of date used and the regularity of her menstrual cycles; birth can normally occur 2 weeks before or after the date or from week 38 to 42. Only 5% of births occur on the EDB.
   b. See Kegel Exercises section and Patient Teaching box Kegel Exercises in Chapter 5.
   c. See Sexuality section and Patient Teaching box Sexuality in Pregnancy; emphasise that intercourse is safe as long as pregnancy is progressing normally and it is comfortable for the woman; sexual expression should be in tune with the woman's changing needs and emotions; inform that spotting can normally occur related to the fragility of the vaginal mucosa and cervix and that changes in positions and activities may be helpful as pregnancy progresses.
   d. See Nursing Care Plan for Discomforts of Pregnancy and Table 11-4; fully assess what she is experiencing; then discuss why it happens, how long it will likely last, and relief measures that are safe and effective (also see Coping With Nutrition-Related Discomforts of Pregnancy section of Chapter 12).

4. See Physical Activity section and Patient Teaching box Exercise Tips for Pregnancy; assess her usual pattern of exercise and activity and consider their safety during pregnancy; discuss precautions and guidelines for safe, effective exercise; emphasise that moderate physical activity benefits her and her baby and will prepare her for the work of labour and birth; caution her to take note of the effects of exercise in terms of temperature, heart rate, and feeling of well-being.

5. a. Risk for urinary tract infection related changes of the renal system during pregnancy (see Preventing UTI section and Table 11-4 Frequency and Urgency):
   - Patient will drink at least 2 to 3 litres of fluids per day; patient will empty bladder at first urge.
   - Explain changes that occur in the renal system during pregnancy; increase fluid intake, use acid-ash forming fluids, void frequently to keep bladder empty, perform good perineal hygiene, use lateral position to enhance renal perfusion and urine formation.
   b. Acute pain in lower back related to needs to be split as neuromuscular changes associated with pregnancy at 23 weeks of gestation (see Table 11-4 Joint Pain, Backache, and Pelvic Pressure):
   - Patient will experience lessening of lower back pain following implementation of suggested relief measures.
   - Explain basis for lower back pain and relief measures, including back massage, pelvic

rock, and posture changes; encourage patient to change footwear for better stability and safety.
   c. Anxiety concerning the process of labour and birth and appropriate measures to cope with the pain and discomfort (see Maternal and Paternal Adaptation—Preparing for Birth, Perinatal Education sections):
   - Couple will enrol in a childbirth education programme in the seventh month of pregnancy.
   - Explain the childbirth process and describe the many nonpharmacological and pharmacological measures to relieve pain; discuss role of partner and possibility of hiring a doula; make a referral to a childbirth education programme and assist with the preparation of a birth plan; discuss childbirth options and prebirth preparations.

6. a. See Fundal Height section; purpose of fundal height: indirect assessment of how foetus is growing.
   b. See Clothing section and Patient Teaching box—Safety During Pregnancy; clothing choices during pregnancy: consider safety and comfort in terms of low-heeled shoe and nonrestrictive clothing.
   c. Gas and constipation: see Table 11-4 Discomforts related to pregnancy, constipation and flatulence section.
   d. Itchiness: if the pregnant patient is experiencing noninflammatory pruritus, use Table 11-4 (Pruritus—Noninflammatory section) for basis of discomfort and relief measures.
   e. Travel during pregnancy: see Travel section; teach the patient that travelling is permitted if the pregnancy is progressing normally; emphasise importance of staying hydrated, wearing seat belt, doing breathing and lower extremities exercises, ambulating every hour for 15 minutes, and voiding every 2 hours.

7. See Emergency box Supine Hypotension for content required to answer each part of this question.

8. a. Assess nipples for eversion; if they are not, the patient may be taught to use a nipple shell to help their nipples protrude although the evidence that this works is not strong; no special exercises are recommended because they could stimulate preterm labour in a susceptible patient as a result of secretion of oxytocin; keep nipples and areola clean and dry; see Preparation for Breastfeeding section.
   b. Ankle edema: see Table 11-4 (ankle oedema to lower extremities); discuss basis of the oedema and encourage use of lower extremities exercises and elevation of legs periodically during the day (Fig. 11-14); emphasise importance of fluid intake.
   c. Leg cramps: see Table 11-4 (leg cramps) and Fig. 11-15; discuss basis of leg cramps, and then

263

demonstrate relief measures such as pressing weight onto foot when standing or dorsiflexing the foot while lying in bed; avoid pointing the toes.

9. a. Anxiety related to perceived risk for preterm labour and birth; patient will identify signs suggestive of preterm labour and the action to take if they occur.
    b. See Recognising Preterm Labour section and Patient Teaching Box - How to Recognise Preterm Labour.
    c. Empty bladder, drink 3 to 4 glasses of water, assume a side-lying position, and count contractions for another hour; if contractions continue, call health care provider.

10. See Sibling Adaptation section and Family-Centred Care Box – Tips for Sibling Preparation, which provide tips for sibling preparation; emphasise importance of considering each child's developmental level; prepare children for prenatal events, time during hospitalization, and the homecoming of the new baby; refer to sibling classes and encourage sibling visitation after birth; suggest books and videos that parents could use to prepare their children for birth; provide opportunities to spend time with newborns/infants if possible.

11. See Maternal Adaptation section and Table 11-4 (psychosocial dynamics, mood swings, and mixed feelings); discuss the basis for the mood swings and experiences during the first trimester including ambivalence; identify measures he can use to support her.

12. See Birth Plans and Birth Setting Choices sections; answer should include:
    • Descriptions of each option along with the criteria for use and the advantages and disadvantages.
    • Onsite visits and interaction with health care providers responsible for care at each site should be encouraged.
    • Speak to couples who gave birth in these settings to get their impressions.
    • Emphasise that the decision is theirs and that they should choose what is comfortable for them; a decision should be made on the basis of a full understanding of each option.
    • Assist couple with creation of a birth plan to facilitate their control over the childbirth process and a more positive birthing experience.

13. See Doula section and Box 11-4 for content required to answer each part of this question.

14. See Home Birth section for content required to answer each part of this question.

15. See Nursing Care section and Table 11-2 for content required for each part of this question.

	Significance	Nursing Action
a. Lower back pain	Normal	b. Teach exercises to help improve comfort
b. HR = 90	Normal	a. Document
c. BP 136/85	Abnormal	c. Reassess BP
d. Fundal height = 34 cm	Normal	a. Document
e. FHR = 170	Abnormal	c. Reassess FHR and assess if there is foetal movement
f. Constipation	Normal	b. Teach to increase fluid, fibre and exercise
g. Voiding every 1-2 hours with burning sensation	Abnormal	c. Assess for UTI
h. States they are anxious and are crying at appointment	Abnormal	c. Assess using a PMD assessment tool
i. Dyspnea when climbing stairs	Normal	b. Education
j. Leukorrhea	Normal	b. Education
k. Nonpitting ankle oedema	Normal	b. Education

CHAPTER 12 MATERNAL NUTRITION

I. Learning Key Terms

1. Low birth weight (LBW)
2. Folate (folic acid); neural tube defects, 0.4 mg (400 mcg)
3. Dietary reference intake (DRI)
4. BMI; underweight, normal weight, overweight, obese
5. Ketonuria
6. Physiological anaemia
7. Lactose intolerance
8. Pica
9. Canada's Food Guide
10. Nausea and vomiting of pregnancy
11. Hyperemesis gravidarum
12. Constipation
13. Pyrosis

II. Reviewing Key Concepts

1. See separate sections for each nutrient in Nutrient Needs During Pregnancy section and Table 12-1 to complete this activity.
2. See Box 12-3 to identify the five risk indicators.
3. See Weight Gain, Pattern of Weight Gain, Hazards of Restricting Adequate Weight Gain, and Excessive Weight Gain sections.
4. See Vegetarian Diets section.
   a. These diets tend to be low in vitamins B12 and B6, iron, calcium, zinc, and perhaps calories; supplements may be needed.
   b. Food needs to be combined to ensure that all essential amino acids are provided.
5. See Table 12-4 for several signs of adequate and inadequate nutrition.
6. See Weight Gain and Pattern of Weight Gain sections and Table 12-2 to determine weight gain patterns based on each woman's BMI; keep in mind that each woman should gain 1 to 2.5 kg in the first trimester; weight gain per week is recommended for the second and third trimester.
   a. Nicole: BMI 21.3 (normal); total 11.5 to 16 kg; 0.4 kg/week
   b. Alice: BMI 29 (overweight); total 7 to 11.5 kg; 0.3 kg/week
   c. Annie: BMI 15.8 (underweight); total 12.5 to 18 kg; 0.5 kg/week
7. b, d, e, and f; Bran, tea, coffee, milk, oxalate-containing vegetables (spinach, Swiss chard), and egg yolks all decrease iron absorption; tomatoes and strawberries contain vitamin C, which enhances iron absorption; meats contain heme iron, which also enhances absorption.
8. c; BMI indicates that this patient is obese; they should not consider a weight loss regimen until healing is complete in the postpartum period; weight gain should be at least 7 kg; increase in calories should reflect energy expenditure of the pregnancy during the third trimester, which would be approximately 462 kcal.

9. b; BMI indicates patient is at a normal weight; total gain should be 11.5 to 16 kg, representing a gain of 0.4 kg/week and 1.6 kg/month during the second and third trimesters.
10. c; Small, frequent meals are better tolerated than large meals that distend the stomach; hunger can worsen nausea; therefore, meals should not be skipped; dry, starchy foods should be eaten in the morning and at other times during the day when nausea occurs; fried, fatty, and spicy foods should be avoided; a bedtime snack is recommended.
11. b, d, and e; Legumes are a good source for folic acid along with whole grains and fortified cereals, oranges, asparagus, liver, and green leafy vegetables; choices a, c, and f are not good sources of folic acid though they do supply other important nutrients for pregnancy (see Box 12-1).

III. Thinking Critically

1. a. Concern regarding amount of recommended weight gain during pregnancy:
   - Identify components of maternal weight gain (see Table 12-2); use Fig. 12-2 to illustrate how the weight gain is distributed over weeks of gestation.
   - Discuss impact of maternal weight gain on foetal growth and development; association between inadequate maternal weight gain and low birth weight and infant mortality.
   - Discuss weight gain total and pattern recommended for a woman with a BMI of 18 (underweight).
   b. Eating for two during pregnancy:
   - Place emphasis on quality of food that meets nutritional requirements, not on the quantity of food.
   - Discuss expected weight gain total and pattern for a woman with a normal BMI.
   - Excessive weight gain during pregnancy may be difficult to lose after pregnancy and could lead to chronic obesity; excessive foetal size and childbirth problems could also result.
   c. Vitamin supplementation during pregnancy: determine what and how much she takes; compare to recommendations for pregnancy; discuss potential problems with toxicity, especially with overuse of fat-soluble vitamins; see Water-Soluble and Fat-Soluble Vitamins sections.
   d. Factors that increase nutritional needs during pregnancy: growth and development of uterine-placental-fetal unit, expansion of maternal blood volume and RBCs, mammary changes, increased basal metabolic rate (BMR); see Nutrients sections and Table 12-1.
   e. Weight reduction diets during pregnancy:
   - BMI indicates overweight status; a gain of 7 to 11.5 kg during pregnancy is recommended.
   - Discuss hazards of inadequate caloric intake during pregnancy in terms of growth and development

265

of foetus and pregnancy-related structures; impact of ketoacidosis.
- Discuss quality of foods and development of good nutritional habits to be used during the postpartum period as part of a sensible weight loss program.
- Discuss importance of exercise and activity during pregnancy.
f. Reduction of water intake: discuss importance of and types of fluid to meet demands of pregnancy-related changes, regulate temperature, and prevent constipation and urinary tract infections (UTIs); consider possible association between dehydration and preterm labour and oligohydramnios; see Fluids section.
g. Lactose intolerance: discuss basis for problem; reduce lactose intake by using lactose-free products, nondairy sources of calcium, and calcium supplements; take lactase supplements; see Calcium section and Box 12-4, Sources of Calcium.

2. See Iron section of Nutrient Needs section, Patient Teaching box Iron Supplementation, and Table 12-1 and Patient Teaching Box, Iron Supplementation.
- Discuss importance of iron.
- Emphasise importance of vitamin C for iron absorption; discuss food sources high in iron and vitamin C; discuss foods to avoid when taking iron.
- Discuss ways to take iron supplements to enhance absorption and minimise side effects including GI upset and constipation.

3. See appropriate section for each nutrition-related discomfort in Coping With Nutritional-Related Discomforts of Pregnancy section.
a. See Nausea and Vomiting section and Patient Teaching Box, Managing Nausea and Vomiting During Pregnancy for several relief measures.
b. See Constipation section; include adequate fluid and roughage/fibre intake, exercise and activity, regular time for elimination.
c. See Pyrosis section; small frequent meals, drink fluids between not with meals, avoid spicy foods, remain upright after eating.

4. See Nursing Care section, Table 12-4, and Box 12-6.
a. Counselling approach:
- Assess her current nutritional status and habits; obtain a diet history.
- Analyze current patterns as a basis for menu planning.
- Discuss weight gain pattern for an underweight woman.
- Use a variety of teaching methods; keep woman actively involved.
- Emphasise importance of good nutrition for herself and her newborn.
b. See Caffeine Consumption section and Box 12-5 for information on caffeine consumption.
c. See Nursing Care section, Safe Food Preparation and Patient Teaching Box, Prevention of Foodborne Illness.

CHAPTER 13 PREGNANCY RISK FACTORS AND ASSESSMENT

I. Learning Key Terms
1. High risk pregnancy
2. Foetal movement counting or kick counts
3. Ultrasound (sonography); transvaginal or abdominal
4. Doppler blood flow analysis
5. Biophysical profile (BPP); ultrasound; foetal breathing movements, foetal body movements, foetal tone, amniotic fluid volume
6. Amniocentesis
7. Percutaneous umbilical blood sampling (PUBS) or cordocentesis
8. Chorionic villus sampling (CVS)
9. Nuchal translucency and maternal serum biochemical markers
10. Cell-free DNA testing
11. Coombs (indirect)
12. Nonstress test
13. Contraction stress test; nipple-stimulated contraction stress, oxytocin-stimulated contraction stress

II. Reviewing Key Concepts
1. See Box 13-1 and Assessment of Risk Factors section, which describe several risk factors in each category listed.
2. See Nursing Role in Assessment for Risk section; answer should emphasise education, support measures, and assisting with or performing the test and follow-up care for each test discussed in the Chapter.
3. See Box 13-3, which lists risk factors for each pregnancy-related problem identified.
4. a; An amniocentesis analyzes amniotic fluid for the L/S ratio and presence of phosphatidylglycerol (Pg) is used to determine pulmonary maturity; choice b refers to a contraction stress test; choice c refers to serial measurements of foetal growth using ultrasound; choice d refers to a non-stress test.
5. c; Food/fluid is not restricted before the test; the test will evaluate the response of the foetal heart rate (FHR) to foetal movement—acceleration is expected; external not internal monitoring is used.
6. b; First trimester screening includes using an ultrasound examination for nuchal translucency, combined with assessment of maternal serum biochemical markers done between 11 and 14 weeks gestation. It is used to screen the pregnant patient for the possibility that the foetus has Down syndrome. Ultrasound examination at 18 to 22 weeks is the screening test for open neural tube defects such as spina bifida; a 1-hour, 50-g glucose test is used to screen for gestational diabetes; amniocentesis and Coombs testing would be used to check for Rh antibodies and sensitization.
7. c; An atypical result is recorded when late decelerations occur with less than 50% of the contractions; a negative test result is recorded when no late decelerations occur during at least three uterine contractions lasting 40 to

266

60 seconds each, within a 10-minute period; a positive test is recorded when there are persistent late decelerations with more than 50% of the contractions; unsatisfactory is the result recorded when there is a failure to achieve adequate uterine contractions.

8. a; A supine position with hips elevated enhances the view of the uterus; a lithotomy position may also be used; a full bladder is not required for the vaginal ultrasound but would be needed for most abdominal ultrasounds; during the test the patient may experience some pressure but medication for pain relief before the test is not required; contact gel is used with the abdominal ultrasound; water-soluble lubricant may be used to ease insertion of the vaginal probe.

III. Thinking Critically

1. See Ultrasound section:
   a. This woman was tested to determine location of gestational sac because PID could have resulted in narrowing of fallopian tube, thereby increasing risk for ectopic pregnancy; in addition, a determination of gestational age and estimation of date of birth would be done related to irregular cycles and unknown date of last menstrual period (LMP).
   b. Explain purpose of test, how it will be performed, and how it will feel; assist her into a lithotomy position or supine position with hips elevated on a pillow; point out structures on monitor as test is performed.

2. See Ultrasound section; instruct patient to come for test with full bladder if appropriate; explain purpose of test and method of examination; assist the patient into a supine position with head and shoulders elevated on pillow and hip slightly tipped to right or left side; observe for supine hypotension during test and orthostatic hypotension when rising to upright position after test; indicate how the foetus is being measured and point out foetus and its movements.

3. See Biophysical Profile section and Tables 13-4 and 13-5 for identification of variables tested; scoring:
   a. Describe how the test will be performed using ultrasound and external electronic foetal monitoring; explain that the purpose of the test is to view the foetus within its environment, to determine the amount of amniotic fluid, and assess the FHR response to foetal activity.
   b. A score of 8 is normal. If a non-stress test is done the test score is out of 10.

4. See Amniocentesis including Safety Alert section and Nurse's Role in Assessment and Management of High Risk Pregnancy section.
   a. Explain procedure, witness informed consent, assess maternal vital signs and health status and FHR before the test; ensure that ultrasound is performed to locate placenta and foetus before the test.
   b. Explain what is happening and what she will be feeling; help her relax; encourage her to ask questions and voice concerns and feelings; assess her reactions.

   c. Monitor maternal vital signs, status, and FHR; tell her when test results should be available and whom to call; administer RhoD immunoglobulin because she is Rh negative; teach her to assess herself for signs of infection, bleeding, rupture of membranes, and uterine contractions; make a follow-up phone call to check her status.

5. See Nonstress Test section.
   a. Test measures response of FHR to foetal activity to determine adequacy of placental perfusion and foetal oxygenation.
   b. Tell her that she can eat before and during the test; schedule test at a time of day that foetus is usually active; assist patient into a semirecumbent or seated position.
   c. Attach tocotransducer to fundus and Doppler transducer at site of point of maximum intensity (PMI); instruct patient to indicate when foetus moves by pushing a button; assess change, if any, in FHR following the movement.
   d. See Figs. 13-10 and 13-11 and Table 13-2 for the criteria to determine the test result.

6. See Contraction Stress Test section.
   a. The test is a way of determining how her foetus will react to the stress of uterine contractions as they would occur during labour; uterine contractions decrease perfusion through the placenta leading to foetal hypoxia; late decelerations during this test could be interpreted as an early warning of foetal compromise.
   b. Assess patient's vital signs, general health status, and contraindications for the test; attach external electronic foetal monitor and assess FHR and uterine activity; assist patient into a lateral, semirecumbent, or seated position.
   c. See Nipple-Stimulated Contraction Stress Test section.
   d. See Oxytocin-Stimulated Contraction Stress Test section.
   e. See Table 13-3 for criteria used to interpret the test results and to document as **negative:** no late decelerations are noted; as **positive:** late decelerations with more than half of the contractions; **atypical:** late decelerations with less than half of the contractions; **equivocal-tachysystole:** decelerations in the presence of contractions more frequent than every 2 min or lasting longer than 90 sec; or **unsatisfactory:** failure to produce three contractions within a 10-min window or inability to trace the foetal heart rate.

CHAPTER 14 PREGNANCY AT RISK: GESTATIONAL CONDITIONS

I. Learning Key Terms

1. Non-severe hypertension
2. Severe hypertension
3. Gestational hypertension
4. Preeclampsia
5. Eclampsia

6. Chronic hypertension
7. Arteriolar vasospasm
8. HELLP syndrome; hemolysis, elevated liver enzymes, low platelets
9. Proteinuria
10. Diuresis and decreased oedema
11. Hyperemesis gravidarum
12. Miscarriage (spontaneous abortion); early pregnancy loss, late pregnancy loss (second trimester loss)
13. Missed miscarriage
14. Recurrent miscarriage (recurrent spontaneous abortion)
15. Cervical insufficiency
16. Cervical cerclage
17. Ectopic pregnancy
18. Gestational trophoblastic disease; hydatidiform mole, invasive mole, choriocarcinoma
19. Complete hydatidiform mole
20. Partial hydatidiform mole
21. Complete placenta previa
22. Marginal placenta previa
23. Placental abruption (premature separation of the placenta)
24. Vasa previa; velamentous insertion of the cord; succenturiate placenta
25. Battledore placenta
26. Disseminated intravascular coagulation (DIC)
27. Von Willebrand's Disease
28. Asymptomatic bacteriuria
29. Cystitis
30. Pyelonephritis
31. Appendicitis
32. Cholelithiasis
33. Cholecystitis

II. Reviewing Key Concepts

1. See Box 14-4 for blood pressure guidelines.
2. See Nursing Care Management—Physical Examination section.
   a. Hyperreflexia and ankle clonus: see Table 14-4, which grades deep tendon reflex (DTR) responses and Fig. 14-3 for illustrations depicting performance of DTRs and ankle clonus.
   b. Proteinuria: describe dipstick and 24-hour urine collection methods to determine level of protein in urine.
3. e   4. c   5. b   6. a   7. d
8. c   9. e   10. a   11. d   12. b
13. f
14. c; The pregnant patient should be seated or in a lateral position and should rest for 5 to 10 minutes, the ideal cuff will have a bladder length that is 80% and a width that is 40% of the arm circumference.
15. b, d, and f; The loading dose should be an IV of 4 g diluted in 100 mL of intravenous fluid; maternal assessment should occur every 15 to 30 minutes and FHR and UC continuously; respirations should be less than 12.

16. b; Magnesium sulphate is a CNS depressant given to prevent seizures.
17. b, d, and e; Magnesium sulphte is administered intravenously in the hospital with preeclampsia; a clean catch, midstream urine specimen should be used to assess urine for protein using a dipstick; fluid intake should be six to eight 240 mL glasses a day along with roughage to prevent constipation; gentle exercise improves circulation and helps preserve muscle tone and a sense of well-being; bed rest is not recommended. Excessively salty food should be avoided.
18. b; Urine would be checked for ketones to assessed for the degree of dehydration. Labetalol is a beta blocker used for hypertension; oral hygiene is important when NPO and after vomiting episodes to maintain the integrity of oral mucosa; taking fluids between, not with, meals reduces nausea, thereby increasing tolerance for oral nutrition.
19. a; The patient is experiencing a threatened abortion; therefore, a conservative approach is attempted first; b reflects management of an inevitable and complete or incomplete abortion; blood tests for HCG and progesterone levels would be done; cerclage or suturing of the cervix is done for recurrent, spontaneous abortion associated with premature dilation of the cervix.
20. c; Choices a, b, and d are appropriate nursing concerns, but deficient fluid is the priority concern, placing the patient's well-being at greatest risk.
21. b; Methotrexate destroys rapidly growing tissue, in this case the foetus and placenta, to avoid rupture of the tube and need for surgery; follow-up with blood tests is needed for 2 to 8 weeks; alcohol and vitamins containing folic acid increase the risk for side effects with this medication or exacerbating the ectopic rupture.
22. c; The clinical manifestations of placenta previa are described; dark red bleeding with pain is characteristic of placental abruption; massive bleeding from many sites is associated with DIC; bleeding is not a sign of preterm labour.
23. a; Haemorrhage is a major potential postpartum complication because the implantation site of the placenta is in the lower uterine segment, which has a limited capacity to contract after birth; infection is another major complication, but it is not the immediate focus of care; b and d are also important but not to the same degree as haemorrhage, which is life threatening.
24. See Screening for Gestational Diabetes Mellitus section.

III. Thinking Critically

1. See Preeclampsia section, Boxes 14-1 and 14-3, Tables 14-1, 14-2, 14-3, and 14-4 for the content required to answer each part of this question.
2. See Pre-eclampsia and HELLP sections, Emergency box Eclampsia, Boxes 14-2, 14-3, 14-5 and

14-5, Tables 14-1, 14-2, 14-3, and 14-4, and 14-5, and Nursing Care Plan for Severe Pre-eclampsia for the content required to answer each part of this question.

3. See Hyperemesis Gravidarum section and Patient Teaching box Diet for Hyperemesis (in Chapter 12) for content required to answer each part of this question.

4. See Ectopic Pregnancy section for content required to answer each part of this question.

5. See Miscarriage section and Table 14-7 for content required to answer both parts of this question.

6. See Miscarriage section, Family-Centred Care box: Discharge Teaching After Pregnancy Loss, and Table 14-7 for content required to answer each part of this question; be sure to determine what she means by a lot of bleeding, and whether she is experiencing any other signs and symptoms related to miscarriage such as pain and cramping; determine the gestational age of her pregnancy and whether there is anyone to bring her to the hospital if inevitable abortion is suspected; priority nursing concern at this time: Deficient fluid volume related to blood loss; acknowledge her loss and provide time for her to express her feelings; inform her about how she may feel (mood swings, depression); refer her for grief counselling, support groups, clergy; make follow-up phone calls.

7. See Hydatidiform Mole section for content required to answer this question.

8. See Placenta Previa and Placental Abruption sections and Table 14-8 to compare findings for each disorder in terms of characteristics of bleeding, uterine tone, pain and tenderness, and ultrasound findings regarding location of placenta and foetal presentation/position; priority nursing diagnoses: consider diagnoses related to major physical problems such as deficient fluid volume related to blood loss, ineffective tissue perfusion (placenta), and risk for foetal injury; major psychosocial nursing diagnoses could include fear/anxiety, interrupted family processes, and anticipatory grieving; comparison of nursing care approaches: consider home care versus hospital care for woman with placenta previa; hospital care is the safest approach for woman experiencing placental abruption; discuss active versus expectant management for each condition; postpartum complications include increased risk for haemorrhage and infection as well as the emotional impact of a major pregnancy-related complication.

9. See Trauma During Pregnancy section, Table 14-9, Emergency box CPR for Pregnant Patients in the Hospital for the content required to answer each part of this question.

10. See Gestational Diabetes Mellitus section, Fig. 14-5, and the Nursing Care Plan for Woman with Gestational Diabetes for the content required to answer each part of this question.

CHAPTER 15 PREGNANCY AT RISK: PRE-EXISTING CONDITIONS

I. Learning Key Terms

1. Diabetes mellitus
2. Hyperglycemia
3. Euglycemia
4. Hypoglycemia
5. Polyuria
6. Polydipsia
7. Polyphagia
8. Glycosuria
9. Ketoacidosis
10. Type 1 diabetes mellitus
11. Type 2 diabetes mellitus
12. Pregestational (Pre-existing) diabetes mellitus
13. Gestational
14. Glycated haemoglobin A_{1c}
15. Macrosomia
16. Hydramnios (polyhydramnios)
17. Glucose metre (glucometer)
18. Cardiac decompensation; 25, 30, childbirth, 24, 72
19. Functional classifications of heart disease; asymptomatic without limitation of physical activity, symptomatic with slight limitation of activity, symptomatic with marked limitation of activity, symptomatic with inability to carry on any physical activity without discomfort
20. Peripartum cardiomyopathy
21. Rheumatic heart disease
22. Mitral valve stenosis; Aortic stenosis
23. Myocardial infarction
24. Infective endocarditis
25. Mitral valve prolapse
26. Anaemia; iron
27. Sickle cell hemoglobinopathy (anaemia)
28. Thalassemia
29. Asthma
30. Cystic fibrosis
31. Pruritus gravidarum
32. Pruritic urticarial papules and plaques of pregnancy (PUPPP)
33. Intrahepatic cholestasis of pregnancy
34. Epilepsy
35. Multiple sclerosis
36. Bell palsy
37. Systemic lupus erythematosus (SLE)

II. Reviewing Key Concepts

1. See Maternal Risks and Complications and Foetal and Neonatal Risks and Complications sections for a list of all major complications.

2. See Thyroid Disorders section for a description of hyperthyroidism and hypothyroidism; consider effects of these disorders on reproductive development, sexuality, fertility in terms of ability to conceive and to sustain a pregnancy to viability, and potential foetal/newborn complications related to maternal treatment of thyroid disorder.

269

3. See Cardiovascular Disorders section; increased risk for miscarriage, preterm labour and birth, IUGR, maternal mortality, and stillbirth.
4. d; The patient is exhibiting signs of DKA; insulin is the required treatment, with the dosage dependent on blood glucose level; intravenous fluids may also be required; choice a is the treatment for hypoglycemia; choices b and c, although they may increase the patient's comfort, are not priorities.
5. c; A 2-hour postprandial blood glucose should be between 5.0–6.6 mmol/L; choices a, b, and d fall within the expected normal ranges.
6. a, b, and c; Fat intake should not be increased and complex carbohydrates are better to maintain blood sugar levels.
7. b, e, and f; Other signs of cardiac compensation include moist, productive, frequent cough, and crackles at bases of lungs; pulse becomes rapid, weak, irregular. See Box 15-3.
8. a; This patient is exhibiting signs of cardiac decompensation; further information regarding cardiac status is required to determine what further action would be needed.
9. c; Furosemide is a diuretic; propranolol is a beta blocker that is used to manage hypertension and tachycardia; although warfarin is an anticoagulant, it can cross the placenta and affect the foetus, whereas heparin, which is a large molecule, does not.
10. b; Bed rest is not recommended for a patient with a class II designation; they will need to avoid heavy exertion and stop activities that cause fatigue and dyspnea; actions in a, c, and d are all appropriate and recommended for class II.

III. Thinking Critically

1. See Preconception Counselling section.
   - Discuss purpose in terms of planning pregnancy for the optimum time when glucose control is established within normal ranges, because this will decrease incidence of congenital anomalies; diagnose any vascular problems; emphasise the importance of her health before the pregnancy, helping to ensure a positive outcome.
   - Discuss how her diabetic management will need to be altered during pregnancy; include her partner, because their help and support during the pregnancy are important.
2. See Table 15-1 and Maternal Risk and Complications section.
3. See Pregestational Diabetes subsections for the content required to answer each part of this question.
4. See Cardiovascular Disorders section, Patient Teaching box The Pregnant Patient at Risk for Cardiac Decompensation, and Box 15-3 for the content required to answer each part of this question.
5. See Epilepsy section including the Safety Alert; inform her that effects of pregnancy on epilepsy are unpredictable; convulsions may injure her or her foetus and lead to miscarriage, preterm labour, or separation of the placenta; medications that will be given in the lowest therapeutic dose must be taken to prevent convulsions; folic acid supplementation is important because anticonvulsants can deplete folic acid stores.
6. See Substance Use section for description of principles to follow; emphasise:
   - Family focus including child care and education and support for parenting
   - Empowerment building
   - A community-based interdisciplinary approach with multiplicity of services, including those related to sexual and physical abuse and lack of social support
   - Continuum of care
   - Pregnancy as a window of opportunity related to motivation for change
   - Harm reduction
7. See Spinal Cord Injury section for the content required to answer each part of the question.

CHAPTER 16 LABOUR AND BIRTH PROCESSES

I. Learning Key Terms

1. Passenger (foetus, placenta), passageway, powers, position of the mother, psychological responses
2. Fontanels
3. Moulding
4. Presentation; cephalic, breech, shoulder
5. Presenting part; occiput, sacrum, scapula
6. Lie; longitudinal (vertical), transverse (horizontal, oblique)
7. Attitude (posture); flexion
8. Biparietal; suboccipitobregmatic
9. Position
10. Engagement
11. Station
12. Bony pelvis, soft tissue
13. Effacement
14. Dilation
15. Lightening
16. Involuntary uterine contractions
17. Bearing down (pushing; contraction of abdominal muscles and diaphragm)
18. Bloody show
19. Mechanism of labour (cardinal movements); engagement, descent, flexion, internal rotation, extension, external rotation (restitution), expulsion
20. Valsalva manoeuvre
21. Latent; Active pushing
22. Labour
23. Ferguson reflex
24. Regular uterine contractions, dilation and effacement; latent, active
25. Dilated and effaced, birth of the baby
26. Birth of the baby, placenta
27. Delivery of the placenta, 2 hours
28. Position, blood pressure, uterine contractions, umbilical cord blood flow
29. Endogenous endorphins

II. Reviewing Key Concepts

1. See separate sections for each of the five factors in Factors of Labour section; consider the factors of passenger, passage, powers, position of mother, psychological response.

2. a, c, d, and e; Station is 1 cm above the ischial spines (–1); 7 cm more to reach full dilation of 10 cm.

3. c, d, e, and f; Systolic blood pressure increases with uterine contractions in the first stage, whereas both systolic and diastolic blood pressures increase during contractions in the second stage; WBC increases.

4. a, d, and e; Quickening refers to the woman's first perception of foetal movement at 16 to 18 weeks of gestation; urinary frequency, lightening, weight loss of 0.5 to 1 kg occur to signal that the onset of labour is near; backache, stronger Braxton Hicks and bloody show are also noted; shortness of breath is relieved once lightening occurs reducing pressure on the diaphragm.

III. Thinking Critically

1. • Examination I: ROP (right occiput posterior, cephalic [vertex] presentation, longitudinal lie, flexed attitude), –1 (station at 1 cm above the ischial spines), 50% effaced, 3 cm dilated.
   • Examination II: RMA (right mentum anterior, cephalic [face] presentation, longitudinal lie, extended attitude), 0 (station at the ischial spines, engaged), 25% effaced, 2 cm dilated.
   • Examination III: LST (left sacrum transverse, breech presentation, longitudinal lie, flexed attitude), +1 (station at 1 cm below the ischial spines), 75% effaced, 6 cm dilated.
   • Examination IV: OA (occiput anterior, cephalic [vertex] presentation, longitudinal lie, flexed attitude), +3 (station at 3 cm below the ischial spines near or on the perineum), 100% effaced, 10 cm (fully dilated).

2. a. See Onset of Labour section of the Process of Labour; explain in simple terms the interaction of maternal and foetal hormones, uterine distention, placental aging, and prostaglandins.
   b. See Signs Preceding Labour section and Box 16-1 for the signs that occur before the onset of labour.
   c. See Positioning of the Labouring Patient section; include the following points in answer:
      • Emphasise that the position of the patient is one of the 5 Ps of labour.
      • Discuss each position and describe its effect.
      • Demonstrate each position and have her practise them with her partner.
      • Emphasise the beneficial effects of ambulation and changing positions on foetus, circulation, comfort, and progress.
   d. Breathing initiation after birth: see Foetal Adaptation, Foetal Respiration section, for a description regarding the onset of newborn breathing.

CHAPTER 17 NURSING CARE OF THE FAMILY DURING LABOUR AND BIRTH

I. Learning Key Terms

1. Regular uterine contractions, effacement, dilation; mucous plug
2. 3, 4, 10
3. Full dilation and effacement, baby's birth
4. Birth of the baby, placenta is expelled, fundus, discoid, globular ovoid, gush of dark blood, lengthening of umbilical cord, vaginal fullness, membranes
5. 2 hours

6. e	7. f	8. h	9. g	10. b
11. k	12. a	13. o	14. i	15. l
16. d	17. m	18. c	19. j	

20. Uterine contractions
21. Increment
22. Acme
23. Decrement
24. Frequency
25. Intensity
26. Duration
27. Resting tone
28. Bearing-down effort

II. Reviewing Key Concepts

1. See First Stage of Labour—Assessment section and Boxes 17-2 for content required to answer each part of this question.
2. See Box 17-9 for content required to answer each part of this question.
3. See Box 17-10 and Fig 17-10, 17-11, and 17-12 and Ambulation and Positioning section for content required to answer each part of this question.
4. See Physical Examination sections that discuss general systems assessment, vital signs, Leopold manoeuvers, assessment of FHR and pattern, assessment of uterine contractions, and vaginal examination; see Boxes 17-5, 17-7, and 17-8 and Tables 17-1 and 17-3 for content required to answer this question.
5. See Laboratory and Diagnostic Tests section for content required to answer this question.
6. See Second Stage of Labour section for content required to answer this question.
7. See Position During Second Stage section for content required to answer this question; include squatting, side-lying, semirecumbent, standing, and hands-and-knees positions in your answer.
8. See Fourth Stage of Labour section for content required to answer this question; discuss how breastfeeding will have positive physiological effects for the mother and enhance attachment and success of breastfeeding.
9. See Second Stage of Labour section; Table 17-4/Box 17-13 for content required to answer this question.
10. a; Although b, c, and d are all important questions, the first question should gather information regarding whether or not the patient is in labour.

271

11. c; pH of amniotic fluid is alkaline at 6.5 or higher, ferning is noted when examining fluid with a microscope, and the fluid is relatively odourless; a strong odour is strongly suggestive of infection.

12. b and d; The only indicators of true labour are cervical change. Other statements are subjective based on maternal perception.

13. c; O or occiput indicates a vertex presentation with the neck fully flexed and the occiput in the transverse section (T) of the woman's pelvis; the station is 2 cm below the ischial spines (+2); the woman is in the active phase of labour as indicated by 6 cm of dilation; the lie is longitudinal (vertical) because the head (cephalic/vertex) is presenting.

14. b; Research has indicated that enemas are not needed during labour; according to research findings a, c, and d have all been found to be beneficial and safe during pregnancy.

III. Thinking Critically

1. See First Stage of Labour—Assessment section and Patient Teaching box How to Distinguish True Labour From Pre-Labour for content required to answer each part of this question.
   a. Determine the status of her labour; if there is any doubt about the information being given or her status, the patient should be advised to come in for evaluation.
   b. Questions should be clear, concise, open ended, and directed toward distinguishing her labour status and determining the basis for action.
   c. Discuss assessment measures, comfort, distraction, emotional support, and who and when to call; it is important that the nurse make follow-up calls to determine how the patient is progressing.

2. a. and b.: See Table 17-3 to determine phase; Denise (active); Teresa (active); Danielle (latent).
   c. See Box 17-4, Tables 17-1 and 17-3, Nursing Care and Supportive Care During Labour and Birth section for care measures required by each woman according to her phase of labour.
   d. See Box 17-12 and Labour Support by the Partner section for several suggested measures the nurse can use to support the support person of the labouring patient.

3. See Box 17-7, Fig. 17-7, and Leopold Manoeuvers and Assessment of Foetal Heart Rate and Pattern sections for content required to answer this question; realise that presentation and position affect location of PMI and the PMI will change as the foetus progresses through the birth canal.

4. See Vaginal Examination section and Box 17-8 for content required to answer each part of this question; explain to the patient the data obtained from monitoring and the vaginal examination and tell her what she can do to decrease her discomfort; privacy and discussion of the results is critical.

5. See Assessment of Amniotic Membranes and Fluid section including the Nursing Alert; immediate assessment of the FHR and pattern (prolapse of the cord could have occurred, compressing the cord and leading to hypoxia and variable deceleration patterns); vaginal examination (status of cervix, check for cord prolapse); assess fluid, document findings and notify primary health care provider; cleanse perineum as soon as possible once status of foetus, mother, and labour are determined; strict infection control measures after rupture because risk for infection increases.

6. See First Stage of Labour—Nursing Care section emphasising supportive care during labour and birth for content required to answer this question.
   • Nursing diagnosis: Anxiety regarding the process of childbirth.
   • Expected outcome: Couple will develop strategies to enhance progress of labour as their anxiety level decreases.
   • Nursing measures: Provide explanations, demonstrate and assist with simple breathing and relaxation techniques; make use of phases of labour to tailor health teaching.

7. See Cultural Factors sections for content required to answer each part of this question.

8. See Ambulation and Positioning and Position During Second Stage sections and Box 17-10 for content required to answer each part of this question.

9. See Mechanism of Birth Vertex Presentation, Immediate Assessment and Care of Newborn, and Fourth Stage sections and Box 17-14, Guidelines for Assistance at the Emergency Birth of a Foetus in the Vertex Presentation, for content required to answer each part of this question.

10. See Bearing-Down Efforts sections for the criteria to use to determine effectiveness of the bearing down technique.

11. See Perineal Trauma related to Childbirth section and Evidence-Informed practise box: When an OASIS Is Not a Scenic Travel Destination: Minimising Anal Sphincter Injury in Childbirth; compare episiotomies with spontaneous lacerations in terms of tissue affected, long-term sequelae, healing process, discomfort; compare reasons given for performing an episiotomy with what research findings demonstrate to be true.

12. See Siblings During Labour and Birth section: Include research findings regarding effect of sibling participation on family and on the sibling; consider the developmental readiness of the child and use developmental principles to prepare him or her for the experience; offer family and sibling classes to prepare them for participation in the birth process; evaluate parental comfort with this option; arrange for a support person to remain with the child during the entire childbirth process.

13. See Fourth Stage of Labour and Family-Newborn Relationships sections and Box 17-17 for content required to answer each section of this question.

CHAPTER 18 MAXIMIZING COMFORT DURING LABOUR AND BIRTH

I. Learning Key Terms

1. Uterine ischemia
2. Visceral
3. Somatic
4. Referred
5. Pain tolerance
6. Gate control theory of pain
7. Beta endorphins
8. Cleansing breath
9. Slow-paced breathing
10. Modified-paced breathing
11. Patterned-paced breathing (pant-blow breathing)
12. Hyperventilation
13. Effleurage
14. Counterpressure
15. Hydrotherapy
16. Transcutaneous electrical nerve stimulation (TENS)
17. Acupressure
18. Acupuncture
19. Biofeedback
20. Aromatherapy
21. Intradermal water block
22. Therapeutic touch

II. Reviewing Key Concepts

1. See Perception of Pain and Factors Influencing the Pain Response sections for content required to answer each part of this question.
2. See Gate Control Theory of Pain section.
3. b   4. f   5. h   6. a   7. g
8. j   9. m   10. d   11. i   12. l
13. c   14. e   15. k   16. n
17. See individual sections for each regional anesthetic listed and Nursing Care section.
18. See Systemic Analgesics section for content required to answer each part of this question.
19. See Nursing Care —Administration of Medications section; onset of action is faster and more reliable and predictable when administered intravenously.
20. d; Patients can and should change their position while in the bath, using lateral and hand-and-knees positioning when indicated; as long as amniotic fluid is clear or only slightly meconium tinged, a whirl-pool can continue; there is no limit to the time they can spend in the water—they can stay as long as they wish. The temperature should be maintained between 35° C/95° F and 37.8° C/100° F.
21. a; Promethazine is a phenothiazine, nalbupine is an opioid agonist-antagonist analgesic; fentanyl is an opioid agonist analgesic.
22. a; Ranitidine (Zantac) is used to neutralise the acidic contents of the stomach. Aspiration of highly acidic gastric contents will damage lung tissue and may occur during a general anaesthetic.
23. c; Administration of Narcan is given to reverse effects of sedation as the patient is experiencing potential symptoms and/or in this case birth is imminent and the provider wants to counteract possible foetal effects as a result of maternal narcotic administration. The nurse should continue to monitor maternal condition for possible side effects of the medication.
24. a, b, d, and f; Spinal headache is rare because the dura is not punctured; using a combined anaesthetic-analgesic and reducing dosage can allow a woman to push when the time is right.
25. a, b, and c; Choices d, e, and f are not associated with opioid abstinence syndrome.
26. b; Changing the patient to a lateral position will enhance cardiac output and raise the blood pressure because compression of the abdominal aorta and vena cava is removed; administering oxygen and notifying the health care provider would follow along with increasing intravenous fluid administration; administration of a vasopressor, if ordered by the health care provider, would follow if the other measures are not sufficient to restore the blood pressure.

III. Thinking Critically

1. See Neurological Origins of Pain section; describe why pain occurs and its very real basis including the types of pain and their origin; discuss how labouring patients experience the pain and factors that influence the experience; identify measures they can use to help their partners reduce and cope with the pain.
2. See Nonpharmacological and Nursing Care sections, Box 18-2 and 18-3, and Nursing Care Plan for content required to answer each part of this question; include the following points in your answer:
   - The choice when and if to use pain medication is based on the labouring patient's decision and the nurse will be available to provide the needed support for the patient
   - There are a variety of nonpharmacological measures that are safe and effective to use during labour and can have beneficial effects on the maternal-Foetal unit and can enhance the progress of labour
3. See Hydrotherapy section for content required to answer each part of this question.
   - Describe the beneficial effects of water therapy and how it can facilitate the labour process thereby decreasing the possibility of Caesarean birth; use research findings to substantiate these claims.
   - Describe the successful experiences of other agencies that have implemented hydrotherapy; state how it has affected the number of births.
   - Use favourable reports of labouring patients who have used hydrotherapy; consider how this could affect other patients preparing for childbirth.
4. See Emergency box Hypotension With Decreased Placental Perfusion for content required to answer each part of this question.
5. See Epidural Analgesia and Anaesthesia section including Nursing Alerts, Figs. 18-9, 18.11, and 18-12, Nursing Care – Administration of Medications and Box 18-6 and 18-8 for content required to answer each part of this question.

273

CHAPTER 19 FETAL HEALTH SURVEILLANCE DURING LABOUR

I. Learning Key Terms
1. Intermittent auscultation (IA)
2. Ultrasound transducer (Doppler ultrasound)
3. Electronic foetal monitoring; external, internal
4. Tocotransducer
5. Spiral electrode
6. Intrauterine pressure catheter (IUPC)
7. Intrauterine resuscitation
8. Scalp stimulation
9. Oligohydramnios
10. Anhydramnios
11. Amnioinfusion
12. Tocolytic therapy

II. Reviewing Key Concepts
1. i	2. j	3. m	4. h	5. g
6. k	7. f	8. c	9. b	10. d
11. e	12. a	13. l		

14. See Foetal Response section and Box 19-1 for a description of each factor that reduces foetal oxygen supply.
15. See Uterine Activity and Foetal Heart Rate Patterns and Table 19-5 for content required to answer each part of this question.
16. See Basis for Monitoring, Nursing Management of Atypical or Abnormal Patterns section, and Box 19-8; include a description of should document all aspects of FHS including the method of monitoring used (IA or EFM), the uterine activity pattern, and the associated FHR features that can be documented as well as the interpretation of the FHS.
17. See Monitoring Techniques section, Evidence-Informed Practise Box, Foetal Monitoring and Table 19-4 for content required to answer each part of this question; be sure to include advantages and disadvantages for each method in answer.
18. See Legal Tip, Foetal Monitoring Standards section; evaluate FHR pattern at frequency that reflects professional standards, agency policy, and condition of maternal-foetal unit; correctly interpret FHR pattern as normal, atypical, or abnormal; take appropriate action; evaluate response to actions taken; notify primary health care provider in a timely fashion; know the chain of command if a dispute about interpretation occurs; document assessment findings, actions, and responses.
19. d; The average resting pressure should be 10 mm Hg; a, b, and c are all findings within the expected ranges.
20. a, c, d, and e; The tocotransducer is always placed over the fundus but the ultrasound transducer, which requires the use of gel, should be repositioned at least hourly; the patient should be encouraged to change positions even though it may mean repositioning the transducers.

21. b; See Nursing Management of Atypical or Abnormal Patterns section.
22. b and d; The baseline rate should be 110 to 160 beats/min; recurrent late deceleration pattern of any magnitude is abnormal.
23. c; The FHR increases as the labouring patient's core body temperature rises; therefore, tachycardia would be the pattern exhibited; it is often a clue of intrauterine infection because fever is often the first sign; diminished variability reflects hypoxia and variable decelerations are characteristic of cord compression; early decelerations are characteristic of head compression and are not considered an abnormal pattern.
24. b; The pattern described is an early deceleration pattern, which is considered to be benign, reassuring, and requiring no action other than documentation of the finding; it is associated with foetal head compression; changing a labouring patient's position and notifying the primary health care provider would be appropriate if atypical or abnormal signs such as late or variable decelerations were occurring; prolapse of cord is associated with variable decelerations as a result of cord compression.

III. Thinking Critically
1. See Monitoring Techniques and Admission Foetal Monitor Strips, Table 19-3, and Box 19-2 for content required to answer each part of this question; include the following points in your answer:
   - Discuss how foetal monitoring is not recommended for patient with no risk factors.
   - Explain the advantages and disadvantages of different types of monitoring.
   - Explain how intermittent auscultation works.
2. See Foetal Heart Rate Patterns section, Box 19-5 and Figs. 19-15, and 19-16 for content required to answer each part of this question; the pattern described is a late deceleration pattern with baseline variability change.
3. See Foetal Heart Rate Patterns section, Boxes 19-6, and Figs. 19-17, 19-18 and 19-18 for content required to answer each part of this question; discuss variable deceleration patterns associated with cord compression.

CHAPTER 20 LABOUR AND BIRTH AT RISK

I. Learning Key Terms
1. Preterm labour
2. Preterm birth
3. Low birth weight (LBW)
4. Foetal fibronectin
5. Cervical length
6. Premature rupture of membranes (PROM)
7. Preterm premature rupture of membranes (PPROM)
8. Chorioamnionitis
9. Dystocia

10. Hypertonic uterine dysfunction
11. Hypotonic uterine dysfunction
12. Pelvic dystocia
13. Soft tissue dystocia
14. Dystocia of foetal origin
15. Cephalopelvic disproportion (CPD) *or* fetopelvic disproportion (FPD)
16. Occipitoposterior
17. Breech
18. Multifoetal pregnancy
19. Prolonged latent phase, protracted active phase—dilation, secondary arrest—no change, protracted descent, arrest of descent, and failure of descent
20. Precipitous labour
21. External cephalic version (ECV)
22. Trial of labour
23. Induction of labour
24. Bishop score
25. Amniotomy
26. Augmentation of labour
27. Cervical ripening
28. Tachysystole
29. Forceps-assisted birth
30. Vacuum-assisted birth *or* vacuum extraction
31. Caesarean birth
32. Postterm, (postdate)
33. Shoulder dystocia; fetopelvic disproportion, excessive foetal size (macrosomia)
34. Prolapse of umbilical cord
35. Amniotic fluid embolism (AFE) *or* anaphylactoid syndrome of pregnancy

II. Reviewing Key Concepts

1. See Spontaneous Versus Indicated Preterm Birth sections and Boxes 20-1 and 20-2 for content required to answer this question.
2. See Activity Restriction section and Box 20-4 for content required to answer this question.
3. b 4. c 5. e 6. a 7. d
8. e 9. c 10. d 11. a 12. f
13. g 14. b
15. See Dystocia section, Table 20-1 and specific sections for each factor for content required to answer this question.
16. See Latent Phase Disorder section and Table 20-1.
   • Purpose: Help patient experiencing hypertonic uterine dysfunction to rest/sleep so active labour can begin usually after a 4- to 6-hour rest period.
   • What: Use shower or warm bath for relaxation, comfort measures, administration of analgesics to inhibit contractions, reduce pain, and encourage rest/sleep and relaxation.
17. See Abnormal Uterine Activity section and Table 20-1 for content required to answer this question.
18. See Oxytocin section and Box 20-10 where several indicators and contraindications are listed.
19. b, c, and e are correct; Previous history of preterm labour and family history increases the risk as does periodontal disease; the BMI represents a normal weight for height.
20. a; Magnesium sulphate is a central nervous system (CNS) depressant; calcium gluconate would be used if toxicity occurs; infusion should be discontinued if respiratory rate is <12.
21. b, c and d; It is inserted into the posterior vaginal fornix; the woman should remain in bed for 2 hours; induction can begin within 30 to 60 minutes of the insert's removal.
22. d; A Bishop score of 9 indicates that the cervix is already sufficiently ripe for successful induction; 10 units of oxytocin is usually mixed in 1 000 mL of an electrolyte solution such as Ringers lactate; the oxytocin solution is piggybacked at the proximal port (port nearest the insertion site).
23. a; Frequency of uterine contractions should not be less than every 2 minutes to allow for an adequate rest period between contractions; b, c, and d are all expected findings within the normal range.
24. c; The presentation of this foetus is breech; the soft buttocks are a less efficient dilating wedge than the foetal head; therefore, labour may be slower; the ultrasound transducer should be placed to the left of the umbilicus at a level at or above it; passage of meconium is an expected finding as a result of pressure on the abdomen during descent; knee-chest position is most often used for occipitoposterior positions.
25. d; The dosage is correct at 12 mg × 2 doses; it should be given intramuscularly; dosages should be spaced 24 hours apart; therefore the next dose should be given at 1 100 the next day.
26. a; The definitive sign of preterm labour is significant change in the cervix.

III. Thinking Critically

1. See Preterm Labour and Birth section and Boxes 20-1, 20-2, and 20-3 for content required to answer this question; keep in mind that many patients go into preterm labour without identifiable risk factors.
2. See Early Recognition and Diagnosis, Prevention, and Suppression of Uterine Activity sections, Boxes 20-5 and 20-6, Family-Centred Care box What to Do If Symptoms of Preterm Labour Occur, and Medication Guides for Tocolytic Therapy and Antenatal Glucocorticoid Therapy with Betamethasone or Dexamethasone for content required to answer each part of this question.
3. See Malposition and Alteration in Secondary Powers section, Table 20-1 and Box 17-10 for the content required to answer this question; LOP indicates that the foetus is in a posterior position—the most common type of malpresentation.
4. See Caesarean Birth sections – Unplanned Caesarean Birth, Nursing Care, and Family Centred Care box – Postpartum Pain Relief after Caesarean Birth for the content required to answer each part of this question.

275

a. Implement typical preoperative care measures as for any major surgery in a calm and professional manner, explaining the purpose of each measure that must be performed; use a family-centred approach.

b. Assess for signs of haemorrhage, pain level, respiratory effort, renal function, circulatory status to extremities, signs of postanesthesia recovery, emotional status, and attachment/reaction to newborn.

c. Measures include assessment of recovery, pain relief, coughing and deep breathing, leg exercises and assistance with ambulation, nutrition and fluid intake (oral, IV); provide opportunities for interaction and care of newborn, assisting her as needed; provide emotional support to help her deal with her disappointment and feelings of failure; help her and her family prepare for discharge, making referrals as needed.

d. Possible decreased self-esteem related to inability to reach goal of a vaginal birth secondary to abnormal foetal heart rate pattern.
   • Discuss and review why Anne needed a Caesarean birth, how she performed during labour, and that she had no control over the abnormal foetal heart rate pattern.
   • Discuss trial of labour after caesarean (TOLAC) and likelihood of it being an option because the reason for her primary Caesarean (abnormal foetal heart rate tracing) may not occur again; discuss TOLAC next time to determine her ability to proceed to vaginal birth.
   • Use follow-up phone calls to assess progress in accepting Caesarean birth.

5. See Malpresentation section, Fig. 20-1 and 20-2; right sacrum anterior (RSA) indicates a breech presentation; consider that descent may be slower, meconium is often expelled, increasing danger of meconium aspiration, and risk for cord prolapse is increased; depending on progress of labour and maternal characteristics, Caesarean or vaginal birth may occur or external cephalic version (ECV) may be attempted.

6. See Induction of Labour section.
   a. See Table 20-2 for factors assessed to determine degree of cervical ripening in preparation for labour process.
   b. Her score should be >9 to ensure a successful induction; cervical ripening will be needed before induction.
   c. See Cervical Ripening Agents section and Medication Guide for guidelines for use and adverse reactions; consider how and where it is inserted, protocol to follow after the insertion, and adverse reactions and what to do if they occur.
   d. See Box 20-9, Procedure: Assisting With Amniotomy; explain what will happen, how it will feel, and why it is being done; assess maternal-fetal unit before and after the procedure; document findings; support woman during procedure telling her what is happening; document procedure and outcomes/reactions appropriately.
   e. Induction protocol:
      1. A
      2. NA (needs to be done frequently)
      3. A
      4. A
      5. A
      6. A
      7. NA (less often 15-30 minutes)
      8. A
      9. NA
      10. NA (1 000 mL in 8 hours)
   f. See Box 20-6—focus on factors related to mother, fetus, and labour process.
   g. See Emergency Measures in Medication Guide - Oxytocin.

7. See Obesity section for content required to answer this question.

CHAPTER 21 POSTPARTUM MATERNAL PHYSIOLOGICAL CHANGES

I. Learning Key Terms
1. Profuse diaphoresis
2. Afterpains
3. Prolactin; oxytocin
4. Episiotomy
5. Excessive postpartal bleeding
6. Hemorrhoid
7. Involution
8. Autolysis
9. Puerperium; fourth trimester
10. Diastasis recti abdominis
11. Lochia
12. Lochia rubra
13. Lochia serosa
14. Lochia alba
15. Engorgement
16. Subinvolution; retained placental fragments, infection
17. Oxytocin
18. Dyspareunia
19. Kegel exercises
20. Colostrum
21. Postpartal diuresis
22. Striae gravidarum

II. Reviewing Key Concepts
1. See Urethra and Bladder section of Urinary System for content required to answer each part of this question.
2. See Gastrointestinal System section for content required to answer this question.
3. See Coagulation Factors section for content required to answer this question.
4. See Box 21-1 for the information to complete your answer.

5. d; Fundus should be at midline; deviation from midline could indicate a full bladder; bright to dark red uterine discharge refers to lochia rubra; oedema and erythema are common shortly after repair of a wound; decreased abdominal muscle tone and enlarged uterus result in abdominal protrusion; separation of the abdominal muscle walls, diastasis rectus abdominis, is common during pregnancy and the postpartum period.

6. b; The patient is describing the normal finding of postpartum diaphoresis, which is the body's attempt to excrete fluid retained during pregnancy; documentation is important but not the first nursing action; infection assessment and health care provider notification are not needed at this time.

7. c; Afterpains are most likely to occur in the following circumstances: multiparity, overdistention of the uterus (macrosomia, multifetal pregnancy, hydramnios), breastfeeding (endogenous oxytocin secretion), and administration of an oxytocic.

III. Thinking Critically

1. a. Afterpains: Breastfeeding with newborn sucking causes the posterior pituitary to secrete oxytocin, stimulating the let-down reflex; uterine contractions are also stimulated, leading to afterpains, which will occur for the first few days postpartum.

   b. See Involution Process section; progress of uterine descent in the abdomen is described.

   c. See Lochia section; discuss characteristics of rubra, serosa, and alba lochia in terms of colour, consistency, amount, odour, and duration.

   d. See Abdomen section for content required to answer question—focus on reason for the occurrence and what can be done to restore abdominal muscle tone safely.

   e. See Fluid Loss section; discuss normalcy of these processes designed to rid the body of fluid retained during pregnancy. Be sure to ask questions regarding characteristics of urine, including amount and any pain with urination, to rule out a bladder infection or urinary retention evidenced by frequent voiding of small amounts of urine (overload).

   f. See Pituitary Hormones and Ovarian Function section; emphasise that breastfeeding can be used as a method of birth control for 6 months if the person is exclusively breastfeeding and their period has not returned (lactational amenorrhea method); discuss appropriate contraceptive methods for a breastfeeding patient, taking care to avoid hormonal-based methods until lactation is well established.

   g. See Nonbreastfeeding Mothers section for content required to answer this question; discuss the process of natural lactation suppression, why it is used now, and what she can do to enhance her comfort and facilitate the process.

   h. See Vagina and Perineum section for content required to answer this question.

CHAPTER 22 NURSING CARE OF THE FAMILY DURING THE POSTPARTUM PERIOD

I. Learning Key Terms

1. Oxytocic
2. Uterine atony
3. Sitz bath
4. Afterpains
5. Splanchnic engorgement, orthostatic hypotension
6. Kegel
7. Engorgement
8. Rubella
9. Rh immune globulin
10. Warm line

II. Reviewing Key Concepts

1. See Promoting Breastfeeding section for the content required to answer this question.

2. See Preventing Bladder Distention section for content required to answer this question.

3. See Promoting Ambulation section including safety alert for content required to answer this question; in addition to activity include the use of support hose (if varicosities are present) and importance of remaining well hydrated.

4. See Suppression of Lactation section for content required to answer this question.

5. See Preventing Excessive Bleeding section; include each measure in your answer:
   • Maintain uterine tone
   • Prevent bladder distention

6. See Box 22-3 and Psychosocial Assessment and Care section for the content required to answer the question.

7. c; The patient should be assisted into a supine position with head and shoulders on a pillow, arms at sides, and knees flexed; this will facilitate relaxation of abdominal muscles and allow deep palpation. The bladder should be emptied first in order to do a proper assessment of the fundus. See Table 22-2.

8. b; A direct and indirect Coombs must be negative, indicating that antibodies have not been formed, before Rh Immune Globulin can be given; it must be given within 72 hours of birth; the newborn needs to be Rh positive; it is often given in the third trimester and then again after birth.

9. d; This is a medical aseptic procedure; therefore, clean, not sterile, equipment is used; the water should be warm at 38° to 40.6 °C; it is often used 2 to 3 times a day for 20 minutes each time.

10. d and e; The sitz bath should be used 2 to 3 times per day for 20 minutes each time; topical medications should be used sparingly only 3 to 4 times per day.

11. b and d; Temperature of 38 °C during the first 24 hours may be related to deficient fluid and is therefore not a concern; fundus should be firm not

277

boggy; saturation of the pad in 15 minutes or less would be a concern; usually postpartum patients have a good appetite after birth; each voiding should be at least 100 mL.

12. c; Approximately 50% to 80% of postpartum patients experience postpartum blues; new parents should be reassured that their skills as parents develop gradually and they should seek help to develop these skills; postpartum blues that are self-limiting and short lived do not require psychotropic medications; support and care of the postpartum patient and their newborn by her partner and family is the most effective prevention and coping strategy; feelings of fatigue from childbirth and meeting demands of newborn can accentuate feelings of depression.

III. Thinking Critically

1. See Promoting Comfort—Nonpharmacological and Pharmacological Interventions sections, assess characteristics of pain and relief measures already tried and effectiveness; use a combination of pharmacological and nonpharmacological measures as indicated by the nature of the pain being experienced; if breastfeeding, administer a systemic analgesic just after a feeding session although some patients may require it prior to the feeding; make sure medication is not contraindicated for breastfeeding patients.

2. See Preventing Excessive Bleeding section and Emergency box Hypovolemic Shock for content required to answer each part of this question.

3. See Rubella vaccination section including Legal Tip for the content required to answer this question.

4. See Prevention of Rh Isoimmunization section including Nursing Alert and Medication Guide for content required to answer this question.

5. See Sexual Activity and Contraception section and the Family Centred Care box Resuming Sexual Activity After Birth for content required to answer this question.

6. a. Nursing diagnosis: Risk for infection of laceration due to possible lack of information about care
   Expected outcome: Laceration will heal without infection.
   Nursing care: See Preventing Infection section and Box 22-2 for full identification of measures to enhance healing and prevent infection.
   b. Nursing diagnosis: Constipation due to inactivity and possible lack of information.
   Expected outcome: Patient will have soft formed bowel movement.
   Nursing care: See Promoting Normal Bowel Function section.
   c. Nursing diagnosis: Acute pain due to episiotomy and hemorrhoids.
   Expected outcome: Patient will experience a reduction in pain following implementation of suggested relief measures.

Nursing care: See Promoting Comfort section and Box 22-2.
   d. Nursing diagnosis: Postpartum blues due to hormonal changes and increased responsibilities following birth
   Expected outcome: Patient will report feeling less emotional and teary following use of recommended coping strategies.
   Nursing care: See Postpartum Blues sections and Patient Teaching box Coping With Postpartum Blues for content required to answer this question.

7. See Preventing Bladder Distention section; most likely basis for finding is bladder distention—discuss implications of bladder distention and measures to facilitate emptying of the bladder.

8. See Promoting Ambulation section including safety alert for content required to answer this question.

9. See Impact of Cultural Diversity for the content required to answer each part of this question.

10. See Table 22-2 for the content required to answer each part of this question.
   a. Position for fundal palpation: supine, head and shoulder on pillow, arms at sides, knees slightly flexed.
   b. Fundal characteristics to assess: consistency (firm or boggy), height (above, at, below umbilicus), location (midline or deviated to the right or left).
   c. Position for assessment of perineum: lateral position with upper leg flexed on hip.
   d. Laceration characteristics to assess: REEDA (redness, edema, ecchymosis, drainage, approximation); presence of haematoma; adequacy of hygiene, including cleanliness, presence of odour, method used to cleanse perineum and to apply topical preparations.
   e. Characteristics of lochia to assess: stage, amount, odour, clots.

11. See Transfer From Recovery Area section for a discussion of essential information that should be reported regarding the patient, the baby, and the significant events and findings from the prenatal and childbirth periods.

12. See Preventing Infection section and Box 22-2 for content required to answer each part of this question.

CHAPTER 23 TRANSITION TO PARENTHOOD

I. Learning Key Terms

1. Attachment; bonding
2. Acquaintance
3. Mutuality
4. Signalling behaviours
5. Claiming
6. En face (face to face)
7. Entrainment
8. Biorhythmicity

9. Reciprocity
10. Synchrony
11. Transition to parenthood
12. Eye contact
13. Adaptation to the parental role
14. Becoming a mother
15. Engrossment
16. Responsivity

II. Reviewing Key Concepts

1. See Parental Attachment, Bonding, and Acquaintance and Assessment of Attachment sections, Tables 23-1, 23-2, and 23-3, and Box 23-1 for content required to answer each part of the question.
2. See Parental Tasks and Responsibilities section for content required to answer this question.
3. See Parent-Infant Contact—Early Contact and Extended Contact section for the content required to answer each part of this question.
4. See Touch section for a description of touch as it progresses from an exploration with fingertips to gentle stroking, patting, and rubbing.
5. Factors influencing parental responses to the birth of their child: see section for each factor in the Diversity in Transition to Parenthood and Parental Sensory Impairment sections.
6. d; Choice a reflects the first phase of identifying likenesses; choice b reflects the second phase of identifying differences; choice c reflects a negative reaction of claiming the infant in terms of pain and discomfort; choice d reflects the third or final stage of identifying uniqueness.
7. b; Early close contact is recommended to initiate and enhance the attachment process.
8. a; Engrossment refers to a father's absorption, preoccupation, and interest in his infant; b represents the claiming process phase I, identifying likeness; c represents reciprocity; d represents en face or face-to-face position with mutual gazing.
9. a, d, and e; See also Table 20.1 Infant Behaviours Affecting Parental Attachment.

III. Thinking Critically

1. See Communication Between Parent and Infant section and Tables 23-1 and 23-2 for the content required to answer each part of this question.
2. See Parental Attachment, Bonding, and Acquaintance and Parent-Infant Contact sections for the content to answer this question; be sure to emphasise that the process of attachment is ongoing and the delay in interacting with the newborn will not affect this process.
   • Help her meet her own physical and emotional needs so that she develops readiness to meet her newborn's needs.
   • Help her get to know her baby and interact with and care for him; point out newborn characteristics, including how the baby is responding to her efforts.
   • Show her how to communicate with her newborn and how her newborn communicates with her.
   • Arrange for follow-up after discharge to assess how attachment is progressing.
3. See Sibling Adaptation section and Family-Centred Care box, which identifies strategies parents can use to help their other children accept a new baby; caution her that adjustment takes time and is strongly related to the developmental level and experiences of the sibling(s); give mother suggestions regarding what she can do now and what she did previously.
4. See Parental Attachment, Bonding, and Acquaintance and Communication Between Parent and Infant sections and Tables 23-1, 23-2, and 23-3 for content required to answer each part of this question; Nursing diagnosis: Risk for impaired parent-infant attachment due to feeling of incompetence regarding newborn care.
5. See Parental Tasks and Responsibilities section; foster attachment, acquaintance, and claiming; help parents get acquainted with the newborn and to reconcile the real child with the fantasy child; discuss the basis of molding, caput succedaneum, and forceps marks and how they will be resolved; be alert for problems with attachment and care so follow-up can be arranged.
6. See Grandparent Adaptation section and Community Focus Box; observe interaction between grandparents and parents taking note of signs of effective interaction and conflict; involve grandparents in teaching sessions as appropriate for this family; spend time with grandparents to help them be supportive without "taking over" or being critical; help the new parents recognise the unique role grandparents can play as parenting role models, nurturers, and providers of respite care.
7. See Becoming a Father section and Table 23-5 to discuss the transition process to fatherhood and nursing measures that provide the father with support, teaching, demonstrations, and practise and interaction time with the newborn.

CHAPTER 24 POSTPARTUM COMPLICATIONS

I. Learning Key Terms

1. Postpartum haemorrhage (PPH); Primary PPH; Secondary PPH
2. Uterine atony
3. Hematoma; vulvar haematomas, vaginal haematomas
4. Placenta accreta
5. Placenta increta
6. Placenta percreta
7. Inversion
8. Subinvolution
9. Haemorrhagic (hypovolemic) shock
10. Immune thrombocytopenic purpura
11. von Willebrand disease
12. Disseminated intravascular coagulation
13. Venous thromboembolism (VTE)
14. Thrombophlebitis

15. Superficial venous thrombosis; Deep vein thrombosis (DVT)
16. Pulmonary embolism
17. Postpartum, puerperal infection
18. Endometritis
19. Mastitis
20. Uterine prolapse
21. Perinatal mood disorders (PMD)
22. Postpartum blues
23. Postpartum depression
24. Postpartum psychosis
25. Detachment
26. Psychotherapy and antidepressants
27. Bipolar disorder
28. Edinburgh Postnatal Depression and the Postpartum Depression Screening Scale
29. Method, availability, specificity, and lethality
30. Generalised anxiety disorder
31. Panic disorder
32. Complicated bereavement

II. Reviewing Key Concepts

1. See haemorrhagic (Hypovolemic) Shock—Collaborative Care section: restore circulating blood volume to enhance perfusion of vital organs and treat the cause of the haemorrhage.
2. See Postpartum Haemorrhage—Nursing Care and Hemorrhagic Shock – Collaborative Care sections and Box 24-1 for content required to answer this question; cite interventions related to improving and monitoring tissue perfusion, treating the cause of the haemorrhage, enhancing healing, supporting the patient and their family, fostering maternal-infant attachment as appropriate, and planning for discharge.
3. See Legal Tip—Standard of Care for Bleeding Emergencies for content required to answer this question.
4. See Nursing Care section of Postpartum Infections and Box 24-3 for a list of prevention measures including good prenatal nutrition to control anaemia and intrapartal haemorrhage perineal hygiene, and adherence to aseptic techniques.
5. See Perinatal Mood Disorders – Nursing Considerations section to answer this question.
6. See Maternal Death section to answer this question.
7. See Perinatal Mood Disorders—Providing Safety sections including the Nursing Alert for the content required to answer each part of this question; identify possibility of a patient harming themselves, their baby, or both of them.
8. b; Although a, and d are correct actions, the patient's hypertensive status would be a contraindicating factor for its use; therefore, the order should be questioned as the nurse's first action. Methylergonovine is administered intravenously and not rectally.
9. d; Carboprost tromethamine is a powerful prostaglandin that is the third-line medication given to treat excessive uterine blood loss or haemorrhage related to uterine atony; it has no action related to pain, infection, or clotting.
10. a; Postpartum infections are infections of the genital tract after birth; pulse will increase, not decrease, in response to fever; lochia characteristics will change, but this will not be the first sign exhibited; WBC count would already be elevated related to pregnancy and birth.
11. b, c, d, and f; Heparin and warfarin (Coumadin) are safe for use by breastfeeding women; heparin, which is administered intravenously or subcutaneously, is the anticoagulant of choice during the acute stage of VTE; warfarin is administered orally, not parenterally.
12. a; Although the other questions are appropriate, the potential for harming themselves or their baby is the most serious and very real concern.
13. c; Carboprost tromethamine is contraindicated in patients with a history of asthma. It can cause bronchoconstriction.
14. d; Tachypnea is a sign and symptom of a pulmonary embolus. All others are not.
15. a, b and c; All are techniques used to manage postpartum haemorrhage.
16. c; St. John's wort.
17. a; Methylergonovine as an oxytocic contracts the uterus, thereby preventing excessive blood loss; lochia will therefore be decreased.

III. Thinking Critically

1. See Postpartum Haemorrhage section, Medication Guide for Drugs Used to Manage Postpartum Haemorrhage, Boxes 24-1 and 24-2, and Emergency box Hemorrhagic Shock for the content required to answer each part of this question.
   a. Risk factors for early postpartum haemorrhage grand multiparity, vaginal full-term twin birth 1 hour ago; hypotonic uterine dysfunction treated with oxytocin; use of forceps for birth; increased manipulation with birth of twins.
   b. Nurse's response to excessive blood loss: Most common cause of the excessive blood loss 1 hour after birth would be uterine atony, especially because woman exhibits several risk factors.
   - Assess fundus for consistency, height, and location; massage if boggy.
   - Express clots, if present, once uterus is firm.
   - Check bladder for distention (distended bladder will reduce uterine contraction); check perineum for swelling and ask woman about experiencing perineal pressure (hematoma formation is possible related to use of forceps for birth).
   c. Guidelines for administering oxytocin IV: Use Medication Guide.
   d. Signs of developing haemorrhagic shock: See Emergency box.

e. Nursing measures to support the patient and family:
- Explain progress, including meaning of findings and need for treatment measures being used, including their purpose and effectiveness.
- Use a calm, professional, organised approach that incorporates periods of uninterrupted rest.
- Initiate comfort measures.
- Provide opportunities for interaction with newborn and updates on newborn's status.

2. See Postpartum Infections section and Box 24-3 for the content required to answer each part of this question.

3. See Mastitis section and Fig. 24-3 for the content required to answer each part of this question; Nursing diagnoses: Acute pain due to inflammation of right breast; Ineffective breastfeeding OR Anxiety due to concerns regarding transmission of infection to newborn; emphasise correction of breastfeeding techniques and breast care measures to prevent recurrence.

4. See Venous Thromboembolic Disorders section for content required to answer each part of this question.
   a. Risk factors: In addition to hypercoagulability of pregnancy continuing into the postpartum period, other risk factors for this patient would be Caesarean birth, obesity, age over 35 years, multiparity, smoker, and varicosities in both legs.
   b. Signs and symptoms indicative of VTE: see Clinical Manifestations section.
   c. Nursing diagnosis: Anxiety due to unexpected development of a postpartum complication.
   d. Expected care management: see Collaborative Care sections including Nursing Alert.
   e. Discharge instructions:
   - How to assess leg and to assess for signs of unusual bleeding
   - Proper use of elastic/support stockings
   - How to take anticoagulant safely and importance of follow-up to assess progress
   - Practises to prevent bleeding while taking an anticoagulant and importance of avoiding pregnancy because warfarin is teratogenic
   - Importance of avoiding aspirin and NSAIDs for pain and food/vitamin supplements that are sources of vitamin K because they can interact with warfarin (Coumadin)

5. See Hematomas section to answer all parts of this section

6. See Perinatal Mood Disorders section, Patient Teaching boxes Signs of Postpartum Blues, Depression, and Psychosis and Preventing Perinatal Mood Disorder, and Box 24-4 for content required to answer each part of this question.

7. See information under Postpartum Haemorrhage related to interprofessional health care teams.

8. See information under Postpartum Infection and Urinary Tract Infection to answer this question.

CHAPTER 25 PHYSIOLOGICAL AND ADAPTATIONS OF THE NEWBORN

I. Learning Key Terms
1. Neutral thermal environment
2. Thermogenesis
3. Nonshivering thermogenesis
4. Convection
5. Radiation
6. Evaporation
7. Conduction
8. Hyperthermia
9. Cold stress
10. Nevus simplex
11. Moulding
12. Caput succedaneum
13. Cephalhematoma
14. Congenital dermal melanocytosis
15. Acrocyanosis
16. Vernix caseosa
17. Milia
18. Jaundice
19. Meconium
20. Erythema toxicum (neonatorum)
21. Uric acid crystals (brick dust)
22. Wink reflex
23. Hydrocele
24. Ecchymosis
25. Murmur
26. Lanugo
27. Subgaleal haemorrhage
28. Desquamation
29. Nevus flammeus (port-wine stain)
30. Infantile hemangioma (strawberry hemangioma)
31. Pseudomenstruation
32. Prepuce
33. Epstein (epithelial) pearls
34. Polydactyly; oligodactyly
35. Syndactyly
36. Sleep-wake states
37. Deep; light; increasing
38. Drowsy, quiet alert, active alert, crying
39. Quiet alert
40. State regulation
41. Habituation
42. Orientation
43. Consolability
44. Temperament
45. Habituation
46. Crying

II. Reviewing Key Concepts
1. See Respiratory System section for a description of how a newborn begins to breathe; include chemical, mechanical, thermal, and sensory factors in your answer.
2. See Transition to Extrauterine Life section at beginning of chapter for identification of each phase and

description of timing/duration and typical newborn behaviours for each phase.

3. a, b, and c; The newborn at 5 hours old is in the second period of reactivity, during which tachycardia, tachypnea, increased muscle tone, skin colour changes, increased mucus production, and passage of meconium are normal findings; temperature should range between 36.5° and 37.2° C, and respiratory rate should range between 30 and 60 BPM; expiratory grunting and nasal flaring and retractions of the sternum are signs of respiratory distress.

4. a; The rash described is erythema toxicum; it is an inflammatory response that has no clinical significance and requires no treatment because it will disappear spontaneously.

5. b; Physiologic jaundice does not appear until after the first 24 hours following birth; further investigation would be needed if it appears during the first 24 hours, because that would be consistent with pathologic jaundice; a, c, and d are all expected findings.

6. d; Choices b and c are common newborn reflexes used to assess integrity of neuromuscular system; syndactyly refers to webbing of the fingers.

7. c; Telangiectatic nevi (nevus simplex) can also appear on the eyelids; milia are plugged sebaceous glands and appear like white pimples; infantile hemangioma or a strawberry mark is a raised, sharply demarcated, bright or dark red swelling; nevus flammeus is a port-wine, flat red to purple lesion that does not blanch with pressure.

III. Thinking Critically

1. See Thermogenesis—Hypothermia and Cold Stress section and Figs. 25.1 and 25.2 for the content required to answer each part of this question. Nursing Diagnosis: Risk for imbalanced body temperature—hypothermia related to adaptation to extrauterine environment associated with newborn status; Expected outcome: newborn's temperature will stabilise between 36.5° and 37.2° C within the first 12 hours of birth.

2. See Integumentary System and Skeletal System sections; discuss each finding in terms of cause, significance for the newborn's health status and adjustment, and how/when it will be resolved; refer to Figs. 25.11 and 25.12 to facilitate parental understanding.

3. See Respiratory System section for the content required to answer this question; consult Table 25.1 for further information.

4. See Sensory Behaviours section including vision, hearing, smell, taste, and touch:
   a. Discuss and demonstrate newborn's capability regarding vision, hearing, touch, taste, and smell.
   b. Face-to-face/eye-to-eye contact, objects (black-and-white changing, complex patterns), sound (talking to infant, music, heartbeat simulator), touch (infant massage, skin-to-skin care).

5. Discuss the characteristics and cause of Congenital Dermal Melanocytosis (see Congenital Dermal Melanocytosis section and Fig. 25.8).

6. See Bilirubin Synthesis and Newborn Jaundice section for the content to compare and contrast each type of jaundice listed.

CHAPTER 26 NURSING CARE OF THE NEWBORN AND FAMILY

I. Learning Key Terms
1. Apgar score; heart rate, respiratory effort, muscle tone, reflex irritability, colour
2. Thermistor probe
3. Ophthalmia neonatorum; Erythromycin
4. Vitamin K
5. New Ballard score
6. Appropriate for gestational age (AGA)
7. Preterm
8. Postterm
9. Post mature
10. Early term
11. Petechiae
12. Bilirubin
13. Physiologic jaundice
14. Kernicterus
15. Transcutaneous bilirubinometer (TcB)
16. Phototherapy
17. Hypoglycemia
18. Hypocalcemia
19. Bradypnea
20. Tachypnea
21. Handwashing (hand hygiene)
22. Bilirubin (fiberoptic) blanket
23. Circumcision

II. Reviewing Key Concepts
Matching:
1. j	2. f	3. b	4. i	5. d
6. h	7. a	8. e	9. g	10. c
11. k				

12. See Protective Environment section; discuss each of the following in your answer:
    a. Environmental modifications
    b. Infection control measures
    c. Safety in terms of security precautions and identification measures
    d. Prevention of newborn falls

13. See Baseline Measurement of Physical Growth section, Table 23.3, Measurements section for content required to answer this question.

14. See Discharge Planning and Teaching section and Home Care boxes Infant Safety and Newborn Bath, Cord Care, Skin Care, Genital Care and Nail Care for content required to answer each part of this question.

15. See Intervention—Airway Maintenance and Box 26-3 Signs of Potential Complications: Abnormal

Newborn Breathing sections for the content required to answer each part of this question.

16. d, e, and f; Thinning of lanugo with bald spots, descent of testes, and absence of scarf sign are consistent with full-term status; pulse and weight are not part of the Ballard scale; the popliteal angle for a full-term newborn would be 90 degrees or less.

17. b; Signs of hypoglycemia include apnea, temperature instability jitteriness, respiratory distress, abnormal cry, poor feeding, lethargy, and seizures.

18. b; Acetaminophen should be given every 4 hours for a maximum of 5 doses in 24 hours; the site should be checked every 15 to 30 minutes for the first hour and then every hour for the next 4 to 6 hours; diaper wipes should not be used on the site because they contain alcohol, which would delay healing and cause discomfort; the yellow exudate is a protective film that forms in 24 hours, and it should not be removed.

19. b, c, and d; Mother does not have to be hepatitis B positive for the vaccine to be given to her newborn;

III. Thinking Critically

1. See Table 26-1 and Apgar Scoring section for the content to answer this question.
   a. Baby Nunez: heart rate: 160 (2); respiratory effort: good, crying (2); muscle tone: flexion, active movement (2); reflex irritability: cry with stimulus (2); colour: acrocyanosis (1); score is 9 and is within normal limits; interpretation: score of 7 to 10 indicates that the infant is not having difficulty adjusting to extrauterine life.
   b. Baby Yoo: heart rate: 102 (2); respiratory effort: slow, irregular, weak cry (1); muscle tone: some flexion (1); reflex irritability: grimace with stimulus (1); colour: pale (0); score is 5; interpretation: score of 4 to 6 indicates moderate difficulty adjusting to extrauterine life.

2. See Discharge Planning and Teaching, Protective Environment, and Promoting Parent-Newborn Interactions sections, Table 23.3, and Family Centred Care box Signs of Illness for the content required to answer each part of this question; by including the parents you have a chance to observe parent-infant interactions and to identify and meet learning needs; foster active involvement in assessment and care of their newborn; encourage discussion of concerns and asking of questions; chance to explain and demonstrate newborn characteristics and capabilities.

3. See Discharge Planning and Parent Education section, Patient Teaching box Care of the Circumcised Newborn at Home, and Home Care box Bathing, Cord Care, Skin Care, *and Nail Care* for the content required to answer each part of this question; Nursing diagnosis: Risk for infection related to removal of foreskin and healing umbilical cord site; Expected outcome: cord and circumcision site will heal without infection.

4. See Phototherapy and Physiological Problems—Hyperbilirubinemia and Parent-Infant Interaction sections and Chapter 22 for a full discussion of the basis for physiologic (nonpathologic) jaundice for the content required to answer each part of this question. Be sure that your answer includes the importance of telling parents in simple terms that their newborn is exhibiting physiologic jaundice, explaining why it occurs, what impact it will have on their newborn's health, and how it will be resolved; in addition, ensure that they are given time to interact with their newborn during feeding times when the infant is out of the lights and even when under the lights.

CHAPTER 27 NEWBORN NUTRITION AND FEEDING

I. Learning Key Terms

1. Lobes
2. Alveoli
3. Milk ducts
4. Nipple erection reflex; inverted (flat)
5. Myoepithelial cells
6. Areola
7. Lactation (lactogenesis)
8. Prolactin
9. Oxytocin
10. Milk ejection reflex
11. Breast (nipple) shell
12. Galactogogue
13. Colostrum
14. Human milk
15. Feeding readiness cues
16. Letdown; milk ejection
17. Rooting reflex
18. Latch (latch-on)
19. Engorgement
20. Football hold
21. Cradle (traditional) hold
22. Lactation consultant
23. Mastitis
24. Tongue-tie
25. Weaning
26. Early onset jaundice (breastfeeding-associated jaundice)
27. Late onset jaundice (breast milk jaundice)

II. Reviewing Key Concepts

1. See Benefits of Breastfeeding, Cultural influences on infant feeding and Lactation and LGBTQ2 families sections and Table 27.1; emphasise the importance and benefits of breastfeeding for infants and family/society.

2. See Effective Latch and Figs. 27.6 and 27.7 for the content required to answer each part of this question.

3. c; Birthweight is regained in 10 to 14 days; meconium stools change to transitional stool by day 2-3; should be fed every 2 to 3 hours for a total of 8 to 10 times per day.

4. d; No soap should be used because it could dry the areola and increase the risk for irritation; vitamin E should not be used because it is a fat-soluble vitamin that the infant could ingest when breastfeeding; lanolin or colostrum/milk are the preferred substances to be applied to the area; plastic liners can trap moisture and lead to sore nipples.

5. b; A combination hormonal oral or injectable contraceptive could decrease the milk supply if given before lactation is well established during the first 6 weeks after birth; after 6 weeks, a progestin-only contraceptive could be used because it is the least likely hormonal contraceptive to affect lactation; exclusive breastfeeding is not considered to be a reliable method because ovulation can occur unexpectedly even before the first menstrual period

6. b; Supplements are not required when using prepared formulas; a 2-week-old infant should consume approximately 90 to 150 mL of formula at each feeding; formula should never be heated in the microwave because it could be overheated or unevenly heated.

7. a, c, and d; Nipples should not be washed using soap; plastic liners can keep nipples and areola moist and increase the risk for tissue breakdown; bring baby to breast, not breast to baby.

III. Thinking Critically

1. See Anatomy of the Lactating Breast, Uniqueness of Human Milk, and Special Considerations sections for the content to answer parts a and b.
   a. Breast size: discuss development of lactation structures during pregnancy; emphasise the importance of this development and not the breast size for successful lactation.
   b. Let-down reflex: explain what it is and why it happens (including physical and emotional triggers); emphasise its importance in providing the infant with hindmilk.
   c. See Indicators of Effective Breastfeeding section and Box 27.2, which identify maternal and newborn indicators of effective breastfeeding; put the indicators in writing and go over each one; provide contact person if mother is concerned.
   d. See Sore Nipples section and Fig. 27.17; discuss and demonstrate measures to prevent and treat sore nipples, including, most importantly, good breastfeeding techniques such as latch-on, removal, and alternating starting breast and positions; discuss effective and recommended breast care measures.
   e. See Engorgement section; begin by describing engorgement, what it is, why and when it occurs, and then discuss prevention and relief measures.
   f. See Lactogenesis section for the content required to answer this question—focus on the impact of oxytocin secretion.
   g. See Breastfeeding and Contraception section; emphasise that breastfeeding is not an effective contraceptive method; although ovulation may be delayed, its return cannot be predicted with accuracy and may occur before the first menstrual period; discuss contraceptive methods that are safe to use with breastfeeding and resuming sexual intercourse during the postpartum period.
   h. See Expressing and Storing Breast Milk, Being Away from the Infant, and Weaning sections; discuss how she can continue breastfeeding if she wishes to do so and how to wean when she is ready emphasising that weaning needs to be a gradual process.

2. See Frequency of Feeding and Sleepy Newborn sections for the content required to answer each part of this question.
   a. Nursing diagnosis: Imbalanced nutrition less than body requirements related to infrequent feeding of newborn.
      Expected outcome: Mother will awaken infant every 2 to 3 hours during the day and every 4 hours at night to feed the infant, achieving at least 8 feedings per day.
   b. Nursing approach: Discuss feeding readiness cues to facilitate proper timing of feedings; discuss techniques to wake sleeping baby and signs indicating adequate intake.

3. See Nursing Care Early Post Partum section and Box 27.2 to determine what to assess; formulate questions that address the assessment factors; in addition ask questions about topics including frequency and duration of feedings, breastfeeding techniques used, how she feels about breastfeeding and how well she feels she is doing, family support for breastfeeding; her ability to rest; and nutrient and fluid intake.

CHAPTER 28 INFANTS WITH GESTATIONAL AGE–RELATED CONDITIONS

I. Learning Key Terms

1. d and h   2. m   3. o   4. p
5. q   6. i   7. a   8. l   9. j
10. k   11. n   12. g   13. c   14. e
15. f   16. b   17. r   18. s   19. t
20. Preterm birth or prematurity
21. Ethical issue
22. Lactic acid
23. Continuous positive airway pressure (CPAP)
24. Mechanical ventilation
25. Polyethylene bag
26. 72
27. 32 to 34 weeks
28. mucosal atrophy
29. Gastrostomy
30. Cycled lighting
31. Periventricular-intraventricular haemorrhage
32. Inhaled nitric oxide
33. Necrotizing enterocolitis
34. Intermittent gavage feeding
35. Respiratory distress syndrome
36. Persistent pulmonary hypertension of the newborn

II. Reviewing Key Concepts

1. Please refer to Transport to a Regional Centre for content related to answer.
2. Please refer to Infants of Diabetic Mothers section for content required to answer
3. Please refer to Preterm Infant and Late Preterm Infant—Nursing Care Management section for content.
4. b, d, and e; Retractions, nasal flaring reflect increased effort and work to breathe; a, c, and f are all expected findings consistent with efficient respiratory effort in the preterm newborn.
5. b; Although a, c, and d are appropriate and important, respiration with adequate gas exchange takes precedence because of the surfactant deficiency which leads to alveolar collapse in preterm infants.
6. c, d; Fracture from trauma is more common in the upper body (e.g., humerus, clavicle); hypocalcemia is common

III. Thinking Critically

1. Please refer Nutritional Support, Infant-led Oral Feeding and Gavage Feeding sections including Figure 28-3 for content.
   a. Observe for ability to suck and swallow and the coordination of each; signs of respiratory distress during the feeding; length of time for the feeding and the amount ingested; presence of regurgitation, vomiting, or abdominal distention after feeding; daily weight gains and losses and elimination patterns.
   b. Emphasise tubing choice and measurement of tubing length, insertion without trauma and securing to maintain placement.
   c. Imbalanced nutrition: less than body requirements related to weak suck associated with premature status.
   d. Initiate measures to prevent aspiration with proper tube insertion andremoval,.
      - instil breast milk or formula by gravity rather than pushing syringe barrel to expedite feeding.
      - Cuddle, swaddle infant during feedings; involve parents; use nonnutritive sucking.
      - Document assessment findings and specifics of the procedure.
   e. Complications include aspiration, obstructed nares, mucous plugs and stomach perforation
2. Please refer to Gavage feeding section for content. Current practise dictates a radiograph as the only certain way to determine nasogastric (NG) tube placement in the stomach. Methods such as auscultation of an air bubble, neck-ear-xiphoid (NEX) measurements for insertion depth, and pH measurements are considered imprecise when used as the only method for determination of placement.
3. See Nursing Care-Developmental Care section
   a. continuous exposure to light and noise; administration of sedatives and pain medications; invasive procedures and medications required for treatment

   b. See Nursing Care-Developmental Care section for content, including supporting skin-to-skin contact, reducing external stimulation, slow controlled handling movements, facilitated tucking, swaddling and nesting.
4. Please refer to Postterm Infant section for content.
   a. Rationale for increased mortality: increased oxygen demands are not met and likelihood for impaired gas exchange occurs, leading to hypoxia and passage of meconium into amniotic fluid; risk for aspiration of meconium into lungs.
   b. Typical assessment findings: thin, emaciated appearance (dysmature) caused by loss of subcutaneous fat and muscle mass; peeling of skin; meconium staining on fingernails; long hair and nails; absence of vernix.
   c. Two major complications: meconium aspiration syndrome and persistent pulmonary hypertension of the newborn (PPHN); see separate sections that describes each complication.
5. Please see Nutritional Support section for content. Minimal enteral (trophic gastrointestinal priming) feedings have been shown to stimulate the infant's gastrointestinal tract, preventing mucosal atrophy and subsequent enteral feeding difficulties. Enteral feedings with as little as 10-15mL/kg/day of mother's own milk or donor breast milk may be given by gavage as soon as the infant is medically stable.
6. See Family Support and Involvement section for content.

CHAPTER 29 THE NEWBORN AT RISK: ACQUIRED AND CONGENITAL CONDITIONS

I. Learning Key Terms
MATCHING

1. J	2. K	3. A	4. C	5. B
6. I	7. E	8. L	9. G	10. M
11. N	12. H	13. O	14. P	15. S
16. F	17. T	18. D	19. Q	20. R

FILL IN THE BLANKS
21. TORCH
22. Herpes Simplex Virus
23. Handwashing
24. Foetal Alcohol Spectrum Disorder
25. Hemolytic Disease of the Newborn
26. Erythroblastosis Fetalis; hydrops fetalis
27. ABO incompatibility
28. Neonatal Abstinence Syndrome
29. Meconium
30. Inborn errors of metabolism
31. Phenylketonuria
32. Galactosemia
33. congenital hypothyroidism
34. low birth weight; preterm
35. THC - tetrahydrocannabinol
36. Cocaine
37. Genetic
38. clavicle

39. phrenic nerve palsy
40. therapeutic hypothermia

II. Reviewing Key Concepts

1. Please see Adverse Exposures Affecting Newborns, Neonatal Abstinence Syndrome and individual substance subsections for content. Details should include: CNS – high pitched cry, difficulties in consoling, tremors, lethargy, poor suck reflex, seizures, sleep distur; GI – poor feeding, abdominal distension, diarrhea; Respiratory – irregular breathing patterns, apnea Please see Nursing Care subsection within Adverse Exposures Affecting Newborns for content; include reducing environmental stimuli, swaddling, rocking and on-demand feeding.
2. Please see Hemotologic Disorders section, Rh and ABO Incompatibility subsections for content. Include specifics related to Rh negative pregnant women and Rh positive Foetus and/or foetal blood group A or B in women with blood group O.
3. Please see subsection Human Immunodeficiency Virus for content.
   Correct answer includes b, c, d; isolating the newborn is not necessary.
'

III. Thinking Critically

1. Please refer to ABO incompatibility, Prevention, Management and Nursing Care subsections for content. Include the following in your answer: vital sign monitoring, maintaining neutral thermal environment, supporting practitioner to complete procedure under sterile conditions, completion of blood sampling, maintaining the baby NPO with NG insitu, maintaining patent IV, resuming phototherapy after completion of procedure.
2. Refer to the Peripheral Nervous System Injuries subsection. Include details related to potential implications for feeding.

CHAPTER 30 PEDIATRIC NURSING IN CANADA

I. Learning Key Terms

1. e	2. i	3. a	4. b	5. f
6. c	7. h	8. k	9. g	10. d
11. j	12. m	13. n	14. l	15. o

II. Reviewing Key Concepts

1. b	2. d	3. d	4. c	
5. Please see box 30-2 for content.				
6. d	7. b	8. T	9. F	10. F
11. F	12. F	13. T	14. T	15. T

III. Thinking Critically

1. Refer to the sub-section on Social Determinants of Health in Children's Health in Canada and Table 30.1 to answer this question. Details to include: Type 1 Diabetes care requires a careful balance of food intake, daily activity and insulin administration. Health inequi-

ties exist for children living in low-income families. Family income determines access to quality food, ability to secure transportation for medical appointments and access to medical supplies. Family income may also influence access to organized physical activities. Family income may place Usman at risk for having inconsistent food intake leading to variable blood glucose control. Usman's family may not be able to fully access the regular medical follow-up care required to obtain the health information and education required to care for a chronic illness. Inconsistent daily blood glucose control may lead to short-term and long-term consequences including acute hypoglycemic events, ketoacidosis, hypertension, retinopathy or neuropathy.
2. Research indicates that Indigenous adolescents with ties to a strong cultural continuity of their band including women leaders, living in a setting with culture-designated buildings, community control of child services, and band-based community services including school, health, fire and police services protect Indigenous youth from suicide. Exploring cultural ties, gender identity and sexual orientation provides insight into possible risk for death by suicide for 15 year old Adlartok.

CHAPTER 31 FAMILY, SOCIAL, AND CULTURAL INFLUENCES ON CHILDREN'S HEALTH

I. Learning Key Terms

1. d	2. e	3. c	4. b	5. f
6. g	7. a	8. k	9. l	10. i
11. j	12. h			

II. Reviewing Key Concepts

1. d	2. c	3. d	4. e	5. c
6. b	7. a	8. b	9. d	10. T
11. F	12. T	13. T	14. F	15. T
16. T				

III. Thinking Critically

1. a. First determine Noemi's knowledge and understanding of English and determine if a translator is needed. Questions which may be asked include but are not limited to the following:
   "How do you feel about immunizations for your children?" "How did you travel to the clinic?" "Do you prefer written instructions in English or your first language?" "Who usually cares for the children during the day?" "Are your children in a day care or are they cared for in your home?"

CHAPTER 32 DEVELOPMENTAL INFLUENCES ON CHILD HEALTH PROMOTION

I. Learning Key Terms

1. m	2. f	3. a	4. h	5. j
6. k	7. b	8. e	9. d	10. n
11. o	12. c	13. i	14. g	15. l

II. Reviewing Key Concepts

1. c	2. a	3. c	4. b	5. d
6. b	7. b	8. c	9. d	10. d
11. c	12. T	13. F	14. T	15. T
16. F	17. T	18. F	19. T	20. T
21. g	22. d	23. c	24. e	25. f
26. j	27. b	28. a	29. i	30. h

III. Thinking Critically

1. a. Factors should include watching television for 4 to 5 hours a day, family history of heart disease, aggressiveness, overweight, and elevated cholesterol.
   b. Strategies should be described that restrict the child's viewing of violent programs, increase the parents' awareness of the content of the shows that are viewed, help the child correlate consequences with the actions, point out subtle messages, and help the child explore alternatives to aggressive conflict resolution.
   c. Outcomes described should include the child selecting more healthful snacks, watching television for about 1 hour per day, increasing physical activity, and exploring the possibility of adding out-of-the-home activities, such as scouting, sports, and music.

CHAPTER 33 PEDIATRIC HEALTH ASSESSMENT

I. Learning Key Terms

1. e	2. a	3. b	4. c	5. d
6. m	7. o	8. v	9. k	10. u
11. n	12. t	13. h	14. l	15. s
16. j	17. r	18. g	19. q	20. f
21. p	22. i			

II. Reviewing Key Concepts

1. b	2. d	3. T	4. T	5. T

6. Please see the History Taking section for content; include identifying information, presenting health issue or concern, present illness, history, family health history, family structure, psychosocial history, review of systems, reproductive health history; it also may include a nutritional history.

7. b	8. c	9. a	10. d	11. b
12. c	13. a	14. b	15. b	16. a
17. d	18. Fenton		19. a	20. T
21. T	22. T	23. b		

24. apical, 1 full minute

25. d	26. c	27. a		

28. Pupils Equal, Round, React to Light and Accommodation

29. b	30. b	31. b	32. b	33. c
34. c	35. d			

III. Thinking Critically

1. Please refer to Ears, Inspection of Internal Structures section for content. Describe the differences in direction the ear canal curves and include examination strategies to straighten the ear canal.

2. Please refer to Table 33-7 for content.

CHAPTER 34 PAIN ASSESSMENT AND MANAGEMENT

I. Learning Key Terms

1. c	2. e	3. a	4. l	5. m
6. f	7. h	8. i	9. g	10. j
11. k	12. d	13. b		

II. Reviewing Key Concepts

1. d	2. d	3. a	4. b	5. d
6. T	7. T	8. F	9. T	10. F
11. T	12. F	13. T	14. b	15. T

16. 8
17. Mothers, or fathers or partners or primary caregivers
18. Cognitive impairment
19. Opioids
20. a. Biologically based (foods, special diets, herbal or plant preparations, vitamins, other supplements)
   b. Manipulative treatments (chiropractic, osteopathy, massage)
   c. Energy based (Reiki, bioelectric or magnetic treatments, pulsed fields, alternating and direct currents)
   d. Mind-body techniques (mental healing, expressive treatments, spiritual healing, hypnosis, relaxation)
   e. Alternative medical systems (homeopathy; naturopathy; ayurvedic; and traditional Chinese medicine, which includes acupuncture and moxibustion)

III. Thinking Critically

1. Please see Recurrent Headaches in Children section for content. Consider common factors including tension, dental braces, sinusitis that contribute to recurrent headaches in children. Include information related to biofeedback techniques and pattern recognition/medication as management strategies.
2. Please see the Intranasal (IN) Route section for content.

CHAPTER 35 PROMOTING OPTIMUM HEALTH DURING CHILDHOOD

I. Learning Key Terms

1. s	2. e	3. d	4. j	5. g
6. l	7. m	8. p	9. f	10. b
11. c	12. a	13. v	14. q	15. r
16. u	17. t	18. h	19. o	20. i
21. n	22. k			

II. Reviewing Key Concepts

1. a	2. a	3. b	4. d	5. c
6. c	7. b	8. b	9. a	10. c
11. c	12. d	13. d		

287

14. Convertible car restraint; rear facing
15. a. Foods: hot dogs, nuts, dried beans, pits from fruits
    b. Play objects: anything with small parts
    c. Common household objects: thumbtacks, nails, screws, coins, jewelry, old refrigerators, storage chest
    d. Electrical items: outlets, garage doors, car windows
16. T   17. T   18. F   19. F   20. F
21. F   22. e   23. b   24. c   25. d
26. f   27. a

III. Thinking Critically

1. See Nutrition – Children Over Two Year of Age section for content to answer this question. Incorporate knowledge of Canada's Food Guide and eating together as a meal as part of answer.
2. See Nutrition – Infant section for content to answer this question.
   Vitamin D—All infants (including those exclusively breastfed) should receive a daily supplement of 400 international units of vitamin D beginning in the first few days of life to prevent rickets and vitamin D deficiency.
   Iron— To prevent iron deficiency, at 6 months, iron-rich foods should be introduced to the diet.
3. See section on Vaccine Hesitancy for content to answer this question.
4. See Use of Fluoride section for content to answer this question.
5. See Motor Vehicle Safety section for content to answer this question.

CHAPTER 36 THE INFANT AND FAMILY

I. Learning Key Terms

1. h   2. k   3. j   4. g   5. b
6. e   7. a   8. i   9. f   10. c
11. d

II. Reviewing Key Concepts

1. c   2. b   3. c   4. c   5. b
6. d   7. d   8. a   9. b   10. T
11. F   12. F   13. F

III. Thinking Critically

1. Descriptions should include the following: lifts head off table when supine, sits erect momentarily, bears full weight on feet, transfers objects from hand to hand, rakes at a small object, bangs a cube on the table, produces vowel sounds and chained syllables, vocalises four distinct vowel sounds, plays peek-a-boo, fears strangers when mother disappears, and imitates simple acts.
2. See Sudden Infant Death Syndrome and Family-Centred Care box: Safe Sleep for Infants—Reducing the Incidence of Sudden Infant Death and Table 36-2 for content to answer this question.

   a) Some answers include: low birth weight, male sex, Indigenous infants, socioeconomically disadvantaged family, genetic factors, maternal smoking, prone sleeping, sleeping on a soft surface, sleeping with an adult or child, sleeping on a noninfant bed surface such as a couch
   b) Breastfeeding, room sharing, and supine sleep position, avoid exposure to cigarette smoke
   c) See Positional Plagiocephaly section for content to answer this question. Discuss importance of "tummy time".
3. See Developing a Sense of Trust (Erikson) section for content required to answer this question.

CHAPTER 37 THE TODDLER AND FAMILY

I. Learning Key Terms

1. c   2. e   3. d   4. a   5. b
6. h   7. g   8. f

II. Reviewing Key Concepts

1. d   2. d   3. c   4. a   5. a
6. b   7. d   8. d

III. Thinking Critically

1. See Anticipatory Guidance section and Family-Centred Care box; Guidance During Toddler Years for content to answer this question. A few questions and clinical data from the following areas should be assessed: nutrition, sleep and activity, dental health, injury prevention, temperament, and psychological development.
2. See Gross and Fine Motor Development and Language sections as well as Table 37-1 for content to answer this question.
   a) Gross motor development milestones include the ability to go up and down stairs alone, using both feet on each step; run fairly well with a wide stance; pick up objects without falling; kick a ball forward without overbalancing.
   b) Fine motor development milestones include the ability to build a tower of six to seven cubes; align two or more cubes in a row like a train; turn the pages of a book one at a time; imitate vertical and circular strokes when drawing; turn doorknobs; and unscrew lids.
   c) Language development milestones include having a vocabulary of 300 words; using two- or three-word phrases; using the pronouns *I, me,* and *you;* understanding directional commands; giving first name; verbalising the need for toileting; and talking incessantly.
3. See section on Negativism for content to answer question. Negativism contributes to the toddler's acquisition of a sense of autonomy by the assertion of self-control and serving as an attempt to control the environment and a way to increase independence.
4. See section on Toilet Independence and Guidelines box: Assessing Toilet Learning Readiness for content to answer this question.

CHAPTER 38 THE PRESCHOOLER AND FAMILY

I. Learning Key Terms

1. h	2. i	3. g	4. a	5. c
6. k	7. f	8. b	9. e	10. j
11. d				

II. Reviewing Key Concepts

1. 3, 4	2. 1.8 to 2.7	3. b	4. c
5. d	6. c	7. T	8. c	9. d

III. Thinking Critically

1. a. See Preschool and Kindergarten Experience for content to answer these questions. The child will need some preparation for this new preschool experience. One cannot guarantee that the child will have less trouble adjusting than a child who has never attended day care. A change such as this, although not drastic, could cause disruption because of differences in the programs, as well as differences between the day care "caregiver" and the preschool "teacher" and styles used by each. The amount and quality of the attention may differ from the day care to the preschool. The preschool may have more expectations for the child to be independent and autonomous than the day care centre does.

   b. An example: The mother will verbalise at least five strategies that can be used to help prepare her child for the preschool experience.

   c. Possible responses might include visit the school ahead of time, introduce the child and the teacher, begin to talk about the new school, refer to the new school in a positive way, and maintain confidence on the first day.

   d. Characteristics that indicate that the child is ready for preschool include social maturity, good attention span, and academic readiness.

2. See section on Play for content to answer this question. Include information about limiting screen time to 1 hour per day for preschoolers.

CHAPTER 39 THE SCHOOL-AGE CHILD AND FAMILY

I. Learning Key Terms

1. e	2. f	3. g	4. b	5. d
6. a	7. c	8. h		

II. Reviewing Key Concepts

1. c	2. T	3. F	4. T	5. F
6. 10; 12; 8		7. T	8. a	9. c
10. d	11. d	12. d	13. b	14. T
15. Direct bullying, indirect bullying				

III. Thinking Critically

1. See Family-Centred Care Box: Guidance for Parents During School Years.

a. Response should include nutritional assessment and his knowledge and use of safety precautions when riding his bike.

b. See section on Play and Sports for content to answer this question. Response should include support for the mother by reassuring her that her child is healthy and that playing soccer will allow him to increase strength and develop motor skill performance.

c. Response should outline the information about nutrition related to good lifelong dietary habits.

d. See Psychosocial Development section for answer to this question. Response should include ideas about how to give the child recognition and positive feedback for his accomplishments.

2. See Enuresis section for content to answer these questions.

   a. Organic causes that may be related to enuresis should be ruled out before psychogenic factors are considered.

   b. See Enuresis, Nursing Care section for content to answer this question.

   c. See Enuresis section for content to answer this question.

CHAPTER 40 THE ADOLESCENT AND FAMILY

I. Learning Key Terms

1. e	2. k	3. f	4. j	5. l
6. g	7. d	8. h	9. i	10. c
11. b	12. a			

II. Reviewing Key Concepts

1. 10.5, 15; 12 years, 7 months				
2. d	3. c	4. pubertal delay, 13		
5. b	6. b	7. 5, 20; 7, 25; 10, 30; 7, 30		
8. c	9. T	10. a	11. d	12. c
13. a	14. d	15. T		

III. Thinking Critically

1. See Sex Differences in General Growth Patterns and Eating Habits and Behaviour for content to answer the question. Nonlean body mass, primarily fat, increases in adolescence. Fatty tissue deposition is more pronounced in girls, particularly in the regions over the thigh, hips, buttocks, and breast tissue.

2. See Developing a Sense of Identity for content to answer question. A sense of group identity is essential to the later development of personal identity. Younger adolescents must resolve questions concerning relationships with peer groups before they are able to resolve questions about who they are in relation to the family and society. Peer groups serve as a strong support to the adolescent, individually and collectively, providing a sense of belonging and a feeling of strength and power. They form a transitional world between dependence and autonomy.

3. See Relationships with Parents and Family-Centred Teaching boxes: Communication With Teens: The Art

of Listening Show and Guidance During Adolescence for content to answer this question. Parents need to respect for the adolescent's privacy; show honest and sincere interest in the adolescent's beliefs and feelings; and listen without interrupting the adolescent.

4. Benefits include exercise for growing muscles and interactions with peers; a "socially acceptable" means to enjoy stimulation and conflict.

5. See sections on Body Art and Tanning for content to include in the class. When teaching teens it is important to encourage teens to explore their feelings and, on the basis of their insights, develop solutions for effecting change. Effective education for adolescents must include opportunities to improve communication skills.

6. See Disorders of the Male Reproductive System for content to answer this question.

CHAPTER 41 CARING FOR THE CHILD WITH A CHRONIC ILLNESS AND AT THE END OF LIFE

I. Learning Key Terms

1. b	2. h	3. e	4. g	5. i
6. c	7. d	8. f	9. k	10. a
11. j				

II. Reviewing Key Concepts

1. d   2. e

3. Strategies include education regarding what can reasonably be expected of the child, assistance in identifying the child's strength, praise for a parental job well done, and encouragement to seek respite care so that parents can renew their energies.

4. Adaptive tasks include accept the child's condition; manage the child's condition on a day-to-day basis; meet the child's normal developmental needs; meet the developmental needs of other family members; cope with ongoing stress and periodic crises; assist family members to manage their feelings; educate others about the child's conditions; and establish a support system.

5. d   6. d

7. Shock/denial, adjustment, and reintegration/ acknowledgment

8. b   9. c

10. Possible answers include loss of senses, confusion, muscle weakness, loss of bowel and bladder control, difficulty swallowing, change in respiratory pattern, and weak/slow pulse.

11. d   12. c   13. c   14. d

III. Thinking Critically

1. Please see Trends in Care Section for content. Responses could include the following:
   - Using the development approach emphasises the child's abilities and strengths rather than his or her disability.
   - Collaborative relationships are characterised by communication, dialogue, active listening, awareness, and acceptance of differences.

- The health care team provides honest, clear information and the patient and family shares family values, acknowledges abilities to follow treatment recommendations.
- Families move between the normal of living with the experience of a complex medical conditions and chronic illness, and the normal of the 'outside world'.

2. Please see Grief and Mourning, Sibling Grief section for content. Information to include: children will try to protect their parents and will try not to upset them or ask questions.

3. Please see Nurses' Reactions to Caring for Dying Children section for content. Information to include maintaining good general health, develop well-rounded interests, develop professional and personal support systems, take time off when needed, develop professional practise based on sound theory and observations, participating in shared-remembrance rituals

CHAPTER 42 IMPACT OF INTELLECTUAL DISABILITY OR SENSORY IMPAIRMENT ON THE CHILD AND FAMILY

I. Learning Key Terms

1. u	2. i	3. t	4. j	5. h
6. k	7. g	8. l	9. f	10. m
11. s	12. e	13. n	14. d	15. r
16. c	17. o	18. b	19. p	20. v
21. a	22. q	23. x	24. w	

II. Reviewing Key Concepts

1. d

2. Task analysis is the process of breaking a skill into its components; it is used when teaching children with an intellectual disability to help them master one part of the skill at a time, beginning with the parts the child has mastered already. Each task is separated into its necessary components and each step is taught completely before proceeding to the next activity.

3. c   4. d   5. genetic counselling

6. d   7. b   8. a   9. d   10. d

11. d

12. Please see Visual Impairment, Care for the Child during Hospitalisation section for content; information to include: Talk to child about everything that is occurring; emphasise aspects of procedures that are felt/heard; approach the child with identifying information; explain sounds; encourage parents to room in; encourage parents' participation; bring familiar objects from home; orient child to surroundings. (If the child has sight on admission but will lose sight during hospitalisation [e.g., as a result of eye surgery], point out significant aspects of the room's layout and practise ambulation with eyes closed before the procedure.)

13. d   14. F

III. Thinking Critically

1. Please see Hearing Impairment, Socialisation section for content. Consider including: 1. Encourage background noise be minimised 2. provide suggestions to facilitate lip-reading, 3. group discussion to incorporate a point person to identify each speaker.

2. Please see Autism Spectrum Disorders, Nursing Care sections for content. Consider including decreasing stimulation by avoiding extraneous auditory and visual distractions, minimise physical contact and eye contact, encourage personal possessions be brought from home.

3. Please see Retinoblastoma, Preparing the Family for Diagnostic and Therapeutic Procedures and Home Care for content. Information to include: general wound care; encourage use of eye patch for infants and toddlers even after socket fully healed; protection of unaffected eye by wearing protective eyewear during sports activities.

CHAPTER 43 FAMILY-CENTRED CARE OF THE CHILD DURING ILLNESS AND HOSPITALIZATION

I. Learning Key Terms

1. f	2. b	3. e	4. a	5. c
6. d				

II. Reviewing Key Concepts

1. e	2. b	3. c	4. a	5. T
6. T	7. c	8. a		

9. Please see Box 43-2 for content.

10. e	11. b	12. c	13. a	14. c
15. c				

16. Please see Box 43-4 for content.

17. Please see Caring for the Child Who is Hospitalized, Preventing or Minimising Fear of Bodily Injury sections for content. Consider including cognitively appropriate explanations of medical terminology including equipment and investigations, use of doll or drawing for child to "explain" thoughts about the upcoming procedure, alternate methods of temperature assessment, no rectal temperatures unless indicated; Use of Band-Aids to prevent "leaking" of bodily parts.

III. Thinking Critically

1. Please see Care of the Child and Family in Special Hospital Situations, Critical Care Unit section for content; including explanation of differences in monitoring, provide family tour if possible, support nursing team and family with visits to regular unit setting after transfer out of CCU.

2. Please see Care of the Child and Family in Special Hospital Situations, Ambulatory or Outpatient section for content. Information to include: Typical trajectory of recovery including return to daily activities, what circumstances require more immediate follow-up, methods of pain management including medication administration details, information related to dressing changes.

CHAPTER 44 PEDIATRIC VARIATIONS OF NURSING INTERVENTIONS

I. Learning Key Terms

1. l	2. k	3. c	4. d	5. e
6. b	7. j	8. f	9. i	
10. g	11. a	12. h		

II. Reviewing Key Concepts

1. c	2. b	3. c

4. Please see Box 44-2 for content. Possible supportive strategies include the following: Expect success; involve the child; provide distraction; encourage expression of feelings during and after procedure; provide positive reinforcement; use play in preparation of and after the procedure.

5. e				
6. T	7. T	8. T	9. a	10. d
11. d	12. b	13. d	14. d	15. a
16. T	17. c	18. d	19. b	20. c
21. b	22. d	23. c	24. a	25. d

III. Thinking Critically

1. Please see Therapeutic Holding and Restraints section for content. Information to include:

   Restraints are used for children with an artificial airway or airway adjunct for delivery of oxygen, indwelling catheters, tubes, drains, lines, pacemaker wires, or suture sites. Physical restraints may be instituted for any of the following reasons:
   - Risk for interruption of therapy used to maintain oxygenation or airway patency
   - Risk of harm if indwelling catheter, tube, drain, line, pacemaker wire, or sutures are removed, dislodged, or ruptured
   - Patient confusion, agitation, unconsciousness, or developmental inability to understand direct requests or instructions
   - Chemical restraints are pharmaceutical agents used to keep a patient safe. Environmental restraints provides a physical space with restrictions of entry and exits,

2. Please see Gavage Feeding, Procedures section for content. Radiography provides most accurate confirmation. GI aspirate colour and pH testing can be useful. Nose-ear-mid xiphoid umbilicus span is adapted as best option.

3. Please see Mechanical Ventilation section for content. Information to include: D – displacement, O – obstruction, P – pneumothorax, E – equipment failure.

CHAPTER 45 RESPIRATORY CONDITIONS

I. Learning Key Terms

1. g	2. f	3. p	4. e	5. m
6. k	7. d	8. j	9. b	10. i
11. c	12. h	13. a	14. o	15. n
16. l				

291

II. Reviewing Key Concepts

1. b	2. c	3. d	4. b	5. b
6. c	7. d	8. a	9. c	10. a
11. b	12. a	13. d	14. c	15. d
16. c	17. a	18. b	19. b	20. c
21. a	22. d	23. c	24. d	25. b
26. e	27. d	28. d	29. a	30. d
31. d	32. c	33. d		

34. Restlessness, tachypnea, tachycardia, diaphoresis

35. d	36. h	37. b	38. e	39. c
40. l	41. a	42. d	43. i	44. k
45. j	46. g	47. f		

III. Thinking Critically

1. Please see Status Asthmaticus section including Nursing Alert for content. Include: child sweats profusely, remains sitting upright, and refuses to lie down. A child who suddenly becomes agitated or suddenly becomes quiet may be seriously hypoxic.
2. See Cystic Fibrosis section for content. Include:
   a. Respiratory symptoms include obstruction of bronchioles and bronchi with thick mucoprotein.
   b. Restricted growth and development as a result of decreased absorption of nutrients, including vitamins and fat; increased oxygen demands for pulmonary function; and delayed bone growth; cystic-fibrosis related diabetes mellitus may also impact nutritional status
   c. Female fertility impacted by highly viscous cervical secretions, blocking sperm entry; male fertility impacted by blockage of vas deferens by secretions; decreased sperm production
3. Asymptomatic children can attend school and daycare if receiving pharmacotherapy. Regular activities may resume with adherence to therapy and symptoms diminished.

CHAPTER 46 GASTROINTESTINAL CONDITIONS

I. Learning Key Terms

1. e	2. d	3. k	4. j	5. i
6. c	7. h	8. b	9. l	10. g
11. a	12. f			

II. Reviewing Key Concepts

1. a	2. d	3. c	4. c	5. c
6. c	7. d			

8. Isotonic
9. hypotonic, less
10. hypertonic; loss, intake; greater
11. b
12. Please see Dehydration, Nursing Care section for content; Include comprehensive and accurate measured intake (oral and parenteral) and output (urine, stools, vomitus, presence/absence of sweating), vital signs; assessment of skin characteristics, mucous membranes, body weight changes, fontanel (infants), sensory alterations

13. c	14. c	15. d	16. b	17. d
18. c	19. a	20. d		
21. handwashing		22. rotavirus		
23. a	24. b	25. e	26. d	27. c
28. b	29. d	30. Pruritis		
31. c	32. b	33. d	34. d	35. a
36. a	37. c	38. a	39. b	40. d
41. d	42. c	43. d	44. b	

45. Please see Dehydration, Therapeutic Management, Parenteral Fluid Therapy subsection for content. Include:
   Phase 1 – Expand volume quickly with isotonic electrolyte solution bolus.
   Phase 2 – Replace deficits and ongoing losses and provide maintenance fluid and electrolyte requirements.
   Phase 3 – Resume oral feedings if possible.

III. Thinking Critically

1. Please see Malrotation and Volvulus and Short Bowel Syndrome sections for content. Include Intestinal malrotation is a serious form of obstruction because the malpositioned bowel may twist or "volve" around itself, which will impair the blood supply causing intestinal ischemia and necrosis. Without urgent diagnosis and surgical intervention, large segments of bowel death may occur. Short bowel syndrome may result and may require years of therapy to allow for intestinal adaptation to occur.
2. Please see section on for content. Include: Ulcerative colitis (UC) is a chronic inflammatory reaction involving the mucosa and submucosa of the large intestine. Mucosa becomes hyperemic and edematous with patchy granulation that bleeds easily and leads to superficial ulceration. Crohn disease (CD) affects the terminal ileum and involves all layers of the bowel wall. Oedema and inflammation progress to deep ulceration with fissure and obstruction.
   • Rectal bleeding: common in UC; uncommon in CD
   • Diarrhea: often severe in UC; moderate to absent in CD
   • Pain: less frequent in UC; common in CD
   • Anorexia: mild to moderate in UC; can be severe in CD
   • Weight loss: moderate in UC; severe in CD
   • Growth restriction: usually mild in UC; often pronounced in CD

CHAPTER 47 CARDIOVASCULAR CONDITIONS

I. Learning Key Terms

1. o	2. r	3. n	4. p	5. m
6. l	7. q	8. k	9. t	10. e
11. d	12. u	13. f	14. c	15. j
16. a	17. g	18. s	19. b	20. h
21. i				

II. Reviewing Key Concepts

1. b   2. a   3. a   4. e   5. a
6. c   7. b
8. Possible complications include acute haemorrhage, low-grade fever, nausea and vomiting, loss of pulse in the catheterized extremity. Rare complications include stroke, seizures, tamponade, and death.

9. d	10. d	11. b	12. d	13. c
14. b	15. c	16. d	17. c	18. d
19. a	20. b	21. c	22. d	23. c
24. d	25. b	26. c	27. d	28. a
29. d	30. a	31. d	32. b	33. c
34. b	35. b	36. d	37. b	38. a
39. a	40. d	41. d	42. a	43. d
44. b	45. d	46. c		

III. Thinking Critically

1. See Congenital Heart Disease section for content. Include birth parent history of diabetes, alcohol consumption or exposure to environmental toxins and infections; family history of cardiac anomaly; associated with some chromosome abnormalities or genetic syndromes.
2. See Preparing the Child and Family for Invasive Procedures section for content. Answer to include details related to information provision and specifics related to coping skills training.

CHAPTER 48 HEMATOLOGICAL AND IMMUNOLOGICAL CONDITIONS

I. Learning Key Terms

1. o   2. c   3. k   4. f   5. m
6. d   7. n   8. H   9. I   10. J
11. A   12. L   13. B   14. G   15. e

II. Reviewing Key Concepts

1. a
2. iron deficiency
3. a
4. Administer between meals; administer with a fruit juice; administer through a straw or with a medication syringe
5. a   6. d   7. d   8. d   9. b
10. d   11. immune thrombocytopenia
12. T   13. 90-100 g/L   14. d   15. c
16. *Pneumocystis carinii* pneumonia
17. d   18. d   19. a   20. T
21. colony stimulating factors
22. 50 to 100 x 10^9/L
23. Administer anti-emetic before chemotherapy begins to prevent development of anticipatory symptoms.
24. Interventions include bland, moist, soft diet; use of a "sponge" toothette instead of a regular toothbrush; frequent rinsing with chlorhexidine, normal saline or sodium bicarbonate mouth rinses, use of local anaesthetics without alcohol; use of a gauze soaked in saline or plain water to cleanse the gums, palate, and inner checks. This should be done before and after feeding and every 2 to 4 hours as needed to cleanse mouth of debris.
25. F
26. Strategies include liberal oral or IV fluid intake, frequent voiding, administration of the drug early in the day to allow for sufficient fluid intake and frequent voiding to occur, administration of Mesna.
27. d   28. F
29. Bone marrow dysfunction includes anemia, bleeding, infection.
30. T   31. d
32. Central Nervous System by leukemic cells; CNS intrathecal prophylactic therapy
33. a

III. Thinking Critically

1. Mild-moderate pain may respond to nonsteroidal anti-inflammatory medication or acetaminophen; opioids may be added; regular IV administration may be required for severe pain; patient-controlled analgesia (PCA) may provide increased flexibility in managing a crisis.
2. Ensure medical identification is worn; educate child to recognise potential risk situations and develop comfort with self-disclosure of condition; avoid aspirin or aspirin-containing compounds.
3. Please see Technological Management of Haematological and Immunological Disorders, Blood Transfusion Therapy section and Table 48-3 for content. Information to include:
   - Vital sign monitoring before, during and after the transfusion.
   - Review patient and donor blood group and type
   - Administer the first 20% of transfusion slowly. Ensure normal saline piggyback infusion setup.
   - Administer transfusion with appropriate filter to eliminate particles.
   - Utilise blood aliquot within 30 minutes of arrival to care setting; complete transfusion within 4 hours.
   - Monitor for transfusion reaction symptoms; if present, stop the transfusion and maintain IV with normal saline while notifying the practitioner of patient's reaction
4. Please see Technological Management of Haematological and Immunological Disorders, Hematopoietic Stem Cell (Bone Marrow) Transplantation section for content. Information to include: Annalise will undergo intensive high-dose combination chemotherapy +/- total body irradiation to fully suppress her own immune system and prevent rejection. Harvested stem cells are administered intravenously and will "repopulate" Annalise's bone marrow to provide a new blood-forming organ. A suitable donor with a "good" haplotype match will be necessary to prevent graft-versus-host disease.

293

CHAPTER 49 GENITOURINARY CONDITIONS

I. Learning Key Terms
1. p	2. a	3. j	4. i	5. l
6. h	7. b	8. o	9. k	10. c
11. n	12. f	13. d	14. m	15. g
16. e				

II. Reviewing Key Concepts
1. d	2. Uncircumcised	3. d	4. a	
5. b	6. b	7. corticosteroid	8. a	
9. c	10. c	11. c	12. b	13. a
14. c	15. e	16. c	17. b	18. b

19. hemodialysis, peritoneal dialysis, hemofiltration
20. Haemodialysis
21. Peritoneal
22. a

III. Thinking Critically
1. Please see Nephrotic Syndrome, Nursing Care section for content. Interventions should include the following: Offer a nutritious diet; limit salt during the oedema phase and while on steroid therapy; enlist the aid of the child and parents in formulation of a diet; provide special and preferred foods; serve food in an attractive manner; serve small quantities.
2. Please see Urinary Tract Infection and Vesicoureteral Reflux sections for content. Information to include: Description of retrograde flow of urine; Reflux does not cause UTIs but when UTI occurs in the context of an infant/child with VUR, kidney scarring/renal injury can occur; daily antibiotic prophylaxis is indicated in infants with VUR; symptoms of UTI in infants require review
3. Please see External Defects, Hydrocele and Cryptorchidism sections for content. Information to include: Advise parents that swelling, discolouration of scrotum resolves spontaneously; pain management strategies should be discussed; straddle toys or straddle infant seats should be avoided for 2-4 weeks; dressing can be removed in 2-3 days and a bath may occur after 3 days. Additional information regarding future fertility and cancer risk should be reviewed.

CHAPTER 50 NEUROLOGICAL CONDITIONS

I. Learning Key Terms
1. j	2. f	3. k	4. g	5. m
6. e	7. i	8. l	9. d	10. a
11. c	12. b	13. h		

II. Reviewing Key Concepts
1. b	2. c	3. b	4. c	5. d
6. c	7. b	8. b	9. d	10. c
11. a	12. Meningococcal meningitis			
13. b	14. d	15. b	16. d	17. e
18. d	19. a	20. e	21. f	22. d

III. Thinking Critically
1. Please see Nursing Care of the Unconscious Child section for content. Information should include: Assessment parameters should include vital signs, pupillary reactions, and level of consciousness. Interventions should include the following: elevate head of bed 15 to 30 degrees, avoid positions or activities that increase intracranial pressure (ICP), prevent constipation, prevent or relieve pain, schedule disturbing procedures to take advantage of therapies that reduce ICP, and monitor ICP.
2. Please see Seizure Disorders – Diagnostic Evaluation section for content. Details to include: a description of the child's behaviour before and during a seizure, the age of onset of the first seizure, the usual time at which seizures occur, any factors that precipitate seizures, any sensory phenomena that the child can describe, duration and progression of the seizure, and postictal feelings and behaviour.
3. Please refer to Intracranial Pressure Monitoring section for content. Details to include: Glasgow Coma Scale (GCS) of < 8, GCS evaluation > than 8 with respiratory assistance, deterioration of condition, subjective judgement regarding clinical appearance, and response.

CHAPTER 51 ENDOCRINE CONDITIONS

I. Learning Key Words
1. e	2. j	3. d	4. n	5. i
6. m	7. k	8. c	9. l	10. g
11. b	12. h	13. a	14. f	

II. Reviewing Key Concepts
1. b   2. c
3. Constitutional growth
4. Acromegaly results from hypersecretion of growth hormone that occurs after epiphyseal closure resulting in growth occurring in a transverse direction. If excess secretion of growth hormone occurs before epiphyseal closure, the disorder is called *pituitary hyperfunction*, and is associated with overgrowth of long bones with proportional weight and head circumference.

5. 7, 6; 9	6. c	7. a	8. b	9. b
10. d	11. b	12. c	13. b	14. insulin
15. d	16. b	17. c	18. d	

19. polyuria (increased urination); polydipsia (increased thirst); polyphagia (increased hunger)
20. rapid-acting, intermediate-acting; before breakfast, the evening meal
21. c   22. b

III. Thinking Critically
1. Please see Disorders of Pituitary Function – Hypopituitarism section for content. Details to include: short stature but proportional height and weight,

well-nourished appearance, a tendency to be relatively inactive and to shun aggressive sports, restricted bone-age proportional to height-age, and eruption of permanent teeth is delayed; teeth may be overcrowded and malpositioned. Sexual development is delayed but normal.

2. Please see Diabetes Insipidus section for content. Details to include:
   a. Clinical manifestations: polyuria, possible enuresis; polydipsia, with intense thirst in some children; infants may be irritable; dehydration may occur if unable to drink.
   b. Therapeutic management: Intranasal, oral or parenteral hormone replacement; injectable form also available but requires medication preparation and frequent injections.

3. Please see Diabetes Type 1 and Hypoglycaemia sections for content. Details to include: nervousness, pallor, tremulousness, palpitations, sweating and hunger; weakness, dizziness, headache, drowsiness, irritability, loss of coordination, seizures and coma present as more severe responses.

4. Please see subsection Signs of Hypoglycemia and Emergency box: Hypoglycemia for content. Glucose tablet, dextrose tablet, apple or orange juice, regular soft drink or sweet beverage recommended for mild-moderate hypoglycemia; Glucagon IM then followed with a planned meal or snack when child is able.

CHAPTER 52 INTEGUMENTARY CONDITIONS

I. Learning Key Terms
1. e	2. F	3. A	4. B	5. J
6. G	7. C	8. D	9. H	10. O
11. I	12. K	13. M	14. S	15. P
16. T	17. R	18. N	19. L	20. O

II. Reviewing Key Concepts
1. C	2. B	3. D	4. A	5. C
6. A	7. B	8. C	9. C	10. False
11. True		12. True		13. True
14. False		15. False		

III. Thinking Critically

1. Please see Infections of the Skin, Bacterial Infections Nursing Care and Table 52-1 for content. Information to include:
   a. Maintain vigilant hand hygiene before and after contact with affected child.
   b. Reminders to child to refrain from touching affected area.
   c. Separate washcloths and towels for affected child.
   d. Regularly clean contact surfaces within the home.
   e. Topical application of bactericidal ointment as directed.
   f. Instruction on removal of undermined skin, crust and debris.

2. Please see Skin Disorders Related to Animal Contacts, Bed Bugs section for content. Details to include:

Inspect mattress, frame, and underside of beds; wash linens in hot water, cover pillows and mattress with plastic; seal cracks and crevices, monitor daily using double-sided carpet sticky tape to catch Cimicidae.

CHAPTER 53 MUSCULOSKELETAL OR ARTICULAR CONDITIONS

I. Learning Key Terms
1. g	2. f	3. h	4. m	5. e
6. d	7. i	8. l	9. c	10. k
11. j	12. a	13. b		

II. Reviewing Key Concepts
1. d	2. d	3. B	4. h	5. i
6. a	7. c	8. b	9. d	10. e
11. f	12. g	13. b	14. c	

15. muscle contraction; sports, running, gymnastics and basketball

16. d	17. b	18. d	19. a	20. d
21. b	22. d	23. lordosis, kyphosis		
24. d	25. a	26. b	27. a	28. b
29. d	30. a	31. d	32. a	33. a
34. d				

III. Thinking Critically

1. Please see Pavlik Harness section for content. Details to include: The straps should be checked at the beginning of therapy and every 1 to 2 weeks for adjustments; recommendations regarding bathing, directive to not adjust the harness and maintain the harness on at all times unless instructed by the practitioner. Skin care is an important aspect of the care of an infant in a harness. Instructions include:
   Check frequently (at least two or three times a day) for red areas under the straps and the clothing.
   Gently massage healthy skin under the straps once a day to stimulate circulation. In general, avoid lotions and powders because they can cake and irritate the skin.
   Always place the diaper under the straps.
   Encourage parents to hold the infant with a harness and continue care and nurturing activities.

2. Please see Box 53-3 Compartment Syndrome Evaluation for content. The six Ps of ischaemia from a vascular, soft tissue, nerve, or bone injury should be included in an assessment of any injury.
   1. Pain
   2. Pulselessness
   3. Pallor
   4. Paresthesia
   5. Paralysis
   6. Pressure

3. Please see Nursing Alert within Fractures section for content.
   Compartment syndrome is a serious complication that results from compression of nerves, blood vessels, and muscle inside a closed space. This injury may be devastating, resulting in tissue death and disuse.

295

The signs and symptoms are:

Pain: Severe pain that is not relieved by analgesics or elevation of the limb; movement increases pain.

Pulse: Inability to palpate a pulse distal to the fracture or compartment.

Pallor: Pale-appearing skin, poor perfusion, capillary refill greater than 3 seconds.

Paresthesia: Tingling or burning sensations.

Paralysis: Inability to move extremity or digits.

Pressure: Involved limb or digits may feel tense and warm; skin is tight, shiny; pressure within the compartment is elevated.

CHAPTER 54 NEUROMUSCULAR OR MUSCULAR CONDITIONS

I. Learning Key Terms

1. g   2. c   3. f   4. d   5. b
6. a   7. e

II. Reviewing Key Concepts

1. a   2. e   3. b   4. d   5. d
6. b   7. d   8. a   9. b
10. latex allergy; latex sensitivity
11. b   12. a   13. c   14. c   15. a

III. Thinking Critically

1. Please see Duchenne Muscular Dystrophy – Therapeutic Management and Nursing Care sections for content. Details include encouragement of age-appropriate independence, housing and transportation to support mobility devices, socialisation and support opportunities for children, long-term care, advance directives and palliative care options.

2. Please see Guillain-Barre Syndrome – Nursing Care section for content. Details to include: Observe for difficulty swallowing and respiratory involvement; monitor vital signs frequently; monitor level of consciousness; maintain meticulous oral and hypopharynx care; change position frequently; perform passive reange of motion routinely; ensure adequate nutrition; provide bowel and bladder care to prevent constipation and urine retention.

3. Please see Spinal Cord Injuries – Nursing Care section for content. Details to include: Stabilise the entire spinal column with a rigid cervical collar with supportive blocks on a rigid backboard;ensure airway patency and continually assess neurologic function to prevent further deterioration; monitor haemodynamic status and administer inotropic support as indicated;

ensure vital signs including temperature are closely monitored; monitor skin integrity; pain management; provision of information for adolescent and parents about regarding status; encourage expression of feelings, anticipate denial, shock.

4. Please see for content, Details to include: phenomenon is caused by noxious stimuli below the level of the lesion, commonly precipitated by distension of the bowel or bladder. Sensory impulses are triggered and travel to the cord lesion, where they are blocked, which causes activation of sympathetic reflex action with disturbed central inhibitory control. Hallmark clinical sign is a drastic increase in systemic blood pressure, accompanied by other symptoms including headache, bradycardia, profuse diaphoresis, cardiac arrhythmias, flushing above the level of the lesion, piloerection and pallor below the level of the lesion, blurred vision, photophobia and visual field cuts, nasal congestion, anxiety; phenomenon is life threatening if noxious stimuli not removed.

CHAPTER 55 CARING FOR THE MENTAL, EMOTIONAL, AND BEHAVIOURAL HEALTH NEEDS OF CHILDREN AND ADOLESCENTS

I. Learning Key Terms

1. h   2. I   3. C   4. B   5. D
6. E   7. A   8. F   9. J.   10. g

II. Reviewing Key Concepts

1. T   2. T   3. F   4. F   5. T
6. A   7. D   8. D   9. C   10. A

III. Thinking Critically

1. Please see Disturbances in Eating Related Behaviours section and Box 55-8 for content. Three major goals for treating and managing eating disorders include 1) restitution of healthy nutritional intake, 2) resolution of disturbed patterns of family interaction and 3) individual psychotherapy to facility optimal psychological functioning. Questions to facilitate assessment of eating-related behaviours: a. Do you worry about losing control when you eat? b. How would you describe your appearance? c. Do you prefer to eat alone?

2. Please see Box 55-5 for content. Consider including a. sudden change in school performance or resists/refuses to go to school, b. social withdrawal from friends, activities, interests that were previously enjoyed, c. wants to give away cherished possessions, d. talks of own death or desire to die.